EUROPEAN PHARMACOPOEIA - SUPPLEMENT 6.5 TO THE 6th EDITION
published 1 January 2009

The 6th Edition of the European Pharmacopoeia consists of volumes 1 and 2 of the publication 6.0, and Supplements 6.1 to 6.5. These will be complemented by **non-cumulative supplements** that are to be kept for the duration of the 6th Edition. 3 supplements will be published in each of the years 2008 and 2009. A cumulative list of reagents was published in Supplement 6.4 and will be published again in Supplement 6.7.

To use the 6th Edition correctly, make sure that you have all the published supplements and consult the index of the most recent supplement to ensure that you use the latest versions of the monographs and general chapters.

EUROPEAN PHARMACOPOEIA - ELECTRONIC VERSION

The 6th Edition is also available in an electronic format (CD-ROM and online version) containing all of the monographs and general chapters found in the printed version. With the publication of each supplement the electronic version is replaced by a new, fully updated, cumulative version.

In addition to the official English and French online versions, a partial Spanish online version (6th Edition) is also available for the convenience of users.

PHARMEUROPA
Quarterly Forum Publication

Pharmeuropa contains preliminary drafts of all new and revised monographs proposed for inclusion in the European Pharmacopoeia and gives an opportunity for all interested parties to comment on the specifications before they are finalised. Pharmeuropa also contains information on the work programme and articles of general interest. Pharmeuropa is available on subscription from the EDQM. The subscription also includes Pharmeuropa Bio and Pharmeuropa Scientific Notes (containing scientific articles on pharmacopoeial matters). Pharmeuropa Online is also available as a complementary service for subscribers to the printed version of Pharmeuropa.

INTERNATIONAL HARMONISATION

See the information given in chapter *5.8. Pharmacopoeial Harmonisation*.

WEBSITE

http://www.edqm.eu
http://www.edqm.eu/store (for prices and orders)

HELPDESK

To send a question or to contact the EDQM, use the HELPDESK, accessible through the EDQM website (visit http://www.edqm.eu/site/FAQ_Helpdesk-521.html).

KNOWLEDGE

Consult KNOWLEDGE, the new free database at http://www.edqm.eu to obtain information on the work programme of the European Pharmacopoeia, the volume of Pharmeuropa and of the European Pharmacopoeia in which a text has been published, trade names of the reagents (for example, chromatography columns) that were used at the time of the elaboration of the monographs, the history of the revisions of a text since its publication in the 5th Edition, representative chromatograms, the list of reference standards used, and the list of certificates granted.

COMBISTATS

CombiStats is a computer program for the statistical analysis of data from biological assays in agreement with chapter *5.3* of the 6th Edition of the European Pharmacopoeia. For more information, visit the website (http://www.edqm.eu/combistats).

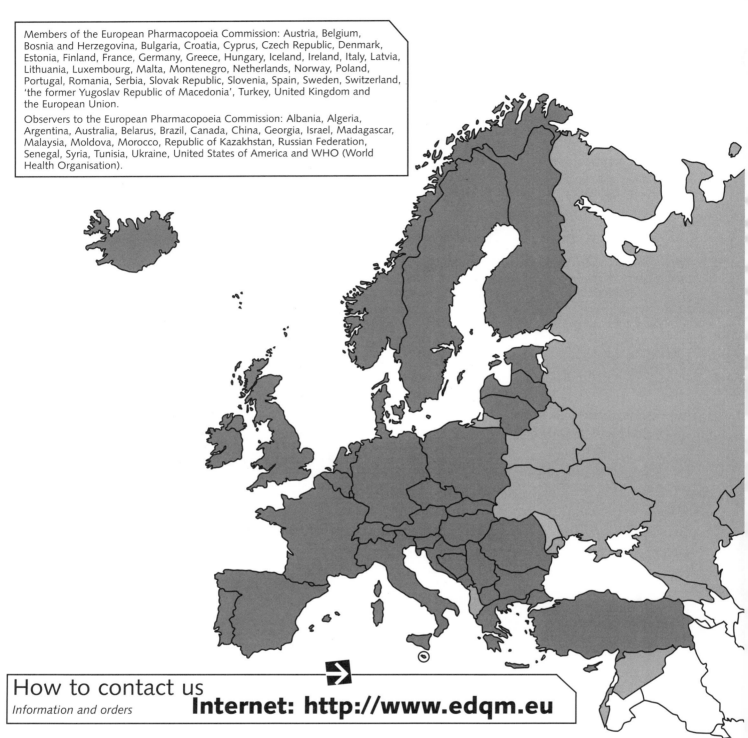

Members of the European Pharmacopoeia Commission: Austria, Belgium, Bosnia and Herzegovina, Bulgaria, Croatia, Cyprus, Czech Republic, Denmark, Estonia, Finland, France, Germany, Greece, Hungary, Iceland, Ireland, Italy, Latvia, Lithuania, Luxembourg, Malta, Montenegro, Netherlands, Norway, Poland, Portugal, Romania, Serbia, Slovak Republic, Slovenia, Spain, Sweden, Switzerland, 'the former Yugoslav Republic of Macedonia', Turkey, United Kingdom and the European Union.

Observers to the European Pharmacopoeia Commission: Albania, Algeria, Argentina, Australia, Belarus, Brazil, Canada, China, Georgia, Israel, Madagascar, Malaysia, Moldova, Morocco, Republic of Kazakhstan, Russian Federation, Senegal, Syria, Tunisia, Ukraine, United States of America and WHO (World Health Organisation).

How to contact us
Information and orders   **Internet: http://www.edqm.eu**

European Directorate for the Quality of Medicines & HealthCare (EDQM)
Council of Europe - 7 allée Kastner
CS 30026, F-67081 STRASBOURG, FRANCE
Tel: +33 (0)3 88 41 30 30*
Fax: +33 (0)3 88 41 27 71*
Do not dial 0 if calling from outside of France

Correspondence ....Via the online HELPDESK (http://www.edqm.eu/site/FAQ_Helpdesk-521.html)

How to place an order

Publications ....https://www.edqm.eu/store
Reference standards .... http://www.edqm.eu
    Reference standards online order form...................................http://www.edqm.eu/site/EDQM_Reference_standards-649.html

Further information, including answers to the most frequently asked questions regarding ordering, is available via the HELPDESK.

All other matters ....info@edqm.eu

All reference standards required for application of the monographs are available from the EDQM.
A catalogue of reference standards can be consulted on the EDQM website and printed directly. The list of newly released reference standards (new reference standards and new batches) is available by clicking on the link 'News' on the page http://crs.edqm.eu/.

EUROPEAN PHARMACOPOEIA

SIXTH EDITION

Supplement 6.5

Published in accordance with the
Convention on the Elaboration of a European Pharmacopoeia
(European Treaty Series No. 50)

edqm
European Directorate for the
Quality of Medicines & HealthCare

Council of Europe

Strasbourg

The European Pharmacopoeia is published by the Directorate for the Quality of Medicines & HealthCare
of the Council of Europe (EDQM).

ISBN: 978-92-871-6316-5

CONTENTS

Note: on the first page of each chapter/section there is a list of contents.

CONTENTS OF SUPPLEMENT 6.5

A vertical line in the margin indicates where part of a text has been revised or corrected. A horizontal line in the margin indicates where part of a text has been deleted. It is to be emphasised that these indications, which are not necessarily exhaustive, are given for information and do not form an official part of the texts. Editorial changes are not indicated. Individual copies of texts will not be supplied.

NEW TEXTS

GENERAL CHAPTERS

2.9.45. Wettability of porous solids including powders

MONOGRAPHS

The monographs below appear for the first time in the European Pharmacopoeia. They will be implemented on 1 July 2009 at the latest.

Vaccines for veterinary use

Porcine enzootic pneumonia vaccine (inactivated) (2448)

Radiopharmaceutical preparations

Medronic acid for radiopharmaceutical preparations (2350)

Monographs

Bitter-fennel herb oil (2380)

Ceftazidime pentahydrate with sodium carbonate for injection (2344)

Dandelion herb with root (1851)

Drospirenone (2404)

Gestodene (1726)

Iopromide (1753)

Rifaximin (2362)

Spike lavender oil (2419)

Vedaprofen for veterinary use (2248)

Zinc gluconate (2164)

REVISED TEXTS

GENERAL CHAPTERS

1.   General notices

2.6.12. Microbiological examination of non-sterile products: microbial enumeration tests

2.6.13. Microbiological examination of non-sterile products: test for specified micro-organisms

2.6.24. Avian viral vaccines: tests for extraneous agents in seed lots

2.6.26. Test for anti-D antibodies in human immunoglobulin for intravenous administration

2.7.9. Test for Fc function of immunoglobulin

2.7.25. Assay of human plasmin inhibitor

2.9.34. Bulk density and tapped density of powders

4.   Reagents (*new, revised, corrected*)

5.2.5. Substances of animal origin for the production of immunological veterinary medicinal products

MONOGRAPHS

The monographs below have been technically revised since their last publication in the European Pharmacopoeia. They will be implemented on 1 July 2009.

General monographs

Substances for pharmaceutical use (2034)

Vaccines for veterinary use

Infectious chicken anaemia vaccine (live) (2038)

Homoeopathic preparations

Herbal drugs for homoeopathic preparations (2045)

Monographs

Aceclofenac (1281)

Benzyl alcohol (0256)

Buprenorphine (1180)

Buprenorphine hydrochloride (1181)

Caffeine monohydrate (0268)

Carboplatin (1081)

Ceftazidime pentahydrate (1405)

Cyproheptadine hydrochloride (0817)

Desmopressin (0712)

Dimenhydrinate (0601)

Etacrynic acid (0457)

Frangula bark dry extract, standardised (1214)

Ginkgo leaf (1828)

Guaiacol (1978)

Hydrocortisone (0335)

Lactose, anhydrous (1061)

Lactose monohydrate (0187)

Magnesium stearate (0229)

Maltodextrin (1542)

Methyldopa (0045)

Methylergometrine maleate (1788)

Mirtazapine (2338)

Oxolinic acid (1353)

Paraffin, white soft (1799)

Penicillamine (0566)

Pentaerythrityl tetranitrate, diluted (1355)

Polysorbate 80 (0428)

Povidone (0685)

Pyrrolidone (2180)

Red poppy petals (1881)

Sodium picosulfate (1031)

Stearic acid (1474)

Sucrose monopalmitate (2319)

Sucrose stearate (2318)

Tenoxicam (1156)

Tolnaftate (1158)

Zidovudine (1059)

CORRECTED TEXTS

*The texts below have been corrected and are republished in their entirety. These corrections are to be taken into account from the publication date of Supplement 6.5 (**1 January 2009**).*

GENERAL CHAPTERS

5.10.   Control of impurities in substances for pharmaceutical use

MONOGRAPHS

Monographs

Amantadine hydrochloride (0463)

Bifonazole (1395)

Bismuth subgallate (1493)

Cefaclor (0986)

Cefadroxil monohydrate (0813)

Chitosan hydrochloride (1774)

Cholecalciferol concentrate (oily form) (0575)

Cholecalciferol concentrate (powder form) (0574)

Cholecalciferol concentrate (water-dispersible form) (0598)

Croscarmellose sodium (0985)

Flurbiprofen (1519)

Foscarnet sodium hexahydrate (1520)

Imipramine hydrochloride (0029)

Interferon beta-1a concentrated solution (1639)

Lactitol monohydrate (1337)

Levomethadone hydrochloride (1787)

Magnesium carbonate, heavy (0043)

Molsidomine (1701)

Moxidectin for veterinary use (1656)

Piperazine citrate (0424)

Tamsulosin hydrochloride (2131)

Tetrazepam (1738)

Tiamulin for veterinary use (1660)

TEXTS WHOSE TITLE HAS CHANGED

The title of the following texts has been changed in Supplement 6.5.

GENERAL CHAPTERS

5.2.5.   Substances of animal origin for the production of immunological veterinary medicinal products *(previously Substances of animal origin for the production of veterinary vaccines)*

MONOGRAPHS

Monographs

Ceftazidime pentahydrate (1405) *(previously Ceftazidime)*

DELETED TEXTS

*The following texts are deleted as of **1 April 2009**.*

GENERAL CHAPTERS

2.9.15. Apparent volume

MONOGRAPHS

Monographs

Lindane (0772)

*The following text was deleted on **1 April 2008**.*

MONOGRAPHS

Vaccines for human use

Pertussis vaccine (0160)

1. GENERAL NOTICES

07/2009:10000

1. GENERAL NOTICES

1.1. GENERAL STATEMENTS

The General Notices apply to all monographs and other texts of the European Pharmacopoeia.

The official texts of the European Pharmacopoeia are published in English and French. Translations in other languages may be prepared by the signatory States of the European Pharmacopoeia Convention. In case of doubt or dispute, the English and French versions are alone authoritative.

In the texts of the European Pharmacopoeia, the word 'Pharmacopoeia' without qualification means the European Pharmacopoeia. The official abbreviation Ph. Eur. may be used to indicate the European Pharmacopoeia.

The use of the title or the subtitle of a monograph implies that the article complies with the requirements of the relevant monograph. Such references to monographs in the texts of the Pharmacopoeia are shown using the monograph title and reference number in *italics*.

A preparation must comply throughout its period of validity; a distinct period of validity and/or specifications for opened or broached containers may be decided by the competent authority. The subject of any other monograph must comply throughout its period of use. The period of validity that is assigned to any given article and the time from which that period is to be calculated are decided by the competent authority in light of experimental results of stability studies.

Unless otherwise indicated in the General Notices or in the monographs, statements in monographs constitute mandatory requirements. General chapters become mandatory when referred to in a monograph, unless such reference is made in a way that indicates that it is not the intention to make the text referred to mandatory but rather to cite it for information.

The active substances, excipients, pharmaceutical preparations and other articles described in the monographs are intended for human and veterinary use (unless explicitly restricted to one of these uses). An article is not of Pharmacopoeia quality unless it complies with all the requirements stated in the monograph. This does not imply that performance of all the tests in a monograph is necessarily a prerequisite for a manufacturer in assessing compliance with the Pharmacopoeia before release of a product. The manufacturer may obtain assurance that a product is of Pharmacopoeia quality from data derived, for example, from validation studies of the manufacturing process and from in-process controls. Parametric release in circumstances deemed appropriate by the competent authority is thus not precluded by the need to comply with the Pharmacopoeia.

The tests and assays described are the official methods upon which the standards of the Pharmacopoeia are based. With the agreement of the competent authority, alternative methods of analysis may be used for control purposes, provided that the methods used enable an unequivocal decision to be made as to whether compliance with the standards of the monographs would be achieved if the official methods were used. In the event of doubt or dispute, the methods of analysis of the Pharmacopoeia are alone authoritative.

Certain materials that are the subject of a pharmacopoeial monograph may exist in different grades suitable for different purposes. Unless otherwise indicated in the monograph, the requirements apply to all grades of the material. In some monographs, particularly those on excipients, a list of functionality-related characteristics that are relevant to the use of the substance may be appended to the monograph for information. Test methods for determination of one or more of these characteristics may be given, also for information.

Quality systems. The quality standards represented by monographs are valid only where the articles in question are produced within the framework of a suitable quality system.

General monographs. Substances and preparations that are the subject of an individual monograph are also required to comply with relevant, applicable general monographs. Cross-references to applicable general monographs are not normally given in individual monographs.

General monographs apply to all substances and preparations within the scope of the Definition section of the general monograph, except where a preamble limits the application, for example to substances and preparations that are the subject of a monograph of the Pharmacopoeia.

General monographs on dosage forms apply to all preparations of the type defined. The requirements are not necessarily comprehensive for a given specific preparation and requirements additional to those prescribed in the general monograph may be imposed by the competent authority.

General monographs and individual monographs are complementary. If the provisions of a general monograph do not apply to a particular product, this is expressly stated in the individual monograph.

Validation of pharmacopoeial methods. The test methods given in monographs and general chapters have been validated in accordance with accepted scientific practice and current recommendations on analytical validation. Unless otherwise stated in the monograph or general chapter, validation of the test methods by the analyst is not required.

Conventional terms. The term 'competent authority' means the national, supranational or international body or organisation vested with the authority for making decisions concerning the issue in question. It may, for example, be a national pharmacopoeia authority, a licensing authority or an official control laboratory.

The expression 'unless otherwise justified and authorised' means that the requirements have to be met, unless the competent authority authorises a modification or an exemption where justified in a particular case.

Statements containing the word 'should' are informative or advisory.

In certain monographs or other texts, the terms 'suitable' and 'appropriate' are used to describe a reagent, micro-organism, test method etc.; if criteria for suitability are not described in the monograph, suitability is demonstrated to the satisfaction of the competent authority.

Medicinal product. (a) Any substance or combination of substances presented as having properties for treating or preventing disease in human beings and/or animals; or (b) any substance or combination of substances that may be used in or administered to human beings and/or animals with a view either to restoring, correcting or modifying physiological functions by exerting a pharmacological, immunological or metabolic action, or to making a medical diagnosis.

Active substance. Any substance intended to be used in the manufacture of a medicinal product and that, when so used, becomes an active ingredient of the medicinal product. Such substances are intended to furnish a pharmacological activity or other direct effect in the diagnosis, cure, mitigation, treatment or prevention of disease, or to affect the structure and function of the body.

Excipient (auxiliary substance). Any constituent of a medicinal product that is not an active substance. Adjuvants, stabilisers, antimicrobial preservatives, diluents, antioxidants, for example, are excipients.

Interchangeable methods. Certain general chapters contain a statement that the text in question is harmonised with the corresponding text of the Japanese Pharmacopoeia and/or the United States Pharmacopeia and that these texts are interchangeable. This implies that if a substance or preparation is found to comply with a requirement using an interchangeable method from one of these pharmacopoeias it complies with the requirements of the European Pharmacopoeia. In the event of doubt or dispute, the text of the European Pharmacopoeia is alone authoritative.

References to regulatory documents. Monographs and general chapters may contain references to documents issued by regulatory authorities for medicines, for example directives and notes for guidance of the European Union. These references are provided for information for users for the Pharmacopoeia. Inclusion of such a reference does not modify the status of the documents referred to, which may be mandatory or for guidance.

1.2. OTHER PROVISIONS APPLYING TO GENERAL CHAPTERS AND MONOGRAPHS

Quantities. In tests with numerical limits and assays, the quantity stated to be taken for examination is approximate. The amount actually used, which may deviate by not more than 10 per cent from that stated, is accurately weighed or measured and the result is calculated from this exact quantity. In tests where the limit is not numerical, but usually depends upon comparison with the behaviour of a reference substance in the same conditions, the stated quantity is taken for examination. Reagents are used in the prescribed amounts.

Quantities are weighed or measured with an accuracy commensurate with the indicated degree of precision. For weighings, the precision corresponds to plus or minus 5 units after the last figure stated (for example, 0.25 g is to be interpreted as 0.245 g to 0.255 g). For the measurement of volumes, if the figure after the decimal point is a zero or ends in a zero (for example, 10.0 ml or 0.50 ml), the volume is measured using a pipette, a volumetric flask or a burette, as appropriate; otherwise, a graduated measuring cylinder or a graduated pipette may be used. Volumes stated in microlitres are measured using a micropipette or microsyringe.

It is recognised, however, that in certain cases the precision with which quantities are stated does not correspond to the number of significant figures stated in a specified numerical limit. The weighings and measurements are then carried out with a sufficiently improved accuracy.

Apparatus and procedures. Volumetric glassware complies with Class A requirements of the appropriate International Standard issued by the International Organisation for Standardisation.

Unless otherwise prescribed, analytical procedures are carried out at a temperature between 15 °C and 25 °C.

Unless otherwise prescribed, comparative tests are carried out using identical tubes of colourless, transparent, neutral glass with a flat base; the volumes of liquid prescribed are for use with tubes having an internal diameter of 16 mm, but tubes with a larger internal diameter may be used provided the volume of liquid used is adjusted (*2.1.5*). Equal volumes of the liquids to be compared are examined down the vertical axis of the tubes against a white background, or if necessary against a black background. The examination is carried out in diffuse light.

Any solvent required in a test or assay in which an indicator is to be used is previously neutralised to the indicator, unless a blank test is prescribed.

Water-bath. The term 'water-bath' means a bath of boiling water unless water at another temperature is indicated. Other methods of heating may be substituted provided the temperature is near to but not higher than 100 °C or the indicated temperature.

Drying and ignition to constant mass. The terms 'dried to constant mass' and 'ignited to constant mass' mean that 2 consecutive weighings do not differ by more than 0.5 mg, the 2nd weighing following an additional period of drying or of ignition respectively appropriate to the nature and quantity of the residue.

Where drying is prescribed using one of the expressions 'in a desiccator' or '*in vacuo*', it is carried out using the conditions described in chapter *2.2.32. Loss on drying*.

Reagents. The proper conduct of the analytical procedures described in the Pharmacopoeia and the reliability of the results depend, in part, upon the quality of the reagents used. The reagents are described in general chapter *4*. It is assumed that reagents of analytical grade are used; for some reagents, tests to determine suitability are included in the specifications.

Solvents. Where the name of the solvent is not stated, the term 'solution' implies a solution in water.

Where the use of water is specified or implied in the analytical procedures described in the Pharmacopoeia or for the preparation of reagents, water complying with the requirements of the monograph *Purified water (0008)* is used, except that for many purposes the requirements for bacterial endotoxins (*Purified water in bulk*) and microbial contamination (*Purified water in containers*) are not relevant. The term 'distilled water' indicates purified water prepared by distillation.

The term 'ethanol' without qualification means anhydrous ethanol. The term 'alcohol' without qualification means ethanol (96 per cent). Other dilutions of ethanol are indicated by the term 'ethanol' or 'alcohol' followed by a statement of the percentage by volume of ethanol (C_2H_6O) required.

Expression of content. In defining content, the expression 'per cent' is used according to circumstances with one of 2 meanings:

— per cent *m/m* (percentage, mass in mass) expresses the number of grams of substance in 100 grams of final product;

— per cent *V/V* (percentage, volume in volume) expresses the number of millilitres of substance in 100 millilitres of final product.

The expression 'parts per million' (or ppm) refers to mass in mass, unless otherwise specified.

Temperature. Where an analytical procedure describes temperature without a figure, the general terms used have the following meaning:

— in a deep-freeze: below – 15 °C;

— in a refrigerator: 2 °C to 8 °C;

— cold or cool: 8 °C to 15 °C;

— room temperature: 15 °C to 25 °C.

1.3. GENERAL CHAPTERS

Containers. Materials used for containers are described in general chapter *3.1*. General names used for materials, particularly plastic materials, each cover a range of products varying not only in the properties of the principal constituent but also in the additives used. The test methods and limits for materials depend on the formulation and are therefore applicable only for materials whose formulation is covered by the preamble to the specification. The use of materials with different formulations, and the test methods and limits applied to them, are subject to agreement by the competent authority.

The specifications for containers in general chapter *3.2* have been developed for general application to containers of the stated category, but in view of the wide variety of containers available and possible new developments, the publication of a specification does not exclude the use, in justified circumstances, of containers that comply with other specifications, subject to agreement by the competent authority.

Reference may be made within the monographs of the Pharmacopoeia to the definitions and specifications for containers provided in chapter *3.2. Containers*. The general monographs for pharmaceutical dosage forms may, under the heading Definition/Production, require the use of certain types of container; certain other monographs may, under the heading Storage, indicate the type of container that is recommended for use.

1.4. MONOGRAPHS

TITLES

Monograph titles are in English and French in the respective versions and there is a Latin subtitle.

RELATIVE ATOMIC AND MOLECULAR MASSES

The relative atomic mass (A_r) or the relative molecular mass (M_r) is shown, as and where appropriate, at the beginning of each monograph. The relative atomic and molecular masses and the molecular and graphic formulae do not constitute analytical standards for the substances described.

CHEMICAL ABSTRACTS SERVICE (CAS) REGISTRY NUMBER

CAS registry numbers are included for information in monographs, where applicable, to provide convenient access to useful information for users. CAS Registry Number® is a Registered Trademark of the American Chemical Society.

DEFINITION

Statements under the heading Definition constitute an official definition of the substance, preparation or other article that is the subject of the monograph.

Limits of content. Where limits of content are prescribed, they are those determined by the method described under Assay.

Herbal drugs. In monographs on herbal drugs, the definition indicates whether the subject of the monograph is, for example, the whole drug or the drug in powdered form. Where a monograph applies to the drug in several states, for example both to the whole drug and the drug in powdered form, the definition states this.

PRODUCTION

Statements under the heading Production draw attention to particular aspects of the manufacturing process but are not necessarily comprehensive. They constitute mandatory requirements for manufacturers, unless otherwise stated. They may relate, for example, to source materials; to the manufacturing process itself and its validation and control;

to in-process testing; or to testing that is to be carried out by the manufacturer on the final article, either on selected batches or on each batch prior to release. These statements cannot necessarily be verified on a sample of the final article by an independent analyst. The competent authority may establish that the instructions have been followed, for example, by examination of data received from the manufacturer, by inspection of manufacture or by testing appropriate samples.

The absence of a Production section does not imply that attention to features such as those referred to above is not required.

Choice of vaccine strain, Choice of vaccine composition. The Production section of a monograph may define the characteristics of a vaccine strain or vaccine composition. Unless otherwise stated, test methods given for verification of these characteristics are provided for information as examples of suitable methods. Subject to approval by the competent authority, other test methods may be used without validation against the method shown in the monograph.

CHARACTERS

The statements under the heading Characters are not to be interpreted in a strict sense and are not requirements.

Solubility. In statements of solubility in the Characters section, the terms used have the following significance, referred to a temperature between 15 °C and 25 °C.

Descriptive term	Approximate volume of solvent in millilitres per gram of solute		
Very soluble	less than	1	
Freely soluble	from	1	to 10
Soluble	from	10	to 30
Sparingly soluble	from	30	to 100
Slightly soluble	from	100	to 1000
Very slightly soluble	from	1000	to 10 000
Practically insoluble	more than		10 000

The term 'partly soluble' is used to describe a mixture where only some of the components dissolve. The term 'miscible' is used to describe a liquid that is miscible in all proportions with the stated solvent.

IDENTIFICATION

Scope. The tests given in the Identification section are not designed to give a full confirmation of the chemical structure or composition of the product; they are intended to give confirmation, with an acceptable degree of assurance, that the article conforms to the description on the label.

First and second identifications. Certain monographs have subdivisions entitled 'First identification' and 'Second identification'. The test or tests that constitute the 'First identification' may be used in all circumstances. The test or tests that constitute the 'Second identification' may be used in pharmacies provided it can be demonstrated that the substance or preparation is fully traceable to a batch certified to comply with all the other requirements of the monograph.

Certain monographs give two or more sets of tests for the purpose of the first identification, which are equivalent and may be used independently. One or more of these sets usually contain a cross-reference to a test prescribed in the Tests section of the monograph. It may be used to simplify the work of the analyst carrying out the identification and the prescribed tests. For example, one identification set cross-refers to a test for enantiomeric purity while the other set gives a test for specific optical rotation: the intended purpose of the two is the same, that is, verification that the correct enantiomer is present.

Powdered herbal drugs. Monographs on herbal drugs may contain schematic drawings of the powdered drug. These drawings complement the description given in the relevant identification test.

TESTS AND ASSAYS

Scope. The requirements are not framed to take account of all possible impurities. It is not to be presumed, for example, that an impurity that is not detectable by means of the prescribed tests is tolerated if common sense and good pharmaceutical practice require that it be absent. See also below under Impurities.

Calculation. Where the result of a test or assay is required to be calculated with reference to the dried or anhydrous substance or on some other specified basis, the determination of loss on drying, water content or other property is carried out by the method prescribed in the relevant test in the monograph. The words 'dried substance' or 'anhydrous substance' etc. appear in parentheses after the result.

Limits. The limits prescribed are based on data obtained in normal analytical practice; they take account of normal analytical errors, of acceptable variations in manufacture and compounding and of deterioration to an extent considered acceptable. No further tolerances are to be applied to the limits prescribed to determine whether the article being examined complies with the requirements of the monograph.

In determining compliance with a numerical limit, the calculated result of a test or assay is first rounded to the number of significant figures stated, unless otherwise prescribed. The last figure is increased by one when the part rejected is equal to or exceeds one half-unit, whereas it is not modified when the part rejected is less than a half-unit.

Indication of permitted limit of impurities. For comparative tests, the approximate content of impurity tolerated, or the sum of impurities, may be indicated for information only. Acceptance or rejection is determined on the basis of compliance or non-compliance with the stated test. If the use of a reference substance for the named impurity is not prescribed, this content may be expressed as a nominal concentration of the substance used to prepare the reference solution specified in the monograph, unless otherwise described.

Herbal drugs. For herbal drugs, the sulphated ash, total ash, water-soluble matter, alcohol-soluble matter, water content, content of essential oil and content of active principle are calculated with reference to the drug that has not been specially dried, unless otherwise prescribed in the monograph.

Equivalents. Where an equivalent is given, for the purposes of the Pharmacopoeia only the figures shown are to be used in applying the requirements of the monograph.

Culture media. The culture media described in monographs and general chapters have been found to be satisfactory for the intended purpose. However, the components of media, particularly those of biological origin, are of variable quality, and it may be necessary for optimal performance to modulate the concentration of some ingredients, notably:

— peptones and meat or yeast extracts, with respect to their nutritive properties;

— buffering substances;

— bile salts, bile extract, deoxycholate, and colouring matter, depending on their selective properties;

— antibiotics, with respect to their activity.

STORAGE

The information and recommendations given under the heading Storage do not constitute a pharmacopoeial requirement but the competent authority may specify particular storage conditions that must be met.

The articles described in the Pharmacopoeia are stored in such a way as to prevent contamination and, as far as possible, deterioration. Where special conditions of storage are recommended, including the type of container (see section 1.3. General chapters) and limits of temperature, they are stated in the monograph.

The following expressions are used in monographs under Storage with the meaning shown.

In an airtight container means that the product is stored in an airtight container (*3.2*). Care is to be taken when the container is opened in a damp atmosphere. A low moisture content may be maintained, if necessary, by the use of a desiccant in the container provided that direct contact with the product is avoided.

Protected from light means that the product is stored either in a container made of a material that absorbs actinic light sufficiently to protect the contents from change induced by such light, or in a container enclosed in an outer cover that provides such protection, or is stored in a place from which all such light is excluded.

LABELLING

In general, labelling of medicines is subject to supranational and national regulation and to international agreements. The statements under the heading Labelling are not therefore comprehensive and, moreover, for the purposes of the Pharmacopoeia only those statements that are necessary to demonstrate compliance or non-compliance with the monograph are mandatory. Any other labelling statements are included as recommendations. When the term 'label' is used in the Pharmacopoeia, the labelling statements may appear on the container, the package, a leaflet accompanying the package, or a certificate of analysis accompanying the article, as decided by the competent authority.

WARNINGS

Materials described in monographs and reagents specified for use in the Pharmacopoeia may be injurious to health unless adequate precautions are taken. The principles of good quality control laboratory practice and the provisions of any appropriate regulations are to be observed at all times. Attention is drawn to particular hazards in certain monographs by means of a warning statement; absence of such a statement is not to be taken to mean that no hazard exists.

IMPURITIES

A list of all known and potential impurities that have been shown to be detected by the tests in a monograph may be given. See also chapter *5.10. Control of impurities in substances for pharmaceutical use*. The impurities are designated by a letter or letters of the alphabet. Where a letter appears to be missing, the impurity designated by this letter has been deleted from the list during monograph development prior to publication or during monograph revision.

FUNCTIONALITY-RELATED CHARACTERISTICS OF EXCIPIENTS

Monographs on excipients may have a section on functionality-related characteristics. The characteristics, any test methods for determination and any tolerances are not mandatory requirements; they may nevertheless be relevant for use of the excipient and are given for information (see also section 1.1. General statements).

REFERENCE STANDARDS

Certain monographs require the use of reference standards (chemical reference substances, biological reference preparations, reference spectra). See also chapter *5.12. Reference standards.* The European Pharmacopoeia Commission establishes the official reference standards, which are alone authoritative in case of arbitration. These reference standards are available from the European Directorate for the Quality of Medicines & HealthCare (EDQM). Information on the available reference standards and a batch validity statement can be obtained via the EDQM website.

1.5. ABBREVIATIONS AND SYMBOLS

A	Absorbance
$A_{1\,cm}^{1\,per\,cent}$	Specific absorbance
A_r	Relative atomic mass
$[\alpha]_D^{20}$	Specific optical rotation
bp	Boiling point
BRP	Biological reference preparation
CRS	Chemical reference substance
d_{20}^{20}	Relative density
IU	International Unit
λ	Wavelength
M	Molarity
M_r	Relative molecular mass
mp	Melting point
n_D^{20}	Refractive index
Ph. Eur. U.	European Pharmacopoeia Unit
ppm	Parts per million
R	Substance or solution defined under *4. Reagents*
R_F	Retardation factor (see chapter *2.2.46*)
R_{st}	Used in chromatography to indicate the ratio of the distance travelled by .a substance to the distance travelled by a reference substance
RV	Substance used as a primary standard in volumetric analysis (chapter *4.2.1*)

Abbreviations used in the monographs on immunoglobulins, immunosera and vaccines

LD_{50}	The statistically determined quantity of a substance that, when administered by the specified route, may be expected to cause the death of 50 per cent of the test animals within a given period
MLD	Minimum lethal dose
L+/10 dose	The smallest quantity of a toxin that, in the conditions of the test, when mixed with 0.1 IU of antitoxin and administered by the specified route, causes the death of the test animals within a given period
L+ dose	The smallest quantity of a toxin that, in the conditions of the test, when mixed with 1 IU of antitoxin and administered by the specified route, causes the death of the test animals within a given period
lr/100 dose	The smallest quantity of a toxin that, in the conditions of the test, when mixed with 0.01 IU of antitoxin and injected intracutaneously causes a characteristic reaction at the site of injection within a given period
Lp/10 dose	The smallest quantity of toxin that, in the conditions of the test, when mixed with 0.1 IU of antitoxin and administered by the specified route, causes paralysis in the test animals within a given period
Lo/10 dose	The largest quantity of a toxin that, in the conditions of the test, when mixed with 0.1 IU of antitoxin and administered by the specified route, does not cause symptoms of toxicity in the test animals within a given period
Lf dose	The quantity of toxin or toxoid that flocculates in the shortest time with 1 IU of antitoxin
$CCID_{50}$	The statistically determined quantity of virus that may be expected to infect 50 per cent of the cell cultures to which it is added
EID_{50}	The statistically determined quantity of virus that may be expected to infect 50 per cent of the fertilised eggs into which it is inoculated
ID_{50}	The statistically determined quantity of a virus that may be expected to infect 50 per cent of the animals into which it is inoculated
PD_{50}	The statistically determined dose of a vaccine that, in the conditions of the test, may be expected to protect 50 per cent of the animals against a challenge dose of the micro-organisms or toxins against which it is active
ED_{50}	The statistically determined dose of a vaccine that, in the conditions of the test, may be expected to induce specific antibodies in 50 per cent of the animals for the relevant vaccine antigens
PFU	Pock-forming units or plaque-forming units
SPF	Specified-pathogen-free

Collections of micro-organisms

ATCC	American Type Culture Collection 10801 University Boulevard Manassas, Virginia 20110-2209, USA
C.I.P.	Collection de Bactéries de l'Institut Pasteur B.P. 52, 25 rue du Docteur Roux 75724 Paris Cedex 15, France
IMI	International Mycological Institute Bakeham Lane Surrey TW20 9TY, Great Britain
I.P.	Collection Nationale de Culture de Microorganismes (C.N.C.M.) Institut Pasteur 25, rue du Docteur Roux 75724 Paris Cedex 15, France

NCIMB	National Collection of Industrial and Marine Bacteria Ltd
	23 St Machar Drive
	Aberdeen AB2 1RY, Great Britain
NCPF	National Collection of Pathogenic Fungi
	London School of Hygiene and Tropical Medicine
	Keppel Street
	London WC1E 7HT, Great Britain
NCTC	National Collection of Type Cultures
	Central Public Health Laboratory
	Colindale Avenue
	London NW9 5HT, Great Britain
NCYC	National Collection of Yeast Cultures
	AFRC Food Research Institute
	Colney Lane
	Norwich NR4 7UA, Great Britain
S.S.I.	Statens Serum Institut
	80 Amager Boulevard, Copenhagen, Denmark

1.6. UNITS OF THE INTERNATIONAL SYSTEM (SI) USED IN THE PHARMACOPOEIA AND EQUIVALENCE WITH OTHER UNITS

INTERNATIONAL SYSTEM OF UNITS (SI)

The International System of Units comprises 3 classes of units, namely base units, derived units and supplementary units[1]. The base units and their definitions are set out in Table 1.6-1.

The derived units may be formed by combining the base units according to the algebraic relationships linking the corresponding quantities. Some of these derived units have special names and symbols. The SI units used in the Pharmacopoeia are shown in Table 1.6-2.

Some important and widely used units outside the International System are shown in Table 1.6-3.

The prefixes shown in Table 1.6-4 are used to form the names and symbols of the decimal multiples and submultiples of SI units.

NOTES

1. In the Pharmacopoeia, the Celsius temperature is used (symbol t). This is defined by the following equation:

$$t = T - T_0$$

where T_0 = 273.15 K by definition. The Celsius or centigrade temperature is expressed in degrees Celsius (symbol °C). The unit 'degree Celsius' is equal to the unit 'kelvin'.

2. The practical expressions of concentrations used in the Pharmacopoeia are defined in the General Notices.

3. The radian is the plane angle between two radii of a circle that cut off on the circumference an arc equal in length to the radius.

4. In the Pharmacopoeia, conditions of centrifugation are defined by reference to the acceleration due to gravity (g):

$$g = 9.806\ 65\ m \cdot s^{-2}$$

5. Certain quantities without dimensions are used in the Pharmacopoeia: relative density (*2.2.5*), absorbance (*2.2.25*), specific absorbance (*2.2.25*) and refractive index (*2.2.6*).

6. The microkatal is defined as the enzymic activity that, under defined conditions, produces the transformation (e.g. hydrolysis) of 1 micromole of the substrate per second.

Table 1.6.-1. − *SI base units*

Quantity		Unit		Definition
Name	Symbol	Name	Symbol	
Length	l	metre	m	The metre is the length of the path travelled by light in a vacuum during a time interval of 1/299 792 458 of a second.
Mass	m	kilogram	kg	The kilogram is equal to the mass of the international prototype of the kilogram.
Time	t	second	s	The second is the duration of 9 192 631 770 periods of the radiation corresponding to the transition between the two hyperfine levels of the ground state of the caesium-133 atom.
Electric current	I	ampere	A	The ampere is that constant current which, maintained in two straight parallel conductors of infinite length, of negligible circular cross-section and placed 1 metre apart in vacuum would produce between these conductors a force equal to 2×10^{-7} newton per metre of length.
Thermodynamic temperature	T	kelvin	K	The kelvin is the fraction 1/273.16 of the thermodynamic temperature of the triple point of water.
Amount of substance	n	mole	mol	The mole is the amount of substance of a system containing as many elementary entities as there are atoms in 0.012 kilogram of carbon-12*.
Luminous intensity	I_v	candela	cd	The candela is the luminous intensity in a given direction of a source emitting monochromatic radiation with a frequency of 540×10^{12} hertz and whose energy intensity in that direction is 1/683 watt per steradian.

* When the mole is used, the elementary entities must be specified and may be atoms, molecules, ions, electrons, other particles or specified groups of such particles.

---

(1) The definitions of the units used in the International System are given in the booklet 'Le Système International d'Unités (SI)', published by the Bureau International des Poids et Mesures, Pavillon de Breteuil, F-92310 Sèvres.

Table 1.6.-2. – *SI units used in the European Pharmacopoeia and equivalence with other units*

Quantity		Unit				Conversion of other units into SI units
Name	Symbol	Name	Symbol	Expression in SI base units	Expression in other SI units	
Wave number	ν	one per metre	1/m	m^{-1}		
Wavelength	λ	micrometre	μm	$10^{-6}m$		
		nanometre	nm	$10^{-9}m$		
Area	A, S	square metre	m^2	m^2		
Volume	V	cubic metre	m^3	m^3		$1\ ml = 1\ cm^3 = 10^{-6}\ m^3$
Frequency	ν	hertz	Hz	s^{-1}		
Density	ρ	kilogram per cubic metre	kg/m^3	$kg{\cdot}m^{-3}$		$1\ g/ml = 1\ g/cm^3 = 10^3\ kg{\cdot}m^{-3}$
Velocity	v	metre per second	m/s	$m{\cdot}s^{-1}$		
Force	F	newton	N	$m{\cdot}kg{\cdot}s^{-2}$		$1\ dyne = 1\ g{\cdot}cm{\cdot}s^{-2} = 10^{-5}\ N$
						$1\ kp = 9.806\ 65\ N$
Pressure	p	pascal	Pa	$m^{-1}{\cdot}kg{\cdot}s^{-2}$	$N{\cdot}m^{-2}$	$1\ dyne/cm^2 = 10^{-1}\ Pa = 10^{-1}\ N{\cdot}m^{-2}$
						$1\ atm = 101\ 325\ Pa = 101.325\ kPa$
						$1\ bar = 10^5\ Pa = 0.1\ MPa$
						$1\ mm\ Hg = 133.322\ 387\ Pa$
						$1\ Torr = 133.322\ 368\ Pa$
						$1\ psi = 6.894\ 757\ kPa$
Dynamic viscosity	η	pascal second	Pa·s	$m^{-1}{\cdot}kg{\cdot}s^{-1}$	$N{\cdot}s{\cdot}m^{-2}$	$1\ P = 10^{-1}\ Pa{\cdot}s = 10^{-1}\ N{\cdot}s{\cdot}m^{-2}$
						$1\ cP = 1\ mPa{\cdot}s$
Kinematic viscosity	ν	square metre per second	m^2/s	$m^2{\cdot}s^{-1}$	$Pa{\cdot}s{\cdot}m^3{\cdot}kg^{-1}$ $N{\cdot}m{\cdot}s{\cdot}kg^{-1}$	$1\ St = 1\ cm^2{\cdot}s^{-1} = 10^{-4}\ m^2{\cdot}s^{-1}$
Energy	W	joule	J	$m^2{\cdot}kg{\cdot}s^{-2}$	$N{\cdot}m$	$1\ erg = 1\ cm^2{\cdot}g{\cdot}s^{-2} =$ $1\ dyne{\cdot}cm = 10^{-7}\ J$ $1\ cal = 4.1868\ J$
Power Radiant flux	P	watt	W	$m^2{\cdot}kg{\cdot}s^{-3}$	$N{\cdot}m{\cdot}s^{-1}$ $J{\cdot}s^{-1}$	$1\ erg/s = 1\ dyne{\cdot}cm{\cdot}s^{-1} =$ $10^{-7}\ W = 10^{-7}\ N{\cdot}m{\cdot}s^{-1} =$ $10^{-7}\ J{\cdot}s^{-1}$
Absorbed dose (of radiant energy)	D	gray	Gy	$m^2{\cdot}s^{-2}$	$J{\cdot}kg^{-1}$	$1\ rad = 10^{-2}\ Gy$
Electric potential, electromotive force	U	volt	V	$m^2{\cdot}kg{\cdot}s^{-3}{\cdot}A^{-1}$	$W{\cdot}A^{-1}$	
Electric resistance	R	ohm	Ω	$m^2{\cdot}kg{\cdot}s^{-3}{\cdot}A^{-2}$	$V{\cdot}A^{-1}$	
Quantity of electricity	Q	coulomb	C	$A{\cdot}s$		
Activity of a radionuclide	A	becquerel	Bq	s^{-1}		$1\ Ci = 37{\cdot}10^9\ Bq = 37{\cdot}10^9\ s^{-1}$
Concentration (of amount of substance), molar concentration	c	mole per cubic metre	mol/m^3	$mol{\cdot}m^{-3}$		$1\ mol/l = 1M = 1\ mol/dm^3 = 10^3\ mol{\cdot}m^{-3}$
Mass concentration	ρ	kilogram per cubic metre	kg/m^3	$kg{\cdot}m^{-3}$		$1\ g/l = 1\ g/dm^3 = 1\ kg{\cdot}m^{-3}$

Table 1.6.-3. – *Units used with the International System*

Quantity	Unit		Value in SI units
	Name	Symbol	
Time	minute	min	$1\ min = 60\ s$
	hour	h	$1\ h = 60\ min = 3600\ s$
	day	d	$1\ d = 24\ h = 86\ 400\ s$
Plane angle	degree	°	$1° = (\pi/180)\ rad$
Volume	litre	l	$1\ l = 1\ dm^3 = 10^{-3}\ m^3$
Mass	tonne	t	$1\ t = 10^3\ kg$
Rotational frequency	revolution per minute	r/min	$1\ r/min = (1/60)\ s^{-1}$

Table 1.6.-4. – *Decimal multiples and sub-multiples of units*

Factor	Prefix	Symbol	Factor	Prefix	Symbol
10^{18}	exa	E	10^{-1}	deci	d
10^{15}	peta	P	10^{-2}	centi	c
10^{12}	tera	T	10^{-3}	milli	m
10^{9}	giga	G	10^{-6}	micro	μ
10^{6}	mega	M	10^{-9}	nano	n
10^{3}	kilo	k	10^{-12}	pico	p
10^{2}	hecto	h	10^{-15}	femto	f
10^{1}	deca	da	10^{-18}	atto	a

2.6. BIOLOGICAL TESTS

2. Methods of analysis

07/2009:20612

2.6.12. MICROBIOLOGICAL EXAMINATION OF NON-STERILE PRODUCTS: MICROBIAL ENUMERATION TESTS

1. INTRODUCTION

The tests described hereafter will allow quantitative enumeration of mesophilic bacteria and fungi that may grow under aerobic conditions.

The tests are designed primarily to determine whether a substance or preparation complies with an established specification for microbiological quality. When used for such purposes follow the instructions given below, including the number of samples to be taken, and interpret the results as stated below.

The methods are not applicable to products containing viable micro-organisms as active ingredients.

Alternative microbiological procedures, including automated methods, may be used, provided that their equivalence to the Pharmacopoeia method has been demonstrated.

2. GENERAL PROCEDURES

Carry out the determination under conditions designed to avoid extrinsic microbial contamination of the product to be examined. The precautions taken to avoid contamination must be such that they do not affect any micro-organisms that are to be revealed in the test.

If the product to be examined has antimicrobial activity, this is insofar as possible removed or neutralised. If inactivators are used for this purpose, their efficacy and their absence of toxicity for micro-organisms must be demonstrated.

If surface-active substances are used for sample preparation, their absence of toxicity for micro-organisms and their compatibility with inactivators used must be demonstrated.

3. ENUMERATION METHODS

Use the membrane filtration method or the plate-count methods, as prescribed. The most-probable-number (MPN) method is generally the least accurate method for microbial counts, however, for certain product groups with a very low bioburden, it may be the most appropriate method.

The choice of method is based on factors such as the nature of the product and the required limit of micro-organisms. The chosen method must allow testing of a sufficient sample size to judge compliance with the specification. The suitability of the method chosen must be established.

4. GROWTH PROMOTION TEST, SUITABILITY OF THE COUNTING METHOD AND NEGATIVE CONTROLS

4-1. GENERAL CONSIDERATIONS

The ability of the test to detect micro-organisms in the presence of product to be tested must be established.

Suitability must be confirmed if a change in testing performance, or the product, which may affect the outcome of the test is introduced.

4-2. PREPARATION OF TEST STRAINS

Use standardised stable suspensions of test strains or prepare them as stated below. Seed lot culture maintenance techniques (seed-lot systems) are used so that the viable micro-organisms used for inoculation are not more than 5 passages removed from the original master seed-lot. Grow each of the bacterial and fungal test strains separately as described in Table 2.6.12.-1.

Use buffered sodium chloride-peptone solution pH 7.0 or phosphate buffer solution pH 7.2 to make test suspensions; to suspend *A. niger* spores, 0.05 per cent of polysorbate 80 may be added to the buffer. Use the suspensions within 2 h or within 24 h if stored at 2-8 °C. As an alternative to preparing and then diluting a fresh suspension of vegetative cells of *A. niger* or *B. subtilis*, a stable spore suspension is prepared and then an appropriate volume of the spore suspension is used for test inoculation. The stable spore suspension may be maintained at 2-8 °C for a validated period of time.

4-3. NEGATIVE CONTROL

To verify testing conditions, a negative control is performed using the chosen diluent in place of the test preparation. There must be no growth of micro-organisms. A negative control is also performed when testing the products as described in section 5. A failed negative control requires an investigation.

4-4. GROWTH PROMOTION OF THE MEDIA

Test each batch of ready-prepared medium and each batch of medium, prepared either from dehydrated medium or from the ingredients described.

Inoculate portions/plates of casein soya bean digest broth and casein soya bean digest agar with a small number (not more than 100 CFU) of the micro-organisms indicated in Table 2.6.12.-1, using a separate portion/plate of medium for each. Inoculate plates of Sabouraud-dextrose agar with a small number (not more than 100 CFU) of the micro-organisms indicated in Table 2.6.12.-1, using a separate plate of medium for each. Incubate in the conditions described in Table 2.6.12.-1.

For solid media, growth obtained must not differ by a factor greater than 2 from the calculated value for a standardised inoculum. For a freshly prepared inoculum, growth of the micro-organisms comparable to that previously obtained with a previously tested and approved batch of medium occurs. Liquid media are suitable if clearly visible growth of the micro-organisms comparable to that previously obtained with a previously tested and approved batch of medium occurs.

4-5. SUITABILITY OF THE COUNTING METHOD IN THE PRESENCE OF PRODUCT

4-5-1. **Preparation of the sample.** The method for sample preparation depends upon the physical characteristics of the product to be tested. If none of the procedures described below can be demonstrated to be satisfactory, an alternative procedure must be developed.

Water-soluble products. Dissolve or dilute (usually a 1 in 10 dilution is prepared) the product to be examined in buffered sodium chloride-peptone solution pH 7.0, phosphate buffer solution pH 7.2 or casein soya bean digest broth. If necessary, adjust to pH 6-8. Further dilutions, where necessary, are prepared with the same diluent.

Non-fatty products insoluble in water. Suspend the product to be examined (usually a 1 in 10 dilution is prepared) in buffered sodium chloride-peptone solution pH 7.0, phosphate buffer solution pH 7.2 or casein soya bean digest broth. A surface-active agent such as 1 g/l of polysorbate 80 may be added to assist the suspension of poorly wettable substances. If necessary, adjust to pH 6-8. Further dilutions, where necessary, are prepared with the same diluent.

Table 2.6.12.-1. – *Preparation and use of test micro-organisms*

Micro-organism	Preparation of test strain	Growth promotion		Suitability of counting method in the presence of the product	
		Total aerobic microbial count	Total yeasts and moulds count	Total aerobic microbial count	Total yeasts and moulds count
Staphylococcus aureus such as: ATCC 6538 NCIMB 9518 CIP 4.83 NBRC 13276	Casein soya bean digest agar and casein soya bean digest broth 30-35 °C 18-24 h	Casein soya bean digest agar and casein soya bean digest broth ≤ 100 CFU 30-35 °C ≤ 3 days	-	Casein soya bean digest agar/MPN casein soya bean digest broth ≤ 100 CFU 30-35 °C ≤ 3 days	-
Pseudomonas aeruginosa such as: ATCC 9027 NCIMB 8626 CIP 82.118 NBRC 13275	Casein soya bean digest agar or casein soya bean digest broth 30-35 °C 18-24 h	Casein soya bean digest agar and casein soya bean digest broth ≤ 100 CFU 30-35 °C ≤ 3 days	-	Casein soya bean digest agar/MPN casein soya bean digest broth ≤ 100 CFU 30-35 °C ≤ 3 days	-
Bacillus subtilis such as: ATCC 6633 NCIMB 8054 CIP 52.62 NBRC 3134	Casein soya bean digest agar or casein soya bean digest broth 30-35 °C 18-24 h	Casein soya bean digest agar and casein soya bean digest broth ≤ 100 CFU 30-35 °C ≤ 3 days	-	Casein soya bean digest agar/MPN casein soya bean digest broth ≤ 100 CFU 30-35 °C ≤ 3 days	-
Candida albicans such as: ATCC 10231 NCPF 3179 IP 48.72 NBRC 1594	Sabouraud-dextrose agar or Sabouraud-dextrose broth 20-25 °C 2-3 days	Casein soya bean digest agar ≤ 100 CFU 30-35 °C ≤ 5 days	Sabouraud-dextrose agar ≤ 100 CFU 20-25 °C ≤ 5 days	Casein soya bean digest agar ≤ 100 CFU 30-35 °C ≤ 5 days MPN: not applicable	Sabouraud-dextrose agar ≤ 100 CFU 20-25 °C ≤ 5 days
Aspergillus niger such as: ATCC 16404 IMI 149007 IP 1431.83 NBRC 9455	Sabouraud-dextrose agar or potato-dextrose agar 20-25 °C 5-7 days, or until good sporulation is achieved	Casein soya bean digest agar ≤ 100 CFU 30-35 °C ≤ 5 days	Sabouraud-dextrose agar ≤ 100 CFU 20-25 °C ≤ 5 days	Casein soya bean digest agar ≤ 100 CFU 30-35 °C ≤ 5 days MPN: not applicable	Sabouraud-dextrose agar ≤ 100 CFU 20-25 °C ≤ 5 days

Fatty products. Dissolve in isopropyl myristate, sterilised by filtration or mix the product to be examined with the minimum necessary quantity of sterile polysorbate 80 or another non-inhibitory sterile surface-active agent, heated if necessary to not more than 40 °C, or in exceptional cases to not more than 45 °C. Mix carefully and if necessary maintain the temperature in a water-bath. Add sufficient of the pre-warmed chosen diluent to make a 1 in 10 dilution of the original product. Mix carefully whilst maintaining the temperature for the shortest time necessary for the formation of an emulsion. Further serial tenfold dilutions may be prepared using the chosen diluent containing a suitable concentration of sterile polysorbate 80 or another non-inhibitory sterile surface-active agent.

Fluids or solids in aerosol form. Aseptically transfer the product into a membrane filter apparatus or a sterile container for further sampling. Use either the total contents or a defined number of metered doses from each of the containers tested.

Transdermal patches. Remove the protective cover sheets ('release liners') of the transdermal patches and place them, adhesive side upwards, on sterile glass or plastic trays. Cover the adhesive surface with a sterile porous material, for example sterile gauze, to prevent the patches from sticking together, and transfer the patches to a suitable volume of the chosen diluent containing inactivators such as polysorbate 80 and/or lecithin. Shake the preparation vigorously for at least 30 min.

4-5-2. **Inoculation and dilution**. Add to the sample prepared as described above (4-5-1) and to a control (with no test material included) a sufficient volume of the microbial suspension to obtain an inoculum of not more than 100 CFU. The volume of the suspension of the inoculum should not exceed 1 per cent of the volume of diluted product.

To demonstrate acceptable microbial recovery from the product, the lowest possible dilution factor of the prepared sample must be used for the test. Where this is not possible due to antimicrobial activity or poor solubility, further appropriate protocols must be developed. If inhibition of growth by the sample cannot otherwise be avoided, the aliquot of the microbial suspension may be added after neutralisation, dilution or filtration.

4-5-3. **Neutralisation/removal of antimicrobial activity**. The number of micro-organisms recovered from the prepared sample diluted as described in 4-5-2 and incubated following the procedure described in 4-5-4, is compared to the number of micro-organisms recovered from the control preparation.

If growth is inhibited (reduction by a factor greater than 2), then modify the procedure for the particular enumeration test to ensure the validity of the results. Modification of the procedure may include, for example, (1) an increase in the volume of the diluent or culture medium, (2) incorporation of specific or general neutralising agents into the diluent, (3) membrane filtration, or (4) a combination of the above measures.

Neutralising agents. Neutralising agents may be used to neutralise the activity of antimicrobial agents (Table 2.6.12.-2). They may be added to the chosen diluent or the medium preferably before sterilisation. If used, their efficacy and their absence of toxicity for micro-organisms must be demonstrated by carrying out a blank with neutraliser and without product.

Table 2.6.12.-2. – *Common neutralising agents for interfering substances*

Interfering substance	Potential neutralising method
Glutaraldehyde, mercurials	Sodium hydrogensulphite (sodium bisulphite)
Phenolics, alcohol, aldehydes, sorbate	Dilution
Aldehydes	Glycine
Quaternary Ammonium Compounds (QACs), parahydroxybenzoates (parabens), bis-biguanides	Lecithin
QACs, iodine, parabens	Polysorbate
Mercurials	Thioglycollate
Mercurials, halogens, aldehydes	Thiosulphate
EDTA (edetate)	Mg^{2+} or Ca^{2+} ions

If no suitable neutralising method can be found, it can be assumed that the failure to isolate the inoculated organism is attributable to the microbicidal activity of the product. This information serves to indicate that the product is not likely to be contaminated with the given species of the micro-organism. However, it is possible that the product only inhibits some of the micro-organisms specified herein, but does not inhibit others not included amongst the test strains or for which the latter are not representative. Then, perform the test with the highest dilution factor compatible with microbial growth and the specific acceptance criterion.

4-5-4. **Recovery of micro-organism in the presence of product**. For each of the micro-organisms listed, separate tests are performed. Only micro-organisms of the added test strain are counted.

4-5-4-1. *Membrane filtration*. Use membrane filters having a nominal pore size not greater than 0.45 μm. The type of filter material is chosen such that the bacteria-retaining efficiency is not affected by the components of the sample to be investigated. For each of the micro-organisms listed, one membrane filter is used.

Transfer a suitable amount of the sample prepared as described under 4-5-1 to 4-5-3 (preferably representing 1 g of the product, or less if large numbers of CFU are expected) to the membrane filter, filter immediately and rinse the membrane filter with an appropriate volume of diluent.

For the determination of total aerobic microbial count (TAMC), transfer the membrane filter to the surface of casein soya bean digest agar. For the determination of total combined yeasts/moulds count (TYMC), transfer the membrane to the surface of Sabouraud-dextrose agar. Incubate the plates as indicated in Table 2.6.12.-1. Perform the counting.

4-5-4-2. *Plate-count methods*. Perform plate-count methods at least in duplicate for each medium and use the mean count of the result.

4-5-4-2-1. Pour-plate method

For Petri dishes 9 cm in diameter, add to the dish 1 ml of the sample prepared as described under 4-5-1 to 4-5-3 and 15-20 ml of casein soya bean digest agar or Sabouraud-dextrose agar, both media being at not more than 45 °C. If larger Petri dishes are used, the amount of agar medium is increased accordingly. For each of the micro-organisms listed in Table 2.6.12.-1, at least 2 Petri dishes are used. Incubate the plates as indicated in Table 2.6.12.-1. Take the arithmetic mean of the counts per medium and calculate the number of CFU in the original inoculum.

4-5-4-2-2. Surface-spread method

For Petri dishes 9 cm in diameter, add 15-20 ml of casein soya bean digest agar or Sabouraud-dextrose agar at about 45 °C to each Petri dish and allow to solidify. If larger Petri dishes are used, the volume of the agar is increased accordingly. Dry the plates, for example in a laminar-air-flow cabinet or an incubator. For each of the micro-organisms listed in Table 2.6.12.-1, at least 2 Petri dishes are used. Spread a measured volume of not less than 0.1 ml of the sample prepared as described under 4-5-1 to 4-5-3 over the surface of the medium. Incubate and count as prescribed under 4-5-4-2-1.

4-5-4-3. *Most-probable-number (MPN) method*. The precision and accuracy of the MPN method is less than that of the membrane filtration method or the plate-count method. Unreliable results are obtained particularly for the enumeration of moulds. For these reasons the MPN method is reserved for the enumeration of TAMC in situations where no other method is available. If the use of the method is justified, proceed as follows.

Prepare a series of at least 3 serial tenfold dilutions of the product as described under 4-5-1 to 4-5-3. From each level of dilution, 3 aliquots of 1 g or 1 ml are used to inoculate 3 tubes with 9-10 ml of casein soya bean digest broth. If necessary, a surface-active agent such as polysorbate 80 or an inactivator of antimicrobial agents may be added to the medium. Thus, if 3 levels of dilution are prepared, 9 tubes are inoculated.

Incubate all tubes at 30-35 °C for not more than 3 days. If reading of the results is difficult or uncertain owing to the nature of the product to be examined, subculture in the same broth, or in casein soya bean digest agar, for 1-2 days at the same temperature and use these results. Determine the most probable number of micro-organisms per gram or millilitre of the product to be examined from Table 2.6.12.-3.

4-6. *RESULTS AND INTERPRETATION*

When verifying the suitability of the membrane filtration method or the plate-count method, a mean count of any of the test organisms not differing by a factor greater than 2 from the value of the control defined in 4-5-2 in the absence of the product must be obtained. When verifying the suitability of the MPN method the calculated value from the inoculum must be within 95 per cent confidence limits of the results obtained with the control.

If the above criteria cannot be met for one or more of the organisms tested with any of the described methods, the method and test conditions that come closest to the criteria are used to test the product.

5. TESTING OF PRODUCTS

5-1. *AMOUNT USED FOR THE TEST*

Unless otherwise prescribed, use 10 g or 10 ml of the product to be examined taken with the precautions referred to above. For fluids or solids in aerosol form, sample 10 containers. For transdermal patches, sample 10 patches.

The amount to be tested may be reduced for active substances that will be formulated in the following conditions: the amount per dosage unit (e.g. tablet, capsule, injection) is less than or equal to 1 mg or the amount per gram or millilitre (for preparations not presented in dose units) is less than 1 mg. In these cases, the amount to be tested is not less than the amount present in 10 dosage units or 10 g or 10 ml of the product.

For materials used as active substances where sample quantity is limited or batch size is extremely small (i.e. less than 1000 ml or 1000 g), the amount tested shall be 1 per cent of the batch unless a lesser amount is prescribed or justified and authorised.

For products where the total number of entities in a batch is less than 200 (e.g. samples used in clinical trials), the sample size may be reduced to 2 units, or 1 unit if the size is less than 100.

Select the sample(s) at random from the bulk material or from the available containers of the preparation. To obtain the required quantity, mix the contents of a sufficient number of containers to provide the sample.

5-2. *EXAMINATION OF THE PRODUCT*

5-2-1. Membrane filtration

Use a filtration apparatus designed to allow the transfer of the filter to the medium. Prepare the sample using a method that has been shown suitable as described in section 4 and transfer the appropriate amount to each of 2 membrane filters and filter immediately. Wash each filter following the procedure shown to be suitable.

For the determination of TAMC, transfer one of the membrane filters to the surface of casein soya bean digest agar. For the determination of TYMC, transfer the other membrane to the surface of Sabouraud-dextrose agar. Incubate the plate of casein soya bean digest agar at 30-35 °C for 3-5 days and the plate of Sabouraud-dextrose agar at 20-25 °C for 5-7 days. Calculate the number of CFU per gram or per millilitre of product.

When examining transdermal patches, filter 10 per cent of the volume of the preparation described under 4-5-1 separately through each of 2 sterile filter membranes. Transfer one membrane to casein soya bean digest agar for TAMC and the other membrane to Sabouraud-dextrose agar for TYMC.

5-2-2. Plate-count methods

5-2-2-1. Pour-plate method

Prepare the sample using a method that has been shown to be suitable as described in section 4. Prepare for each medium at least 2 Petri dishes for each level of dilution. Incubate the plates of casein soya bean digest agar at 30-35 °C for 3-5 days and the plates of Sabouraud-dextrose agar at 20-25 °C for 5-7 days. Select the plates corresponding to a given dilution and showing the highest number of colonies less than 250 for TAMC and 50 for TYMC. Take the arithmetic mean per culture medium of the counts and calculate the number of CFU per gram or per millilitre of product.

5-2-2-2. Surface-spread method

Prepare the sample using a method that has been shown to be suitable as described in section 4. Prepare at least 2 Petri dishes for each medium and each level of dilution. For incubation and calculation of the number of CFU proceed as described for the pour-plate method.

Table 2.6.12.-3. – *Most-probable-number values of micro-organisms*

Observed combinations of numbers of tubes showing growth in each set			MPN per gram or per millilitre of product	95 per cent confidence limits
Number of grams or millilitres of product per tube				
0.1	0.01	0.001		
0	0	0	< 3	0-9.4
0	0	1	3	0.1-9.5
0	1	0	3	0.1-10
0	1	1	6.1	1.2-17
0	2	0	6.2	1.2-17
0	3	0	9.4	3.5-35
1	0	0	3.6	0.2-17
1	0	1	7.2	1.2-17
1	0	2	11	4-35
1	1	0	7.4	1.3-20
1	1	1	11	4-35
1	2	0	11	4-35
1	2	1	15	5-38
1	3	0	16	5-38
2	0	0	9.2	1.5-35
2	0	1	14	4-35
2	0	2	20	5-38
2	1	0	15	4-38
2	1	1	20	5-38
2	1	2	27	9-94
2	2	0	21	5-40
2	2	1	28	9-94
2	2	2	35	9-94
2	3	0	29	9-94
2	3	1	36	9-94
3	0	0	23	5-94
3	0	1	38	9-104
3	0	2	64	16-181
3	1	0	43	9-181
3	1	1	75	17-199
3	1	2	120	30-360
3	1	3	160	30-380
3	2	0	93	18-360
3	2	1	150	30-380
3	2	2	210	30-400
3	2	3	290	90-990
3	3	0	240	40-990
3	3	1	460	90-1980
3	3	2	1100	200-4000
3	3	3	> 1100	

5-2-3. **Most-probable-number method**

Prepare and dilute the sample using a method that has been shown to be suitable as described in section 4. Incubate all tubes at 30-35 °C for 3-5 days. Subculture if necessary, using the procedure shown to be suitable. Record for each level of dilution the number of tubes showing microbial growth. Determine the most probable number of micro-organisms per gram or millilitre of the product to be examined from Table 2.6.12.-3.

5-3. *INTERPRETATION OF THE RESULTS*

The total aerobic microbial count (TAMC) is considered to be equal to the number of CFU found using casein soya bean digest agar; if colonies of fungi are detected on this medium, they are counted as part of the TAMC. The total combined yeasts/mould count (TYMC) is considered to be equal to the number of CFU found using Sabouraud-dextrose agar; if colonies of bacteria are detected on this medium, they are counted as part of the TYMC. When the TYMC is expected to exceed the acceptance criterion due to the bacterial growth, Sabouraud-dextrose agar containing antibiotics may be used. If the count is carried out by the MPN method the calculated value is the TAMC.

When an acceptance criterion for microbiological quality is prescribed it is interpreted as follows:

— 10^1 CFU: maximum acceptable count = 20;

— 10^2 CFU: maximum acceptable count = 200;

— 10^3 CFU: maximum acceptable count = 2000, and so forth.

The recommended solutions and media are described in general chapter *2.6.13*.

07/2009:20613

2.6.13. MICROBIOLOGICAL EXAMINATION OF NON-STERILE PRODUCTS: TEST FOR SPECIFIED MICRO-ORGANISMS

1. INTRODUCTION

The tests described hereafter will allow determination of the absence or limited occurrence of specified micro-organisms that may be detected under the conditions described.

The tests are designed primarily to determine whether a substance or preparation complies with an established specification for microbiological quality. When used for such purposes, follow the instructions given below, including the number of samples to be taken, and interpret the results as stated below.

Alternative microbiological procedures, including automated methods, may be used, provided that their equivalence to the Pharmacopoeia method has been demonstrated.

2. GENERAL PROCEDURES

The preparation of samples is carried out as described in general chapter *2.6.12*.

If the product to be examined has antimicrobial activity, this is insofar as possible removed or neutralised as described in general chapter *2.6.12*.

If surface-active substances are used for sample preparation, their absence of toxicity for micro-organisms and their compatibility with inactivators used must be demonstrated as described in general chapter *2.6.12*.

3. GROWTH-PROMOTING AND INHIBITORY PROPERTIES OF THE MEDIA, SUITABILITY OF THE TEST AND NEGATIVE CONTROLS

The ability of the test to detect micro-organisms in the presence of the product to be tested must be established. Suitability must be confirmed if a change in testing performance, or the product, which may affect the outcome of the test is introduced.

3-1. *PREPARATION OF TEST STRAINS*

Use standardised stable suspensions of test strains or prepare them as stated below. Seed lot culture maintenance techniques (seed-lot systems) are used so that the viable micro-organisms used for inoculation are not more than 5 passages removed from the original master seed-lot.

3-1-1. **Aerobic micro-organisms**. Grow each of the bacterial test strains separately in casein soya bean digest broth or on casein soya bean digest agar at 30-35 °C for 18-24 h. Grow the test strain for *Candida albicans* separately on Sabouraud-dextrose agar or in Sabouraud-dextrose broth at 20-25 °C for 2-3 days.

— *Staphylococcus aureus* such as ATCC 6538, NCIMB 9518, CIP 4.83 or NBRC 13276;

— *Pseudomonas aeruginosa* such as ATCC 9027, NCIMB 8626, CIP 82.118 or NBRC 13275;

— *Escherichia coli* such as ATCC 8739, NCIMB 8545, CIP 53.126 or NBRC 3972;

— *Salmonella enterica* subsp. *enterica* serovar Typhimurium, such as ATCC 14028 or, as an alternative, *Salmonella enterica* subsp. *enterica* serovar Abony such as NBRC 100797, NCTC 6017 or CIP 80.39;

— *Candida albicans* such as ATCC 10231, NCPF 3179, IP 48.72 or NBRC 1594.

Use buffered sodium chloride-peptone solution pH 7.0 or phosphate buffer solution pH 7.2 to make test suspensions. Use the suspensions within 2 h or within 24 h if stored at 2-8 °C.

3-1-2. **Clostridia**. Use *Clostridium sporogenes* such as ATCC 11437 (NBRC 14293, NCIMB 12343, CIP 100651) or ATCC 19404 (NCTC 532 or CIP 79.03) or NBRC 14293. Grow the clostridial test strain under anaerobic conditions in reinforced medium for clostridia at 30-35 °C for 24-48 h. As an alternative to preparing and then diluting down a fresh suspension of vegetative cells of *Cl. sporogenes*, a stable spore suspension is used for test inoculation. The stable spore suspension may be maintained at 2-8 °C for a validated period.

3-2. *NEGATIVE CONTROL*

To verify testing conditions, a negative control is performed using the chosen diluent in place of the test preparation. There must be no growth of micro-organisms. A negative control is also performed when testing the products as described in section 4. A failed negative control requires an investigation.

3-3. *GROWTH PROMOTION AND INHIBITORY PROPERTIES OF THE MEDIA*

Test each batch of ready-prepared medium and each batch of medium prepared either from dehydrated medium or from ingredients.

Verify suitable properties of relevant media as described in Table 2.6.13.-1.

Test for growth promoting properties, liquid media: inoculate a portion of the appropriate medium with a small number (not more than 100 CFU) of the appropriate micro-organism. Incubate at the specified temperature for not more than the shortest period of time specified

Table 2.6.13.-1 − *Growth promoting, inhibitory and indicative properties of media*

	Medium	Property	Test strains
Test for bile-tolerant gram-negative bacteria	Enterobacteria enrichment broth-Mossel	Growth promoting	*E. coli* *P. aeruginosa*
		Inhibitory	*S. aureus*
	Violet red bile glucose agar	Growth promoting + indicative	*E. coli* *P. aeruginosa*
Test for *Escherichia coli*	MacConkey broth	Growth promoting	*E. coli*
		Inhibitory	*S. aureus*
	MacConkey agar	Growth promoting + indicative	*E. coli*
Test for *Salmonella*	Rappaport Vassiliadis *Salmonella* enrichment broth	Growth promoting	*Salmonella enterica* subsp. *enterica* serovar Typhimurium or *Salmonella enterica* subsp. *enterica* serovar Abony
		Inhibitory	*S. aureus*
	Xylose, lysine, deoxycholate agar	Growth promoting + indicative	*Salmonella enterica* subsp. *enterica* serovar Typhimurium or *Salmonella enterica* subsp. *enterica* serovar Abony
Test for *Pseudomonas aeruginosa*	Cetrimide agar	Growth promoting	*P. aeruginosa*
		Inhibitory	*E. coli*
Test for *Staphylococcus aureus*	Mannitol salt agar	Growth promoting + indicative	*S. aureus*
		Inhibitory	*E. coli*
Test for clostridia	Reinforced medium for clostridia	Growth promoting	*Cl. sporogenes*
	Columbia agar	Growth promoting	*Cl. sporogenes*
Test for *Candida albicans*	Sabouraud dextrose broth	Growth promoting	*C. albicans*
	Sabouraud dextrose agar	Growth promoting + indicative	*C. albicans*

in the test. Clearly visible growth of the micro-organism comparable to that previously obtained with a previously tested and approved batch of medium occurs.

Test for growth promoting properties, solid media: perform the surface-spread method, inoculating each plate with a small number (not more than 100 CFU) of the appropriate micro-organism. Incubate at the specified temperature for not more than the shortest period of time specified in the test. Growth of the micro-organism comparable to that previously obtained with a previously tested and approved batch of medium occurs.

Test for inhibitory properties, liquid or solid media: inoculate the appropriate medium with at least 100 CFU of the appropriate micro-organism. Incubate at the specified temperature for not less than the longest period of time specified in the test. No growth of the test micro-organism occurs.

Test for indicative properties: perform the surface-spread method, inoculating each plate with a small number (not more than 100 CFU) of the appropriate micro-organism. Incubate at the specified temperature for a period of time within the range specified in the test. Colonies are comparable in appearance and indication reactions to those previously obtained with a previously tested and approved batch of medium.

3-4. *SUITABILITY OF THE TEST METHOD*

For each product to be tested, perform the sample preparation as described in the relevant paragraph in section 4. Add each test strain at the time of mixing, in the prescribed growth medium. Inoculate the test strains individually. Use a number of micro-organisms equivalent to not more than 100 CFU in the inoculated test preparation. Perform the test as described in the relevant paragraph in section 4 using the shortest incubation period prescribed. The specified micro-organisms must be detected with the indication reactions as described in section 4.

Any antimicrobial activity of the product necessitates a modification of the test procedure (see 4-5-3 of general chapter *2.6.12*).

If for a given product the antimicrobial activity with respect to a micro-organism for which testing is prescribed cannot be neutralised, then it is to be assumed that the inhibited micro-organism will not be present in the product.

4. TESTING OF PRODUCTS

4-1. *BILE-TOLERANT GRAM-NEGATIVE BACTERIA*

4-1-1. **Sample preparation and pre-incubation**. Prepare a sample using a 1 in 10 dilution of not less than 1 g of the product to be examined as described in general chapter *2.6.12*, but using casein soya bean digest broth as the chosen diluent, mix and incubate at 20-25 °C for a time sufficient to resuscitate the bacteria but not sufficient to encourage multiplication of the organisms (usually 2 h but not more than 5 h).

4-1-2. **Test for absence**. Unless otherwise prescribed, use the volume corresponding to 1 g of the product, as prepared in 4-1-1, to inoculate enterobacteria enrichment broth-Mossel. Incubate at 30-35 °C for 24-48 h. Subculture on plates of violet red bile glucose agar. Incubate at 30-35 °C for 18-24 h.

The product complies with the test if there is no growth of colonies.

4-1-3. **Quantitative test**

4-1-3-1. *Selection and subculture*. Inoculate suitable quantities of enterobacteria enrichment broth-Mossel with the preparation as described under 4-1-1 and/or dilutions of it containing respectively 0.1 g, 0.01 g and 0.001 g (or 0.1 ml, 0.01 ml and 0.001 ml) of the product to be examined. Incubate at 30-35 °C for 24-48 h. Subculture each of the cultures on a plate of violet red bile glucose agar. Incubate at 30-35 °C for 18-24 h.

4-1-3-2. *Interpretation*. Growth of colonies constitutes a positive result. Note the smallest quantity of the product that gives a positive result and the largest quantity that gives a negative result. Determine from Table 2.6.13.-2 the probable number of bacteria.

Table 2.6.13.-2 – *Interpretation of results*

Results for each quantity of product			Probable number of bacteria per gram or millilitre of product
0.1 g or 0.1 ml	0.01 g or 0.01 ml	0.001 g or 0.001 ml	
+	+	+	$> 10^3$
+	+	−	$< 10^3$ and $> 10^2$
+	−	−	$< 10^2$ and > 10
−	−	−	< 10

4-2. *ESCHERICHIA COLI*

4-2-1. **Sample preparation and pre-incubation**. Prepare a sample using a 1 in 10 dilution of not less than 1 g of the product to be examined as described in general chapter *2.6.12*, and use 10 ml or the quantity corresponding to 1 g or 1 ml to inoculate a suitable amount (determined as described under 3-4) of casein soya bean digest broth, mix and incubate at 30-35 °C for 18-24 h.

4-2-2. **Selection and subculture**. Shake the container, transfer 1 ml of casein soya bean digest broth to 100 ml of MacConkey broth and incubate at 42-44 °C for 24-48 h. Subculture on a plate of MacConkey agar at 30-35 °C for 18-72 h.

4-2-3. **Interpretation**. Growth of colonies indicates the possible presence of *E. coli*. This is confirmed by identification tests.

The product complies with the test if no colonies are present or if the identification tests are negative.

4-3. *SALMONELLA*

4-3-1. **Sample preparation and pre-incubation**. Prepare the product to be examined as described in general chapter *2.6.12*, and use the quantity corresponding to not less than 10 g or 10 ml to inoculate a suitable amount (determined as described under 3-4) of casein soya bean digest broth, mix and incubate at 30-35 °C for 18-24 h.

4-3-2. **Selection and subculture**. Transfer 0.1 ml of casein soya bean digest broth to 10 ml of Rappaport Vassiliadis *Salmonella* enrichment broth and incubate at 30-35 °C for 18-24 h. Subculture on plates of xylose, lysine, deoxycholate agar. Incubate at 30-35 °C for 18-48 h.

4-3-3. **Interpretation**. The possible presence of *Salmonella* is indicated by the growth of well-developed, red colonies, with or without black centres. This is confirmed by identification tests.

The product complies with the test if colonies of the types described are not present or if the confirmatory identification tests are negative.

4-4. *PSEUDOMONAS AERUGINOSA*

4-4-1. **Sample preparation and pre-incubation**. Prepare a sample using a 1 in 10 dilution of not less than 1 g of the product to be examined as described in general chapter *2.6.12*, and use 10 ml or the quantity corresponding to 1 g or 1 ml to inoculate a suitable amount (determined as described under 3-4) of casein soya bean digest broth and mix. When testing transdermal patches, filter the volume of sample corresponding to 1 patch of the preparation described under 4-5-1 in general chapter *2.6.12* through a sterile filter membrane and place in 100 ml of casein soya bean digest broth. Incubate at 30-35 °C for 18-24 h.

4-4-2. **Selection and subculture**. Subculture on a plate of cetrimide agar and incubate at 30-35 °C for 18-72 h.

4-4-3. **Interpretation**. Growth of colonies indicates the possible presence of *P. aeruginosa*. This is confirmed by identification tests.

The product complies with the test if colonies are not present or if the confirmatory identification tests are negative.

4-5. *STAPHYLOCOCCUS AUREUS*

4-5-1. **Sample preparation and pre-incubation**. Prepare a sample using a 1 in 10 dilution of not less than 1 g of the product to be examined as described in general chapter *2.6.12*, and use 10 ml or the quantity corresponding to 1 g or 1 ml to inoculate a suitable amount (determined as described under 3-4) of casein soya bean digest broth and mix. When testing transdermal patches, filter the volume of sample corresponding to 1 patch of the preparation described under 4-5-1 in general chapter *2.6.12* through a sterile filter membrane and place in 100 ml of casein soya bean digest broth. Incubate at 30-35 °C for 18-24 h.

4-5-2. **Selection and subculture**. Subculture on a plate of mannitol salt agar and incubate at 30-35 °C for 18-72 h.

4-5-3. **Interpretation**. The possible presence of *S. aureus* is indicated by the growth of yellow/white colonies surrounded by a yellow zone. This is confirmed by identification tests.

The product complies with the test if colonies of the types described are not present or if the confirmatory identification tests are negative.

4-6. *CLOSTRIDIA*

4-6-1. **Sample preparation and heat treatment**. Prepare a sample using a 1 in 10 dilution (with a minimum total volume of 20 ml) of not less than 2 g or 2 ml of the product to be examined as described in general chapter *2.6.12*. Divide the sample into 2 portions of at least 10 ml. Heat 1 portion at 80 °C for 10 min and cool rapidly. Do not heat the other portion.

4-6-2. **Selection and subculture**. Use 10 ml or the quantity corresponding to 1 g or 1 ml of the product to be examined of both portions to inoculate suitable amounts (determined as described under 3-4) of reinforced medium for clostridia. Incubate under anaerobic conditions at 30-35 °C for 48 h. After incubation, make subcultures from each container on Columbia agar and incubate under anaerobic conditions at 30-35 °C for 48-72 h.

4-6-3. **Interpretation**. The occurrence of anaerobic growth of rods (with or without endospores) giving a negative catalase reaction indicates the presence of clostridia. This is confirmed by identification tests.

The product complies with the test if colonies of the types described are not present or if the confirmatory identification tests are negative.

4-7. *CANDIDA ALBICANS*

4-7-1. **Sample preparation and pre-incubation**. Prepare the product to be examined as described in general chapter *2.6.12*, and use 10 ml or the quantity corresponding to not less than 1 g or 1 ml to inoculate 100 ml of Sabouraud-dextrose broth and mix. Incubate at 30-35 °C for 3-5 days.

4-7-2. **Selection and subculture**. Subculture on a plate of Sabouraud-dextrose agar and incubate at 30-35 °C for 24-48 h.

4-7-3. Interpretation. Growth of white colonies may indicate the presence of *C. albicans*. This is confirmed by identification tests.

The product complies with the test if such colonies are not present or if the confirmatory identification tests are negative.

The following section is given for information.

5. RECOMMENDED SOLUTIONS AND CULTURE MEDIA

The following solutions and culture media have been found to be satisfactory for the purposes for which they are prescribed in the test for microbial contamination in the Pharmacopoeia. Other media may be used provided that their suitability can be demonstrated.

Stock buffer solution. Place 34 g of potassium dihydrogen phosphate in a 1000 ml volumetric flask, dissolve in 500 ml of purified water, adjust to pH 7.2 ± 0.2 with sodium hydroxide, dilute to 1000.0 ml with purified water and mix. Dispense into containers and sterilise. Store at 2-8 °C.

Phosphate buffer solution pH 7.2. Prepare a mixture of stock buffer solution and purified water (1:800 *V/V*) and sterilise.

Buffered sodium chloride-peptone solution pH 7.0

Potassium dihydrogen phosphate	3.6 g
Disodium hydrogen phosphate dihydrate	7.2 g, equivalent to 0.067 M phosphate
Sodium chloride	4.3 g
Peptone (meat or casein)	1.0 g
Purified water	1000 ml

Sterilise in an autoclave using a validated cycle.

Casein soya bean digest broth

Pancreatic digest of casein	17.0 g
Papaic digest of soya bean	3.0 g
Sodium chloride	5.0 g
Dipotassium hydrogen phosphate	2.5 g
Glucose monohydrate	2.5 g
Purified water	1000 ml

Adjust the pH so that after sterilisation it is 7.3 ± 0.2 at 25 °C. Sterilise in an autoclave using a validated cycle.

Casein soya bean digest agar

Pancreatic digest of casein	15.0 g
Papaic digest of soya bean	5.0 g
Sodium chloride	5.0 g
Agar	15.0 g
Purified water	1000 ml

Adjust the pH so that after sterilisation it is 7.3 ± 0.2 at 25 °C. Sterilise in an autoclave using a validated cycle.

Sabouraud-dextrose agar

Dextrose	40.0 g
Mixture of peptic digest of animal tissue and pancreatic digest of casein (1:1)	10.0 g
Agar	15.0 g
Purified water	1000 ml

Adjust the pH so that after sterilisation it is 5.6 ± 0.2 at 25 °C. Sterilise in an autoclave using a validated cycle.

Potato dextrose agar

Infusion from potatoes	200 g
Dextrose	20.0 g
Agar	15.0 g
Purified water	1000 ml

Adjust the pH so that after sterilisation it is 5.6 ± 0.2 at 25 °C. Sterilise in an autoclave using a validated cycle.

Sabouraud-dextrose broth

Dextrose	20.0 g
Mixture of peptic digest of animal tissue and pancreatic digest of casein (1:1)	10.0 g
Purified water	1000 ml

Adjust the pH so that after sterilisation it is 5.6 ± 0.2 at 25 °C. Sterilise in an autoclave using a validated cycle.

Enterobacteria enrichment broth-Mossel

Pancreatic digest of gelatin	10.0 g
Glucose monohydrate	5.0 g
Dehydrated ox bile	20.0 g
Potassium dihydrogen phosphate	2.0 g
Disodium hydrogen phosphate dihydrate	8.0 g
Brilliant green	15 mg
Purified water	1000 ml

Adjust the pH so that after heating it is 7.2 ± 0.2 at 25 °C. Heat at 100 °C for 30 min and cool immediately.

Violet red bile glucose agar

Yeast extract	3.0 g
Pancreatic digest of gelatin	7.0 g
Bile salts	1.5 g
Sodium chloride	5.0 g
Glucose monohydrate	10.0 g
Agar	15.0 g
Neutral red	30 mg
Crystal violet	2 mg
Purified water	1000 ml

Adjust the pH so that after heating it is 7.4 ± 0.2 at 25 °C. Heat to boiling; do not heat in an autoclave.

MacConkey broth

Pancreatic digest of gelatin	20.0 g
Lactose monohydrate	10.0 g
Dehydrated ox bile	5.0 g
Bromocresol purple	10 mg
Purified water	1000 ml

Adjust the pH so that after sterilisation it is 7.3 ± 0.2 at 25 °C. Sterilise in an autoclave using a validated cycle.

See the information section on general monographs (cover pages)

MacConkey agar

Pancreatic digest of gelatin	17.0 g
Peptones (meat and casein)	3.0 g
Lactose monohydrate	10.0 g
Sodium chloride	5.0 g
Bile salts	1.5 g
Agar	13.5 g
Neutral red	30.0 mg
Crystal violet	1 mg
Purified water	1000 ml

Adjust the pH so that after sterilisation it is 7.1 ± 0.2 at 25 °C. Boil for 1 min with constant shaking then sterilise in an autoclave using a validated cycle.

Rappaport Vassiliadis *Salmonella* enrichment broth

Soya peptone	4.5 g
Magnesium chloride hexahydrate	29.0 g
Sodium chloride	8.0 g
Dipotassium phosphate	0.4 g
Potassium dihydrogen phosphate	0.6 g
Malachite green	0.036 g
Purified water	1000 ml

Dissolve, warming gently. Sterilise in an autoclave using a validated cycle, at a temperature not exceeding 115 °C. The pH is to be 5.2 ± 0.2 at 25 °C after heating and autoclaving.

Xylose, lysine, deoxycholate agar

Xylose	3.5 g
L-Lysine	5.0 g
Lactose monohydrate	7.5 g
Sucrose	7.5 g
Sodium chloride	5.0 g
Yeast extract	3.0 g
Phenol red	80 mg
Agar	13.5 g
Sodium deoxycholate	2.5 g
Sodium thiosulphate	6.8 g
Ferric ammonium citrate	0.8 g
Purified water	1000 ml

Adjust the pH so that after heating it is 7.4 ± 0.2 at 25 °C. Heat to boiling, cool to 50 °C and pour into Petri dishes. Do not heat in an autoclave.

Cetrimide agar

Pancreatic digest of gelatin	20.0 g
Magnesium chloride	1.4 g
Dipotassium sulphate	10.0 g
Cetrimide	0.3 g
Agar	13.6 g
Purified water	1000 ml
Glycerol	10.0 ml

Heat to boiling for 1 min with shaking. Adjust the pH so that after sterilisation it is 7.2 ± 0.2 at 25 °C. Sterilise in an autoclave using a validated cycle.

Mannitol salt agar

Pancreatic digest of casein	5.0 g
Peptic digest of animal tissue	5.0 g
Beef extract	1.0 g
D-Mannitol	10.0 g
Sodium chloride	75.0 g
Agar	15.0 g
Phenol red	0.025 g
Purified water	1000 ml

Heat to boiling for 1 min with shaking. Adjust the pH so that after sterilisation it is 7.4 ± 0.2 at 25 °C. Sterilise in an autoclave using a validated cycle.

Reinforced medium for clostridia

Beef extract	10.0 g
Peptone	10.0 g
Yeast extract	3.0 g
Soluble starch	1.0 g
Glucose monohydrate	5.0 g
Cysteine hydrochloride	0.5 g
Sodium chloride	5.0 g
Sodium acetate	3.0 g
Agar	0.5 g
Purified water	1000 ml

Hydrate the agar, dissolve by heating to boiling with continuous stirring. If necessary, adjust the pH so that after sterilisation it is 6.8 ± 0.2 at 25 °C. Sterilise in an autoclave using a validated cycle.

Columbia agar

Pancreatic digest of casein	10.0 g
Meat peptic digest	5.0 g
Heart pancreatic digest	3.0 g
Yeast extract	5.0 g
Maize starch	1.0 g
Sodium chloride	5.0 g
Agar, according to gelling power	10.0-15.0 g
Purified water	1000 ml

Hydrate the agar, dissolve by heating to boiling with continuous stirring. If necessary, adjust the pH so that after sterilisation it is 7.3 ± 0.2 at 25 °C. Sterilise in an autoclave using a validated cycle. Allow to cool to 45-50 °C; add, where necessary, gentamicin sulphate corresponding to 20 mg of gentamicin base and pour into Petri dishes.

07/2009:20624

2.6.24. AVIAN VIRAL VACCINES: TESTS FOR EXTRANEOUS AGENTS IN SEED LOTS

GENERAL PROVISIONS

a) In the following tests, chickens and/or chicken material such as eggs and cell cultures shall be derived from chicken flocks free from specified pathogens (SPF) (*5.2.2*).

b) Cell cultures for the testing of extraneous agents comply with the requirements for the master cell seed of chapter *5.2.4. Cell cultures for the production of veterinary vaccines*, with the exception of the karyotype test and the tumorigenicity test, which do not have to be carried out.

c) In tests using cell cultures, precise specifications are given for the number of replicates, monolayer surface areas and minimum survival rate of the cultures. Alternative numbers of replicates and cell surface areas are possible as well, provided that a minimum of 2 replicates are used, the total surface area and the total volume of test substance applied are not less than that prescribed here and the survival rate requirements are adapted accordingly.

d) For a freeze-dried preparation, reconstitute using a suitable liquid. Unless otherwise stated or justified, the test substance must contain a quantity of virus equivalent to at least 10 doses of vaccine in 0.1 ml of inoculum.

e) If the virus of the seed lot would interfere with the conduct and sensitivity of the test, neutralise the virus in the preparation with a monospecific antiserum.

f) Monospecific antiserum and serum of avian origin used for cell culture or any other purpose, in any of these tests, shall be free from antibodies against and free from inhibitory effects on the organisms listed hereafter under 7. Antibody specifications for sera used in extraneous agents testing.

g) Where specified in a monograph or otherwise justified, if neutralisation of the virus of the seed lot is required but difficult to achieve, the *in vitro* tests described below are adapted, as required, to provide the necessary guarantees of freedom from contamination with an extraneous agent.

h) Other types of tests than those indicated may be used provided they are at least as sensitive as those indicated and of appropriate specificity. Nucleic acid amplification techniques (*2.6.21*) give specific detection for many agents and can be used after validation for sensitivity and specificity.

1. TEST FOR EXTRANEOUS AGENTS USING EMBRYONATED HENS' EGGS

Use a test substance, diluted if necessary, containing a quantity of neutralised virus equivalent to at least 10 doses of vaccine in 0.2 ml of inoculum. Suitable antibiotics may be added. Inoculate the test substance into 3 groups of 10 embryonated hens' eggs as follows:

— group 1: 0.2 ml into the allantoic cavity of each 9- to 11-day-old embryonated egg;

— group 2: 0.2 ml onto the chorio-allantoic membrane of each 9- to 11-day-old embryonated egg;

— group 3: 0.2 ml into the yolk sac of each 5- to 6-day-old embryonated egg.

Candle the eggs in groups 1 and 2 daily for 7 days and the eggs in group 3 daily for 12 days. Discard embryos that die during the first 24 h as non-specific deaths; the test is not valid unless at least 6 embryos in each group survive beyond the first 24 h after inoculation. Examine macroscopically for abnormalities all embryos that die more than 24 h after inoculation, or that survive the incubation period. Examine also the chorio-allantoic membranes of these eggs for any abnormality and test the allantoic fluids for the presence of haemagglutinating agents.

Carry out a further embryo passage. Pool separately material from live and from the dead and abnormal embryos. Inoculate each pool into 10 eggs for each route as described above, chorio-allantoic membrane material being inoculated onto chorio-allantoic membranes, allantoic fluids into the allantoic cavity and embryo material into the yolk sac. For eggs inoculated by the allantoic and chorio-allantoic routes, candle the eggs daily for 7 days, proceeding and examining the material as described above. For eggs inoculated by the yolk sac route, candle the eggs daily for 12 days, proceeding and examining the material as described above.

The seed lot complies with the test if no test embryo shows macroscopic abnormalities or dies from causes attributable to the seed lot and if examination of the chorio-allantoic membranes and testing of the allantoic fluids show no evidence of the presence of any extraneous agent.

2. TEST IN CHICKEN KIDNEY CELLS

Prepare 7 monolayers of chicken kidney cells, each monolayer having an area of about 25 cm². Maintain 2 monolayers as negative controls and treat these in the same way as the 5 monolayers inoculated with the test substance, as described below. Remove the culture medium when the cells reach confluence. Inoculate 0.1 ml of the test substance onto each of the 5 monolayers. Allow adsorption for 1 h, add culture medium and incubate the cultures for a total of at least 21 days, subculturing at 4- to 7-day intervals. Each passage is made with pooled cells and fluids from all 5 monolayers after carrying out a freeze-thaw cycle. Inoculate 0.1 ml of pooled material onto each of 5 recently prepared monolayers of about 25 cm² each, at each passage. For the last passage, grow the cells also on a suitable substrate so as to obtain an area of about 10 cm² of cells from each of the monolayers for test A. The test is not valid if less than 80 per cent of the monolayers survive after any passage.

Examine microscopically all the cell cultures frequently throughout the entire incubation period for any signs of cytopathic effect or other evidence of the presence of contaminating agents in the test substance. At the end of the total incubation period, carry out the following procedures.

A. Fix and stain (with Giemsa or haematoxylin and eosin) about 10 cm² of confluent cells from each of the 5 monolayers. Examine the cells microscopically for any cytopathic effect, inclusion bodies, syncytial formation, or other evidence of the presence of contaminating agents from the test substance.

B. Drain and wash about 25 cm² of cells from each of the 5 monolayers. Cover these cells with a 0.5 per cent suspension of washed chicken erythrocytes (using at least 1 ml of suspension for each 5 cm² of cells). Incubate the cells at 4 °C for 20 min and then wash gently in phosphate buffered saline pH 7.4. Examine the cells microscopically for haemadsorption attributable to the presence of a haemadsorbing agent in the test substance.

C. Test individual samples of the fluids from each cell culture using chicken erythrocytes for haemagglutination attributable to the presence of a haemagglutinating agent in the test substance.

The test is not valid if there are any signs of extraneous agents in the negative control cultures. The seed lot complies with the test if there is no evidence of the presence of any extraneous agent.

3. TEST FOR AVIAN LEUCOSIS VIRUSES

Prepare at least 13 replicate monolayers of either DF-1 cells or primary or secondary chick embryo fibroblasts from the tissues of 9- to 11-day-old embryos that are known to be genetically susceptible to subgroups A, B and J of avian leucosis viruses and that support the growth of exogenous but not endogenous avian leucosis viruses (cells from C/E strain chickens are suitable). Each replicate shall have an area of about 50 cm^2.

Remove the culture medium when the cells reach confluence. Inoculate 0.1 ml of the test substance onto each of 5 of the replicate monolayers. Allow adsorption for 1 h, and add culture medium. Inoculate 2 of the replicate monolayers with subgroup A avian leucosis virus (not more than 10 CCID$_{50}$ in 0.1 ml), 2 with subgroup B avian leucosis virus (not more than 10 CCID$_{50}$ in 0.1 ml) and 2 with subgroup J avian leucosis virus (not more than 10 CCID$_{50}$ in 0.1 ml) as positive controls. Maintain not fewer than 2 non-inoculated replicate monolayers as negative controls.

Incubate the cells for a total of at least 9 days, subculturing at 3- to 4-day intervals. Retain cells from each passage level and harvest the cells at the end of the total incubation period. Wash cells from each passage level from each replicate and resuspend the cells at 10^7 cells per millilitre in barbital-buffered saline for subsequent testing by a Complement Fixation for Avian Leucosis (COFAL) test or in phosphate buffered saline for testing by Enzyme-Linked Immunosorbent Assay (ELISA). Then, carry out 3 cycles of freezing and thawing to release any group-specific antigen and perform a COFAL test or an ELISA test on each extract to detect group-specific avian leucosis antigen if present.

The test is not valid if group-specific antigen is detected in fewer than 5 of the 6 positive control replicate monolayers or if a positive result is obtained in any of the negative control monolayers, or if the results for both of the 2 negative control monolayers are inconclusive. If the results for more than 1 of the test replicate monolayers are inconclusive, then further subcultures of reserved portions of the fibroblast monolayers shall be made and tested until an unequivocal result is obtained. If a positive result is obtained for any of the test monolayers, then the presence of avian leucosis virus in the test substance has been detected.

The seed lot complies with the test if there is no evidence of the presence of any avian leucosis virus.

4. TEST FOR AVIAN RETICULOENDOTHELIOSIS VIRUS

Prepare 11 monolayers of primary or secondary chick embryo fibroblasts from the tissues of 9- to 11-day old chick embryos or duck embryo fibroblasts from the tissues of 13- to 14-day-old embryos, each monolayer having an area of about 25 cm^2.

Remove the culture medium when the cells reach confluence. Inoculate 0.1 ml of the test substance onto each of 5 of the monolayers. Allow adsorption for 1 h, and add culture medium. Inoculate 4 of the monolayers with avian reticuloendotheliosis virus as positive controls (not more than 10 CCID$_{50}$ in 0.1 ml). Maintain 2 non-inoculated monolayers as negative controls.

Incubate the cells for a total of at least 10 days, subculturing twice at 3- to 4-day intervals. The test is not valid if fewer than 3 of the 4 positive controls or fewer than 4 of the 5 test monolayers or neither of the 2 negative controls survive after any passage.

For the last subculture, grow the fibroblasts on a suitable substrate so as to obtain an area of about 10 cm^2 of confluent fibroblasts from each of the original 11 monolayers for the subsequent test: test about 10 cm^2 of confluent fibroblasts derived from each of the original 11 monolayers by immunostaining for the presence of avian reticuloendotheliosis virus. The test is not valid if avian reticuloendotheliosis virus is detected in fewer than 3 of the 4 positive control monolayers or in any of the negative control monolayers, or if the results for both of the 2 negative control monolayers are inconclusive. If the results for more than 1 of the test monolayers are inconclusive then further subcultures of reserved portions of the fibroblast monolayers shall be made and tested until an unequivocal result is obtained.

The seed lot complies with the test if there is no evidence of the presence of avian reticuloendotheliosis virus.

5. TEST FOR CHICKEN ANAEMIA VIRUS

Prepare eleven 20 ml suspensions of the MDCC-MSBI cell line or another cell line of equivalent sensitivity in 25 cm^2 cell culture flasks containing about 5×10^5 cells/ml. Inoculate 0.1 ml of the test substance into each of 5 flasks. Inoculate 4 of the suspensions with 10 CCID$_{50}$ chicken anaemia virus as positive controls. Maintain not fewer than 2 non-inoculated suspensions. Maintain all the cell cultures for a total of at least 24 days, subculturing 8 times at 3- to 4-day intervals. During the subculturing the presence of chicken anaemia virus may be indicated by a metabolic colour change in the infected cultures, the culture fluids becoming red in comparison with the control cultures. Examine the cells microscopically for cytopathic effect. At this time or at the end of the incubation period, centrifuge the cells from each flask at low speed and resuspend at about 10^6 cells/ml and place 25 µl in each of 10 wells of a multi-well slide. Examine the cells by immunostaining.

The test is not valid if chicken anaemia virus is detected in fewer than 3 of the 4 positive controls or in any of the non-inoculated controls. If the results for more than 1 of the test suspensions are inconclusive, then further subcultures of reserved portions of the test suspensions shall be made and tested until an unequivocal result is obtained.

The seed lot complies with the test if there is no evidence of the presence of chicken anaemia virus.

6. TEST FOR EXTRANEOUS AGENTS USING CHICKS

Inoculate each of at least 10 chicks with the equivalent of 100 doses of vaccine by the intramuscular route and with the equivalent of 10 doses by eye-drop. Chicks that are 2 weeks of age are used in the test except that if the seed virus is pathogenic for birds of this age, older birds may be used, if required and justified. In exceptional cases, for inactivated vaccines, the virus may be neutralised by specific antiserum if the seed virus is pathogenic for birds at the age of administration. Repeat these inoculations 2 weeks later. Observe the chicks for a period of 5 weeks from the day of the first inoculation. No antimicrobial agents shall be administered to the chicks during the test period. The test is not valid if fewer than 80 per cent of the chicks survive to the end of the test period.

Collect serum from each chick at the end of the test period. Test each serum sample for antibodies against each of the agents listed below (with the exception of the virus type of the seed lot) using one of the methods indicated for testing for the agent.

Clinical signs of disease in the chicks during the test period (other than signs attributable to the virus of the seed lot) and the detection of antibodies in the chicks after inoculation (with the exception of antibodies to the virus of the seed lot), are classed as evidence of the presence of an extraneous agent in the seed lot.

It is recommended that sera from these birds is retained so that additional testing may be carried out if requirements change.

A. Standard tests

Agent	Type of test
Avian adenoviruses, group 1	SN, EIA, AGP
Avian encephalomyelitis virus	AGP, EIA
Avian infectious bronchitis virus	EIA, HI
Avian infectious laryngotracheitis virus	SN, EIA, IS
Avian leucosis viruses	SN, EIA
Avian nephritis virus	IS
Avian orthoreoviruses	IS, EIA
Avian reticuloendotheliosis virus	AGP, IS, EIA
Chicken anaemia virus	IS, EIA, SN
Egg drop syndrome virus	HI, EIA
Avian infectious bursal disease virus	Serotype 1: AGP, EIA, SN
	Serotype 2: SN
Influenza A virus	AGP, EIA, HI
Marek's disease virus	AGP
Newcastle disease virus	HI, EIA
Turkey rhinotracheitis virus	EIA
Salmonella pullorum	Agg

Agg: agglutination
AGP: agar gel precipitation
EIA: enzyme immunoassay (e.g. ELISA)
HI: haemagglutination inhibition
IS: immunostaining (e.g. fluorescent antibody)
SN: serum neutralisation

B. Additional tests for turkey extraneous agents

If the seed virus is of turkey origin or was propagated in turkey substrates, tests for antibodies against the following agents are also carried out.

Agent	Type of test
Chlamydia spp.	EIA
Avian infectious haemorrhagic enteritis virus	AGP
Avian paramyxovirus 3	HI
Avian infectious bursal disease virus type 2	SN

A test for freedom from turkey lympho-proliferative disease virus is carried out by intraperitoneal inoculation of twenty 4-week-old turkey poults. Observe the poults for 40 days. The test is not valid if more than 20 per cent of the poults die from non-specific causes. The seed lot complies with the test if sections of spleen and thymus taken from 10 poults 2 weeks after inoculation show no macroscopic or microscopic lesions (other than those attributable to the seed lot virus) and no poult dies from causes attributable to the seed lot.

C. Additional tests for duck extraneous agents

If the seed virus is of duck origin or was propagated in duck substrates, tests for antibodies against the following agents are also carried out.

Agent	Type of test
Chlamydia spp.	EIA
Duck and goose parvoviruses	SN, EIA
Duck enteritis virus	SN
Duck hepatitis virus type I	SN

The seed lot complies with the test if there is no evidence of the presence of any extraneous agent.

D. Additional tests for goose extraneous agents

If the seed virus is of goose origin or was prepared in goose substrates, tests for the following agents are also carried out.

Agent	Type of test
Duck and goose parvovirus	SN, EIA
Duck enteritis virus	SN
Goose haemorrhagic polyomavirus	test in goslings shown below or another suitable test

Inoculate subcutaneously the equivalent of at least 10 doses to each of ten 1-day-old susceptible goslings. Observe the goslings for 28 days. The test is not valid if more than 20 per cent of the goslings die from non-specific causes. The seed virus complies with the test if no gosling dies from causes attributable to the seed lot.

7. ANTIBODY SPECIFICATIONS FOR SERA USED IN EXTRANEOUS AGENTS TESTING

All batches of serum to be used in extraneous agents testing, either to neutralise the vaccine virus (seed lot or batch of finished product) or as a supplement for culture media used for tissue culture propagation, shall be shown to be free from antibodies against and free from inhibitory effects on the following micro-organisms by suitably sensitive tests.

Avian adenoviruses
Avian encephalomyelitis virus
Avian infectious bronchitis viruses
Avian infectious bursal disease virus types 1 and 2
Avian infectious haemorrhagic enteritis virus
Avian infectious laryngotracheitis virus
Avian leucosis viruses
Avian nephritis virus
Avian paramyxoviruses 1 to 9
Avian orthoreoviruses
Avian reticuloendotheliosis virus
Chicken anaemia virus
Duck enteritis virus
Duck hepatitis virus type I
Egg drop syndrome virus
Fowl pox virus
Influenza viruses
Marek's disease virus
Turkey herpesvirus
Turkey rhinotracheitis virus

Non-immune serum for addition to culture media can be assumed to be free from antibodies against any of these viruses if the agent is known not to infect the species of origin of the serum and it is not necessary to test the serum for such antibodies. Monospecific antisera for virus neutralisation can be assumed to be free from the antibodies against any of these viruses if it can be shown that the immunising antigen could not have been contaminated with antigens derived from that virus and if the virus is known not to infect the species of origin of the serum; it is not necessary to test the serum for such antibodies. It is not necessary to retest sera obtained from birds from SPF chicken flocks (*5.2.2*).

Batches of sera prepared for neutralising the vaccine virus must not be prepared from any passage level derived from the virus isolate used to prepare the master seed lot or from an isolate cultured in the same cell line.

07/2009:20626

2.6.26. TEST FOR ANTI-D ANTIBODIES IN HUMAN IMMUNOGLOBULIN FOR INTRAVENOUS ADMINISTRATION

MATERIALS

Phosphate-buffered saline (PBS). Dissolve 8.0 g of *sodium chloride R*, 0.76 g of *anhydrous disodium hydrogen phosphate R*, 0.2 g of *potassium chloride R* and 0.2 g of *potassium dihydrogen phosphate R* in *water R* and dilute to 1000 ml with the same solvent. If the solution has to be kept for several days, 0.2 g of *sodium azide R* may be added in order to avoid microbial contamination.

Papain solution. Use serological-grade papain from a commercial source, the activity of which has been validated.

Red blood cells. Use pooled D-positive red blood cells from not fewer than 3 donors, preferably of group OR_2R_2. D-positive red blood cells may also be obtained from OR_1R_1 or OR_1R_2 donors. Mixing phenotypes has not been tested and is therefore not recommended.

Use pooled D-negative red blood cells, preferably from 3 donors of group Orr. When only 1 donor of group Orr is available, D-negative red blood cells from only 1 donor may be used.

Wash the cells 4 times with PBS or until the supernatant is clear. Centrifuge the cells at 1800 *g* for 5 min to pack. Treat the packed cells with papain solution according to the manufacturer's instructions.

Store red blood cells for not more than 1 week in a preservative solution. A preparation of the following composition is appropriate:

Trisodium citrate	8 g/l
D-glucose	20 g/l
Citric acid	0.5 g/l
Sodium chloride	4.2 g/l
Inosine	0.938 g/l
Adenosine triphosphate (ATP)	0.4 g/l
Chloramphenicol	0.34 g/l
Neomycin sulphate	0.1 g/l

Microtitre plates. Use V-bottomed rigid micro-titre plates.

Reference standards. Immunoglobulin (anti-D antibodies test) BRP and *Immunoglobulin (anti-D antibodies test negative control) BRP* are suitable for use as the reference preparation and negative control, respectively.

METHOD

The test described in this chapter is performed at room temperature on the reference solutions, the negative control solutions and the test solutions at the same time and under identical conditions.

Reference solutions and negative control solutions. Reconstitute the reference preparation and the negative control according to instructions. The immunoglobulin G (IgG) concentration is 50 g/l in each of the reconstituted preparations. Make a 2-fold dilution of each reconstituted preparation with PBS containing *bovine albumin R* at 2 g/l, to give solutions containing IgG at 25 g/l. Prepare 7 further serial 2-fold dilutions of each preparation using PBS containing *bovine albumin R* at 2 g/l to extend the dilution range to 1/256 (0.195 g/l IgG). Add 20 µl of each dilution to the microtitre plate.

Test solutions. Dilute the preparation to be examined with PBS containing *bovine albumin R* at 2 g/l to give a starting IgG concentration of 25 g/l. For 50 g/l products, this is a 2-fold dilution; adjust the dilution factor accordingly for samples that are not 50 g/l to give a starting concentration of 25 g/l for testing. This 25 g/l solution is assigned a nominal 2-fold dilution factor for comparison with the reference preparations, even if this does not reflect the true dilution factor used to achieve 25 g/l. Prepare 7 further serial 2-fold dilutions of each preparation using PBS containing *bovine albumin R* at 2 g/l to extend the nominal dilution range to 1/256 (0.195 g/l IgG) for comparison with the reference preparations over the same IgG concentration range. Make 2 independent sets of dilutions. Add 20 µl of each dilution to the microtitre plate.

Prepare 3 per cent *V/V* suspensions of papain-treated D-positive (preferably OR_2R_2, but OR_1R_1 or OR_1R_2 may also be used) and D-negative (Orr) red blood cells in PBS containing *bovine albumin R* at 2 g/l. Add 20 µl of D-positive cells to 1 dilution series of each of the preparation to be examined, the reference preparation and the negative control, and 20 µl of D-negative cells to the other dilution series of each of the preparation to be examined, the reference preparation and the negative control. Mix by shaking the plate on a shaker for 10 s.

Centrifuge the plate at 80 *g* for 1 min to pack the cells. Place the plate at an angle of approximately 70°. Read after at least 3 min and once the cells have streamed in the wells containing the negative control and the wells where the D-negative cells have been added. A cell button at the bottom of the well indicates a positive result. A stream of cells represents a negative result.

Record the endpoint titre as the reciprocal of the highest dilution that gives rise to a positive result.

The negative control must have a titre not greater than 2, otherwise an investigation of the test reagents and conditions has to be performed.

The titre of the preparation to be examined is not greater than the titre of the reference preparation when all preparations are titrated from 25 g/l.

2.7. BIOLOGICAL ASSAYS

07/2009:20709

2.7.9. TEST FOR Fc FUNCTION OF IMMUNOGLOBULIN

The test for Fc function of immunoglobulin is carried out using method A or B. Method B is an adaptation of the procedure of method A for the use of microtitre plates for the measurement of complement-mediated haemolysis. Differences in the test procedures between methods A and B are addressed in the test.

REAGENTS

Stabilised human blood. Collect group O human blood into ACD anticoagulant solution. Store the stabilised blood at 4 °C for not more than 3 weeks.

Phosphate-buffered saline pH 7.2. Dissolve 1.022 g of *anhydrous disodium hydrogen phosphate R*, 0.336 g of *anhydrous sodium dihydrogen phosphate R* and 8.766 g of *sodium chloride R* in 800 ml of *water R* and dilute to 1000 ml with the same solvent.

Magnesium and calcium stock solution. Dissolve 1.103 g of *calcium chloride R* and 5.083 g of *magnesium chloride R* in *water R* and dilute to 25 ml with the same solvent.

Barbital buffer stock solution. Dissolve 207.5 g of *sodium chloride R* and 25.48 g of *barbital sodium R* in 4000 ml of *water R* and adjust to pH 7.3 using *1 M hydrochloric acid*. Add 12.5 ml of magnesium and calcium stock solution and dilute to 5000 ml with *water R*. Store at 4 °C in transparent containers.

Albumin barbital buffer solution. Dissolve 0.150 g of *bovine albumin R* in 20 ml of barbital buffer stock solution and dilute to 100 ml with *water R*. Prepare immediately before use.

Tannic acid solution. Dissolve 10 mg of *tannic acid R* in 100 ml of phosphate-buffered saline pH 7.2. Prepare immediately before use.

Guinea-pig complement. Prepare a pool of serum from the blood of not fewer than 10 guinea-pigs. Separate the serum from the clotted blood by centrifugation at about 4 °C. Store the serum in small amounts below – 70 °C. Immediately before starting complement-initiated haemolysis, dilute to 125-200 CH_{50} per millilitre with albumin barbital buffer solution and store in an ice-bath during the test.

Rubella antigen. Suitable rubella antigen for haemagglutination-inhibition titre (HIT). Titre > 256 HA units.

Preparation of tanned human red blood cells. Separate human red blood cells by centrifuging an appropriate volume of stabilised human blood, wash the cells at least 3 times with phosphate-buffered saline pH 7.2 and suspend at 2 per cent V/V in phosphate-buffered saline pH 7.2. Add 0.2 ml of tannic acid solution to 14.8 ml of phosphate-buffered saline pH 7.2. Mix 1 volume of the freshly prepared dilution with 1 volume of the human red blood cell suspension and incubate at 37 °C for 10 min. Collect the cells by centrifugation (800 g for 10 min), discard the supernatant and wash the cells once with phosphate-buffered saline pH 7.2. Resuspend the tanned cells at 1 per cent V/V in phosphate-buffered saline pH 7.2.

Antigen coating of tanned human red blood cells. Take a suitable volume (V_s) of tanned cells, add 0.2 ml of rubella antigen per 1.0 ml of tanned cells and incubate at 37 °C for 30 min. Collect the cells by centrifugation (800 g for 10 min) and discard the supernatant. Add a volume of albumin barbital buffer solution equivalent to the discarded supernatant, resuspend and collect the cells as described

and repeat the washing procedure. Resuspend with albumin barbital buffer solution using a volume equivalent to 3/4 of V_s, thereby obtaining the initial volume (V_i). Mix 900 µl of albumin barbital buffer solution with 100 µl of V_i, which is thereby reduced to the residual volume (V_r), and determine the initial absorbance at 541 nm (A). Dilute V_r by a factor equal to A using albumin barbital buffer solution, thereby obtaining the final adjusted volume $V_f = V_r \times A$ of sensitised human red blood cells and adjusting A to 1.0 ± 0.1 for a tenfold dilution.

Antibody binding of antigen-coated tanned human red blood cells. Prepare the following solutions in succession and in duplicate, using for each solution a separate half-micro cuvette (for example, disposable type) or test-tube.

(1) *Test solutions.* If necessary, adjust the immunoglobulin to be examined to pH 7.

Where method A is performed, dilute volumes of the preparation to be examined with albumin barbital buffer to obtain 30 mg and 40 mg of immunoglobulin and adjust the volume to 900 µl with albumin barbital buffer.

Where method B is performed, dilute volumes of the preparation to be examined with albumin barbital buffer to obtain 15 mg and 30 mg of immunoglobulin and adjust the volume to 1200 µl with albumin barbital buffer.

(2) *Reference solutions.* Prepare as for the test solutions using *human immunoglobulin BRP*.

(3) *Complement control.* Albumin barbital buffer solution.

Where method A is performed, add to each cuvette/test-tube 100 µl of sensitised human red blood cells and mix well. Allow to stand for 15 min, add 1000 µl of albumin barbital buffer solution, collect the cells by centrifugation (1000 g for 10 min) of the cuvette/test-tube and remove 1900 µl of the supernatant. Replace the 1900 µl with albumin barbital buffer solution and repeat the whole of the washing procedure, finally leaving a volume of 200 µl. Test samples may be stored in sealed cuvettes/test-tubes at 4 °C for not longer than 24 h.

Where method B is performed, add to each test-tube 300 µl of sensitised human red blood cells and mix well (the final immunoglobulin concentration is in the range of 10-20 mg/ml). Allow to stand for 15 min, add 1500 µl of albumin barbital buffer solution and stir gently until homogeneous. Collect the cells by centrifugation (1000 g for 10 min) of the test-tube, remove the supernatant and add approximately 3 ml of albumin barbital buffer solution. Repeat this operation up to 4 times in total, leaving a final volume of 300 µl. Test samples may be stored in sealed test-tubes at 4 °C for not longer than 24 h.

Complement-initiated haemolysis.

To measure haemolysis where method A is performed, add 600 µl of albumin barbital buffer solution warmed to 37 °C to the test sample, resuspend the cells carefully by repeated pipetting (not fewer than 5 times) and place the cuvette in the thermostatted cuvette holder of a spectrophotometer. After 2 min, add 200 µl of diluted guinea-pig complement (125-200 CH_{50}/ml), mix thoroughly by pipetting twice and start immediately after the second pipetting the time-dependent recording of absorbance at 541 nm, using albumin barbital buffer solution as the compensation liquid. Stop the measurement if absorbance as a function of time has clearly passed the inflexion point.

To measure haemolysis where method B is performed, add 900 µl of albumin barbital buffer solution warmed to 37 °C to each test-tube and resuspend the cells carefully by repeated pipetting (not fewer than 5 times). The microtitre plate must be prewarmed to 37 °C before starting the test. Transfer 240 µl of each solution into 4 microtitre plate wells then incubate the microplate at 37 °C for 6 min, stirring gently every 10 s. To each microtitre plate well add 60 µl of diluted guinea-pig complement (150 CH_{50}/ml). Mix for 10 s and immediately start recording the absorbance at 541 nm at 37 °C, measuring every 20 s. Stop the measurement if the absorbance as a function of time has clearly passed the inflexion point.

Evaluation. For each cuvette/test-tube/well, determine the slope (S) of the haemolysis curve at the approximate inflexion point by segmenting the steepest section in suitable time intervals (for example, $\Delta t = 1$ min), and calculate S between adjacent intersection points, expressed as ΔA per minute. The largest value for S serves as S_{exp}. In addition, determine the absorbance at the start of measurement (A_s) by extrapolating the curve, which is almost linear and parallel to the time axis within the first few minutes. Correct S_{exp} using the expression:

$$S' = \frac{S_{exp}}{A_s}$$

Calculate the arithmetic mean of the values of S' for each preparation (test and reference solution). Calculate the index of Fc function (I_{Fc}) from the expression:

$$I_{Fc} = \frac{100 \times \left(\overline{S'} - \overline{S'}_c\right)}{\overline{S'}_s - \overline{S'}_c}$$

$\overline{S'}$ = arithmetic mean of the corrected slope for the preparation to be examined;

$\overline{S'}_s$ = arithmetic mean of the corrected slope for the reference preparation;

$\overline{S'}_c$ = arithmetic mean of the corrected slope for the complement control.

Calculate the index of Fc function for the preparation to be examined: the value is not less than that stated in the leaflet accompanying the reference preparation.

07/2009:20725

2.7.25. ASSAY OF HUMAN PLASMIN INHIBITOR

Human plasmin inhibitor, also called human α_2-antiplasmin, is a plasma protein that inhibits the plasmin (a serine protease) pathway of fibrinolysis by rapidly forming a complex with free plasmin. Furthermore, upon blood coagulation, human plasmin inhibitor is cross-linked to fibrin strands by factor XIII, and interferes with binding of the proenzyme plasminogen to fibrin.

The potency of human plasmin inhibitor is estimated by comparing the ability of the preparation to be examined to inhibit the cleavage of a specific chromogenic substrate by plasmin with the same ability of a reference standard of human plasmin inhibitor. Plasmin cleavage of the chromogenic substrate yields a chromophore that can be quantified spectrophotometrically.

The individual reagents for the assay may be obtained separately or in commercial kits. Both end-point and kinetic methods are available. Procedures and reagents may vary between different kits and the manufacturer's instructions are followed. The essential features of the procedure are described in the following example of a microtitre-plate kinetic method.

REAGENTS

Dilution buffer pH 7.5. According to the manufacturer's instructions, a suitable buffer is used. Adjust the pH (*2.2.3*) if necessary.

Plasmin. A preparation of human plasmin that does not contain significant amounts of other proteases is preferably used. Reconstitute and store according to the manufacturer's instructions.

Plasmin chromogenic substrate. A suitable specific chromogenic substrate for plasmin is used: H-D-cyclohexylalanyl-norvalyl-lysyl-*p*-nitroaniline hydrochloride (H-D-CHA-Nva-Lys-*p*NA.HCl) or L-pyroglutamyl-L-phenylalanyl-L-lysine-*p*-nitroaniline hydrochloride (Glp-Phe-Lys-*p*NA.HCl). Reconstitute in *water R* to give a suitable concentration according to the manufacturer's instructions.

METHOD

Varying quantities of the preparation to be examined are mixed with a given quantity of plasmin and the remaining plasmin activity is determined using a suitable chromogenic substrate.

Reconstitute or thaw the preparation to be examined according to the manufacturer's instructions. Dilute with dilution buffer pH 7.5 and prepare at least 2 independent series of 3 or 4 dilutions for both the preparation to be examined and the reference standard.

Mix 0.020 ml of each dilution with 0.020 ml of dilution buffer pH 7.5 and warm to 37 °C. Add 0.040 ml of a plasmin solution (test concentration in the range of 0.2 nkat/ml to 1.6 nkat/ml) previously heated to 37 °C and leave at 37 °C for 1 min. Add 0.020 ml of the chromogenic substrate solution, previously heated to 37 °C, to each mixture. Immediately start measurement of the change in absorbance at 405 nm (*2.2.25*) using a microtitre plate reader. Calculate the rate of change of absorbance (ΔA/min). Alternatively, an end-point assay might be used by stopping the reaction with acetic acid and measuring the absorbance at 405 nm.

In both cases the duration of the cleavage of the chromogenic substrate should be chosen to produce a linear increase in absorbance at 405 nm, before substrate depletion becomes significant. If the assay is performed in test tubes or cuvettes using a spectrophotometric method, the volumes of reagent solutions are changed proportionally.

Substract the optical density of the blank (prepared with dilution buffer pH 7.5) from the optical density of the preparation to be examined. Check the validity of the assay and calculate the potency of the preparation to be examined by the usual statistical methods (*5.3*).

2.9. PHARMACEUTICAL TECHNICAL PROCEDURES

2. Methods of analysis

07/2009:20934

2.9.34. BULK DENSITY AND TAPPED DENSITY OF POWDERS

Bulk density

The bulk density of a powder is the ratio of the mass of an untapped powder sample to its volume, including the contribution of the interparticulate void volume. Hence, the bulk density depends on both the density of powder particles and the spatial arrangement of particles in the powder bed. The bulk density is expressed in grams per millilitre despite the International Unit being kilogram per cubic metre ($1 \text{ g/ml} = 1000 \text{ kg/m}^3$), because the measurements are made using cylinders. It may also be expressed in grams per cubic centimetre.

The bulking properties of a powder are dependent upon the preparation, treatment and storage of the sample, i.e. how it has been handled. The particles can be packed to have a range of bulk densities and, moreover, the slightest disturbance of the powder bed may result in a changed bulk density. Thus, the bulk density of a powder is often very difficult to measure with good reproducibility and, in reporting the results, it is essential to specify how the determination was made.

The bulk density of a powder is determined either by measuring the volume of a known mass of powder sample, which may have been passed through a sieve, in a graduated cylinder (Method 1), or by measuring the mass of a known volume of powder that has been passed through a volumeter into a cup (Method 2) or has been introduced into a measuring vessel (Method 3).

Methods 1 and 3 are favoured.

METHOD 1: MEASUREMENT IN A GRADUATED CYLINDER

Procedure. Pass a quantity of powder sufficient to complete the test through a sieve with apertures greater than or equal to 1.0 mm, if necessary, to break up agglomerates that may have formed during storage; this must be done gently to avoid changing the nature of the material. Into a dry, graduated, 250 ml cylinder (readable to 2 ml), gently introduce, without compacting, approximately 100 g (m) of the test sample weighed with 0.1 per cent accuracy. If necessary, carefully level the powder without compacting, and read the unsettled apparent volume (V_0) to the nearest graduated unit. Calculate the bulk density in grams per millilitre using the formula m/V_0. Generally, replicate determinations are desirable for the determination of this property.

If the powder density is too low or too high, such that the test sample has an untapped apparent volume of more than 250 ml or less than 150 ml, it is not possible to use 100 g of powder sample. In this case, a different amount of powder is selected as the test sample, such that its untapped apparent volume is between 150 ml and 250 ml (apparent volume greater than or equal to 60 per cent of the total volume of the cylinder); the mass of the test sample is specified in the expression of results.

For test samples having an apparent volume between 50 ml and 100 ml, a 100 ml cylinder readable to 1 ml can be used; the volume of the cylinder is specified in the expression of results.

METHOD 2: MEASUREMENT IN A VOLUMETER

Apparatus. The apparatus (Figure 2.9.34.-1) consists of a top funnel fitted with a 1.0 mm sieve, mounted over a baffle box containing 4 glass baffles over which the powder slides and bounces as it passes. At the bottom of the baffle box is a funnel that collects the powder and allows it to pour into a cup mounted directly below it. The cup may be cylindrical (25.00 ± 0.05 ml volume with an internal diameter of 30.00 ± 2.00 mm) or square (16.39 ± 2.00 ml volume with internal dimensions of 25.4 ± 0.076 mm).

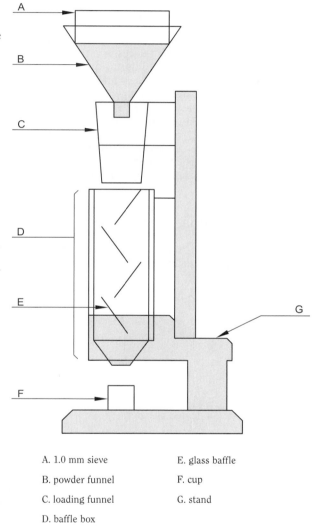

A. 1.0 mm sieve   E. glass baffle

B. powder funnel   F. cup

C. loading funnel   G. stand

D. baffle box

Figure 2.9.34.-1. – *Volumeter*

Procedure. Allow an excess of powder to flow through the apparatus into the sample receiving cup until it overflows, using a minimum of 25 cm³ of powder with the square cup and 35 cm³ of powder with the cylindrical cup. Carefully, scrape excess powder from the top of the cup by smoothly moving the edge of the blade of a spatula perpendicular to and in contact with the top surface of the cup, taking care to keep the spatula perpendicular to prevent packing or removal of powder from the cup. Remove any material from the side of the cup and determine the mass (M) of the powder to the nearest 0.1 per cent. Calculate the bulk density in grams per millilitre using the formula M/V_0 (where V_0 is the volume of the cup) and record the average of 3 determinations using 3 different powder samples.

METHOD 3: MEASUREMENT IN A VESSEL

Apparatus. The apparatus consists of a 100 ml cylindrical vessel of stainless steel with dimensions as specified in Figure 2.9.34.-2.

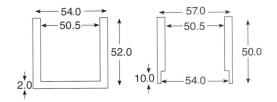

Figure 2.9.34.-2. – *Measuring vessel (left) and cap (right) Dimensions in millimetres*

Procedure. Pass a quantity of powder sufficient to complete the test through a 1.0 mm sieve, if necessary, to break up agglomerates that may have formed during storage, and allow the obtained sample to flow freely into the measuring vessel until it overflows. Carefully scrape the excess powder from the top of the vessel as described under Method 2. Determine the mass (M_0) of the powder to the nearest 0.1 per cent by subtracting the previously determined mass of the empty measuring vessel. Calculate the bulk density in grams per millilitre using the formula $M_0/100$ and record the average of 3 determinations using 3 different powder samples.

Tapped density

The tapped density is an increased bulk density attained after mechanically tapping a receptacle containing the powder sample.

The tapped density is obtained by mechanically tapping a graduated measuring cylinder or vessel containing the powder sample. After observing the initial powder volume or mass, the measuring cylinder or vessel is mechanically tapped, and volume or mass readings are taken until little further volume or mass change is observed. The mechanical tapping is achieved by raising the cylinder or vessel and allowing it to drop, under its own mass, a specified distance by one of 3 methods as described below. Devices that rotate the cylinder or vessel during tapping may be preferred to minimise any possible separation of the mass during tapping down.

METHOD 1

Apparatus. The apparatus (Figure 2.9.34.-3) consists of the following:

– a 250 ml graduated cylinder (readable to 2 ml) with a mass of 220 ± 44 g;

– a settling apparatus capable of producing, per minute, either nominally 250 ± 15 taps from a height of 3 ± 0.2 mm, or nominally 300 ± 15 taps from a height of 14 ± 2 mm. The support for the graduated cylinder, with its holder, has a mass of 450 ± 10 g.

Procedure. Proceed as described above for the determination of the bulk volume (V_0). Secure the cylinder in the support. Carry out 10, 500 and 1250 taps on the same powder sample and read the corresponding volumes V_{10}, V_{500} and V_{1250} to the nearest graduated unit. If the difference between V_{500} and V_{1250} is less than 2 ml, V_{1250} is the tapped volume. If the difference between V_{500} and V_{1250} exceeds 2 ml, repeat in increments of, for example, 1250 taps, until the difference between successive measurements is less than 2 ml. Fewer taps may be appropriate for some powders, when validated. Calculate the tapped density in grams per millilitre using

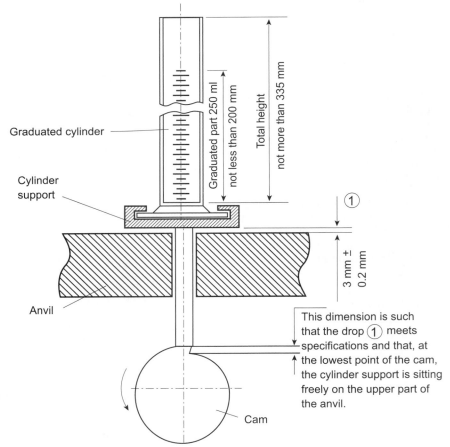

Figure 2.9.34.-3 – *Settling device for powder samples Dimensions in millimetres*

See the information section on general monographs (cover pages)

the formula m/V_f (where V_f is the final tapped volume). Generally, replicate determinations are desirable for the determination of this property. Specify the drop height with the results.

If it is not possible to use a 100 g test sample, use a reduced amount and a suitable 100 ml graduated cylinder (readable to 1 ml) weighing 130 ± 16 g and mounted on a support weighing 240 ± 12 g. Specify the modified test conditions with the results.

METHOD 2

Procedure. Proceed as directed under Method 1 except that the mechanical tester provides a fixed drop of 3 ± 0.2 mm at a nominal rate of 250 taps per minute.

METHOD 3

Procedure. Proceed as described under Method 3 for measuring the bulk density, using the measuring vessel equipped with the cap shown in Figure 2.9.34.-2. The measuring vessel with the cap is lifted 50-60 times per minute by the use of a suitable tapped density tester. Carry out 200 taps, remove the cap and carefully scrape excess powder from the top of the measuring vessel as described under Method 3 for measuring the bulk density. Repeat the procedure using 400 taps. If the difference between the 2 masses obtained after 200 and 400 taps exceeds 2 per cent, repeat the test using 200 additional taps until the difference between successive measurements is less than 2 per cent. Calculate the tapped density in grams per millilitre using the formula $M_f/100$ (where M_f is the mass of powder in the measuring vessel) and record the average of 3 determinations using 3 different powder samples.

Measures of powder compressibility

Because the interparticulate interactions influencing the bulking properties of a powder are also the interactions that interfere with powder flow, a comparison of the bulk and tapped densities can give a measure of the relative importance of these interactions in a given powder. Such a comparison is often used as an index of the ability of the powder to flow, for example the compressibility index or the Hausner ratio.

The compressibility index and Hausner ratio are measures of the propensity of a powder to be compressed as described above. As such, they are measures of the powder's ability to settle, and they permit an assessment of the relative importance of interparticulate interactions. In a free-flowing powder, such interactions are less significant, and the bulk and tapped densities will be closer in value. For more-poorly flowing materials, there are frequently greater interparticulate interactions, and a greater difference between the bulk and tapped densities will be observed. These differences are reflected in the compressibility index and the Hausner ratio.

Compressibility index:

$$\frac{100\,(V_0 - V_f)}{V_0}$$

V_0 = unsettled apparent volume;

V_f = final tapped volume.

Hausner Ratio:

$$\frac{V_0}{V_f}$$

Depending on the material, the compressibility index can be determined using V_{10} instead of V_0.

07/2009:20945

2.9.45. WETTABILITY OF POROUS SOLIDS INCLUDING POWDERS

INTRODUCTION

The wettability of solid surfaces is commonly characterised by direct or indirect contact angle measurements. The contact angle (θ) between a liquid and a solid is the angle naturally formed when a drop of a liquid is placed on a solid surface. This is depicted in Figure 2.9.45.-1. For a given liquid, wettable solids show a low contact angle and non-wettable solids show a contact angle of 90° or more.

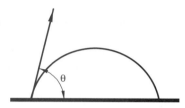

Figure 2.9.45.-1. – *Contact angle (θ) of a sessile drop observed on a non-porous surface*

2 methods for the determination of wettability are described below. The methods are capable of measuring the wettability of porous solids like powders or granules. Both methods express the wettability by a contact angle measurement between the porous solid and a given liquid.

The sessile drop method is based on direct measurement of a contact angle of a sessile drop on a compacted powder disc.

With the Washburn method the contact angle is indirectly measured. The method is based on the capillary effect of the powder pores. The effect (mass gain) is recorded by special electronic balances starting the moment when the powder sample touches the surface of a liquid, preferably not dissolving or poorly dissolving the sample. The measurement has very little or no effect on the state of the powder.

Any pre-treatment of the sample to be examined is disadvantageous, since the properties may be significantly altered. For example, the compaction of a powder as a disc may decrease the surface free energy when the crystalline state of the powder is changed (e.g. metastable forms), or may increase surface free energy by creating crystal defects (disadvantage of the sessile drop method since compacted powder discs are tested).

The methods are usually applied to examine the following parameters:

— batch-to-batch consistency of samples in terms of wettability;

— effect of liquid viscosity on wettability;

— effect of surface tension of a liquid on wettability;

— alteration of surface properties of samples.

SESSILE DROP METHOD

This method may be used to characterise directly the wettability of coatings and compacted formulations such as tablets. Moreover, it is sometimes possible to use the sessile drop instrument in a dynamic measurement (dynamic contact angle measurement, Figure 2.9.45.-2) of porous solid/liquid systems where the contact angle decreases. By taking several contact angle measurements as a function of time, the rate of spreading accompanied by penetration of a liquid droplet into a slightly porous solid may be studied.

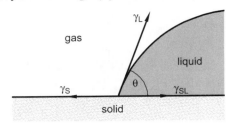

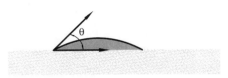

Figure 2.9.45.-2. – *Sessile drop determination with visual inspection of the droplet*

Under equilibrium conditions the contact angle of a sessile drop depends on 3 interrelated surface tensions and is determined using Young's equation (see Figure 2.9.45.-2, 1st part):

$$\gamma_S = \gamma_{SL} + \gamma_L \cos \theta$$

γ_S =   surface tension of the solid with air;

γ_{SL} =   interfacial tension of the solid with the liquid;

γ_L =   surface tension of the liquid with air.

PROCEDURE

Since powders are unable to form a completely flat surface, the powder is usually compacted as a disc in an attempt to make the surface smoother. A liquid drop with a given volume is placed on the disc (see Figure 2.9.45.-2) allowing direct measurement of the contact angle using a goniometer fitted with an eyepiece protractor, or by geometric construction on a photomicrograph. Other physical and mathematical procedures of data analysis may also be appropriate. The drop volume may influence the result. Several determinations of the contact angle (θ) (n = 6) are usually carried out and the average is calculated.

WASHBURN METHOD

The Washburn method is able to measure the contact angle of porous solids with a contact angle in the range of 0-90°.

The tested material is the combination of the sample, the holder and the filter system. Therefore, an estimation or determination of the true value is not possible and only apparent values of the contact angle can be determined. However, the contact angle of the sample is the functional property on which the result is significantly dependent. The outcome of the test is a ranking order listing the wettability of different substances or formulations characterised by an apparent contact angle.

PRINCIPLE

If a porous solid is brought into contact with a liquid, such that the solid is not submerged in the liquid, but rather is just touching the liquid surface, then the rise of liquid into the pores of the solid due to capillary action will be governed by the following equations:

$$m^2 = \frac{t}{A}$$ (1)

m =   mass of liquid sucked into the solid;

t =   time elapsed since the solid and the liquid were brought into contact;

A =   constant, dependent on the properties of the liquid and the solid to be examined, calculated using the following equation:

$$A = \frac{\eta}{c \times \rho^2 \times \gamma \times \cos \theta}$$ (2)

η =   viscosity of the liquid;

ρ =   density of the liquid;

γ =   surface tension of the liquid;

θ =   contact angle between the solid and the liquid;

c =   material constant, dependent on the porous texture of the solid.

Equations (1) and (2) lead to equation (3):

$$\cos \theta = \frac{m^2}{t} \times \frac{\eta}{c \times \rho^2 \times \gamma}$$ (3)

In setting up a Washburn determination, a liquid with known density (ρ), viscosity (η), and surface tension (γ) is used. Under these conditions, when the mass of liquid rising into the porous solid is monitored as a function of time (such that capillary penetration rate ($\frac{m^2}{t}$) is the experimental data), 2 unknowns remain according to equation (3): the contact angle (θ) of the liquid on the solid, and the solid material constant (c).

Determination of the material constant (c). The material constant for a porous solid is determined by the following equation, considering cylindrical pores:

$$\frac{\pi^2 \times r^5 \times N^2}{2}$$ (4)

r =   average capillary radius within the porous solid;

N =   number of capillaries per volumetric unit.

If a Washburn determination is performed with a liquid considered to have a contact angle of 0° (cos 0° = 1) on the solid, then the solid material constant (c) is the only remaining unknown in equation (3) and can thus be determined. *n*-Heptane is the liquid of choice for determining material constants because of its low surface tension (20.14 mN·m⁻¹ at 25 °C). *n*-Hexane may also be used (18.43 mN·m⁻¹ at 25 °C) but is more volatile. If the powder dissolves too quickly in these liquids, hexamethyldisiloxane may be used instead (15.9 mN·m⁻¹ at 25 °C). Replicate determinations are performed (n = 6) and the average value calculated.

Once the material constant (c) has been determined for the solid to be examined, a sample of the solid can be tested for wettability by another liquid. The material constant determined by the *n*-heptane test is used in the Washburn equation, in combination with the capillary penetration rate ($\frac{m^2}{t}$) data obtained while testing the substance to be examined in the prescribed liquid. This allows calculation of the contact angle.

NOTE: if a series of liquids (at least 2 liquids in addition to the liquid used to determine the material constant) is tested against a given solid then the resultant contact angle data can be used to calculate the surface energy of the porous solid.

APPARATUS

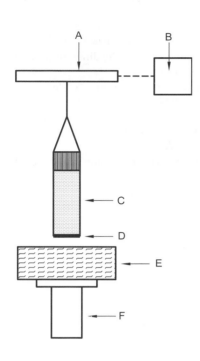

A. electronic balance   C. sample holder   E. immersion liquid

B. computer   D. filter   F. lift

Figure 2.9.45.-3. – *Apparatus for contact angle measurement by the Washburn method*

Figure 2.9.45.-3 shows the principal components of the apparatus. The main device is an electronic balance with a suitable processor ensuring a suitable resolution in force measurement and a suitable resolution in lifting up the immersion liquid towards the sample.

Table 2.9.45.-1 indicates parameters of the electronic balance that are generally considered suitable.

Table 2.9.45.-1. – *Technical parameters of the electronic balance*

	Lift	**Mass measurement**
Range	> 110 mm	0 - 210 g
Resolution	0.1 µm	10 µg
Speed	0.099 - 500 mm/min	-

Sample holders. The sample holder may be a small glass cylinder with a sintered-glass filter at one end.

Powder material holders (see Figure 2.9.45-4) may also be made of aluminium; they are less fragile than those made of glass and have small holes in the bottom that render them easier to clean than a sintered-glass filter. The cover for the cell is equipped with 2 screw threads. One connects it with the sample chamber while the other allows the user to guide a piston down onto the sample itself and compact it. The apparatus is similar to an automatic tensiometer, except for the sample holder.

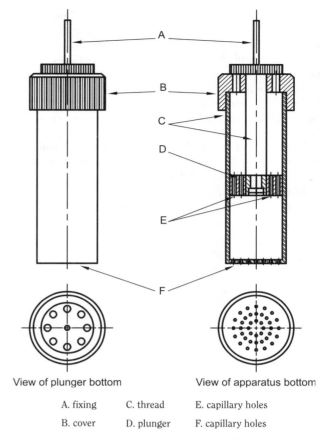

View of plunger bottom   View of apparatus bottom

A. fixing   C. thread   E. capillary holes

B. cover   D. plunger   F. capillary holes

Figure 2.9.45.-4. – *Example of sample holder with plunger for compaction of a powder*

PROCEDURE

Filling of the sample holder. Place a disc of filter paper in the bottom of the aluminium or glass sample holder. This prevents powder from leaking out of the bottom of the cell. The filter does not have to be made of paper, but it must be a material that is easily wetted by the liquid to be tested. A black-band filter (used for reverse osmosis) is recommended because of its high porosity and minimum flow resistance.

Place a known amount of powder into the cell. The reproducibility of material constants and contact angles will depend on the ability to weigh out the same amount of powder for each test when a sufficient and adjusted amount of powder is compacted in a uniform way (i.e. tapping/compaction of the powder).

For most powders, a correct amount is in the range of a few grams, typically filling about 2/3 of the capacity of the holder. Place a second piece of filter paper on top of the powder in the cell. This will prevent powder from rising through the holes in the piston during the compaction process and/or during the determination.

Tapping/compaction of the powder. A bulk powder bed is very porous and thus very sensitive to small influences that can easily alter the porosity and consequently the *c*-constant. Therefore a tapped powder may be advantageous and will show more reproducible results. The appropriate number of taps must first be evaluated: 50-100 taps are usually appropriate.

If the aluminium sample holder is used then it may be mounted in the cylinder of a stamp volumeter, which can run the evaluated number of taps.

If tapping is not appropriate, the powder bed is compacted by screwing the piston of the aluminium sample holder applying a specified pressure.

A further possibility is centrifugation under defined conditions. Where applicable, a compacted disc of the powder sample may also be mounted on the electronic balance. A sample holder is omitted in this case.

After connecting to the balance, the sample holder is positioned with the porous solid just above the surface of the liquid (see Figure 2.9.45.-3), using the lift.

The liquid is raised further until it just touches the bottom of the porous sample. Mass-versus-time data is then collected as liquid penetrates into the solid. Data can be presented in either graphical or tabular format. The apparatus may perform the whole determination automatically.

CRITICAL PARAMETERS

The following points must be considered.

Sample properties:

— water content of the sample;

— crystalline or solid-state properties of the sample (polymorphic form, type of solvate).

Sample preparation:

— homogeneity of any powder blend to be examined;

— particle-size distribution; before testing it is sometimes advisable to sieve the sample (e.g. using a 250 µm sieve);

— the optimal compaction parameters (amount of sample, number of taps or piston mass) must be determined;

— the compaction state of the different powder samples must be uniform;

— the sample holder or, if used, the glass frit must be carefully cleaned;

— uniformity of the results is improved by using a sample holder made of aluminium.

Immersion liquid:

— specifications of the immersion liquid must be indicated.

4. REAGENTS

See the information section on general monographs (cover pages)

07/2009:40101

4.1.1. REAGENTS

Ammonium carbonate. *1005200.*

Ammonium carbonate solution R1. *1005202.*

Dissolve 20 g of *ammonium carbonate R* in 20 ml of *dilute ammonia R1* and dilute to 100 ml with *water R*.

Anise ketone. $C_{10}H_{12}O_2$. (M_r 164.2). *1174700.* [122-84-9]. 1-(4-Methoxyphenyl)propan-2-one.

Bromothymol blue. *1012900.*

Bromothymol blue solution R4. *1012904.*

Dissolve 100 mg of *bromothymol blue R* in a mixture of equal volumes of *ethanol 96 per cent R* and *water R* and dilute to 100 ml with the same mixture of solvents. Filter if necessary.

Butane-1,4-diol. $HO(CH_2)_4OH$. (M_r 90.12). *1174800.* [110-63-4].

Cadmium nitrate tetrahydrate. $Cd(NO_3)_2,4H_2O$. (M_r 308.5). *1174900.* [10022-68-1].

Hygroscopic orthorhombic crystals, very soluble in water, soluble in acetone and in ethanol (96 per cent).

mp: about 59.5 °C.

Cortisone. $C_{21}H_{28}O_5$. (M_r 360.4). *1175000.* [53-06-5].

Content: minimum 95.0 per cent.

mp: 223-228 °C.

Methyldopa, racemic. $C_{10}H_{13}NO_4, 1^1/_2H_2O$. ($M_r$ 238.2). *1175100.*

Mixture of equal volumes of (2S)- and (2R)-2-amino-3-(3,4-dihydroxyphenyl)-2-methylpropanoic acids.

N-Methyl-*m*-toluidine. $C_8H_{11}N$. (M_r 121.2). *1175200.* [696-44-6]. *N*,3-Dimethylaniline. *N*,3-Dimethylbenzenamine. Methyl-*m*-tolylamine.

Content: minimum 97 per cent.

Nickel nitrate hexahydrate. $Ni(NO_3)_2,6H_2O$. (M_r 290.8). *1175300.* [13478-00-7].

Pyridin-2-amine. $C_5H_6N_2$. (M_r 94.1). *1073400.* [504-29-0]. 2-Aminopyridine.

Large crystals soluble in water and in ethanol (96 per cent).

bp: about 210 °C.

mp: about 58 °C.

Reichstein's substance S. $C_{21}H_{30}O_4$. (M_r 346.5). *1175400.* [152-58-9].

Content: minimum 95.0 per cent.

mp: about 208 °C.

Triethylamine. *1093000.*

Triethylamine R2. $C_6H_{15}N$. (M_r 101.2). *1093002.* [121-44-8]. *N,N*-Diethylethanamine.

Complies with the requirements prescribed for *triethylamine R* and with the following additional requirements.

Content: minimum 99.5 per cent, determined by gas chromatography.

Water: maximum 0.2 per cent.

It is suitable for gradient elution in liquid chromatography. *Use freshly distilled or from a freshly opened container.*

4. Reagents

See the information section on general monographs (cover pages)

5.2. GENERAL TEXTS ON BIOLOGICAL PRODUCTS

07/2009:50205

5.2.5. SUBSTANCES OF ANIMAL ORIGIN FOR THE PRODUCTION OF IMMUNOLOGICAL VETERINARY MEDICINAL PRODUCTS

1. SCOPE

Substances of animal origin (for example serum, trypsin and serum albumin) may be used during the manufacture of immunological veterinary medicinal products.

The requirements set out in this chapter apply to substances of animal origin produced on a batch basis, for use at all stages of manufacture, for example in culture media or as added constituents of products during blending. These requirements are not intended for the control of seed materials or substrates of animal origin that are covered by requirements in other pharmacopoeial texts such as the monograph *Vaccines for veterinary use (0062)* and chapter *5.2.4. Cell cultures for the production of veterinary vaccines.*

2. GENERAL PRINCIPLES AND REQUIREMENTS

Substances of animal origin comply with the requirements of the European Pharmacopoeia (where a relevant monograph exists).

Restrictions are placed on the use of substances of animal origin because of safety concerns associated with pathogens that may be present in them and epidemiological and/or regulatory concerns associated with the presence of particular antigens (either live or inactivated).

General principles:

— it is recommended to minimise, wherever practicable, the use of substances of animal origin;

— unless otherwise justified, the use of substances of animal origin as constituents in the formulation of medicinal products is not acceptable except where such substances are subject to a treatment validated for the inactivation of live extraneous agents.

General requirements:

— any batch of substance (after inactivation and/or processing, if relevant) found to contain or suspected of containing any living extraneous agent shall be discarded or used only in exceptional and justified circumstances; to be accepted for use, further processing must be applied that will ensure elimination and/or inactivation of the extraneous agent, and it shall then be demonstrated that the elimination and/or inactivation has been satisfactory;

— any batch of substance that, as concluded from the risk assessment, may induce an unacceptable detectable immune response in the target species as a consequence of contamination with inactivated extraneous agents, must not be used for the manufacture of that particular immunological veterinary medicinal product.

3. RISK MANAGEMENT

No single measure or combination of measures can guarantee the safety of the use of substances of animal origin, but they can reduce the risk from such use. It is therefore necessary for the manufacturer of immunological veterinary medicinal products to take account of this when choosing a substance of animal origin to use in manufacture, and to conduct a risk assessment, taking into account the origin of the substance and the manufacturing steps applied to it.

In addition, risk management procedures must be applied. Any residual risk must be evaluated in relation to the potential benefits derived from the use of the substance for the manufacture of the immunological veterinary medicinal product.

3-1. *RISK ASSESSMENT*

The risk assessment must take account of the animal diseases occurring in the country of origin of the animals used as a source of the substance, the potential infectious diseases occurring in the source species and the likely infectivity in the source organ or tissue. From this information, as part of the risk assessment, a list can be prepared of the extraneous agents that may be present in the substance.

The risk of contamination of the substance and the resultant immunological veterinary medicinal product with living extraneous agents needs to be assessed. The risk of contamination of the substance and the resultant immunological veterinary medicinal product with inactivated extraneous agents may also need to be taken into account. This would be the case if, for example, the contaminant was one from which a European country is officially free and/or is the subject of a specific disease control program in a European country and where the presence of the inactivated agent could lead to the stimulation of a detectable immune response in recipient animals.

As part of the risk assessment, the presence in the substance of antibodies that can interfere with the detection and/or inactivation of living extraneous agents must also be taken into account.

The risk assessment may need to be repeated and the risk management steps described below re-evaluated and revised in order to take account of changes:

— in the incidence of diseases occurring in the country or countries of origin of animals used as the source for the substance, including emerging diseases (new pathogens);

— in the incidence of diseases and of disease control measures applied in the European countries in which immunological veterinary medicinal products manufactured with the substance are used.

3-2. *RISK CONTROL*

For each of the potential extraneous agents identified by the risk assessment, and taking into account the proposed use of the substance, the risk must be controlled by the use of one or a combination of the followings measures:

— placing restrictions on the source of the material and auditing this;

— using validated inactivation procedures;

— demonstrating the ability of a production step to remove or inactivate extraneous agents;

— testing for extraneous agents.

4. CONTROL MEASURES

4-1. *SOURCE*

All substances of animal origin used in the manufacture (including blending) of immunological veterinary medicinal products must be from a known and documented source (including species of origin and country of origin of source animals and tissues).

4-2. *PREPARATION*

Substances of animal origin are prepared from a homogeneous bulk designated with a batch number. A batch may contain substances derived from as many animals as desired but once defined and given a batch number, the batch is not added to or contaminated in any way.

The production method used to prepare the substance of animal origin from the raw material may contribute to the removal and/or inactivation of extraneous agents (see section 4-3).

4-3. *INACTIVATION AND/OR OTHER PROCESSING STEPS FOR REMOVAL OF EXTRANEOUS AGENTS*

The inactivation procedure and/or other processing steps chosen shall have been validated and shown to be capable of reducing the titre of potential extraneous agents described below in the substance concerned by a factor of at least 10^6.

If this reduction in titre cannot be shown experimentally, a maximum pre-treatment titre of the extraneous agent must be set, taking into account the reduction in titre afforded by the inactivation/processing step and including a safety margin factor of 100; each batch of substance must be tested to determine the pre-treatment starting titre and confirm it is no greater than the specified limit, unless proper risk assessment, based on valid and suitable data, shows that titres will always be at least 100-fold below the titre that can effectively be inactivated.

The validation of the procedure(s) is conducted with a suitable representative range of viruses covering different types and sizes (enveloped and non-enveloped, DNA and RNA, single- and double-stranded, temperature- and pH-resistant), including test viruses with different degrees of resistance, taking into account the type of procedure(s) to be applied and the viruses that may be present in the material. The evidence for the efficacy of the procedure may take the form of references to published literature and/or experimental data generated by the manufacturer, but must be relevant to the conditions that will be present during the production and inactivation/processing of the substance.

For inactivated immunological veterinary medicinal products, the method used for inactivation of the active ingredient may also be validated for inactivation of possible contaminants from substances of animal origin used in the manufacture of this active ingredient.

4-4. *TESTS*

Depending on the outcome of the risk assessment and the validation data available for any procedure applied, tests for extraneous agents may be conducted on each batch before and/or after the application of an inactivation/processing step. For examination of the substance for freedom from extraneous agents, any solids are dissolved or suspended in a suitable medium to provide a suitable preparation for testing. A sufficient quantity of the preparation is tested to give a suitably sensitive test, as established in the validation studies.

As well as tests for living extraneous agents, tests may need to be conducted for the presence of inactivated extraneous agents, depending on the risks identified.

Freedom from living extraneous viruses. A sample from each batch of the substance is tested for extraneous viruses by general and specific tests. These tests are validated with respect to sensitivity and specificity for detection of a suitable range of potential extraneous viruses. Suitably sensitive cell cultures are used for the tests for extraneous viruses, including primary cells from the same species as the substance to be examined.

General test. The inoculated cell cultures are observed regularly for 21 days for cytopathic effects. At the end of each 7-day period, a proportion of the original cultures is fixed, stained and examined for cytopathic effects, and a proportion is tested for haemadsorbing agents.

Specific tests. A proportion of the cells available at the end of the general test is tested for specific viruses. The specific viruses to be tested for are potential extraneous viruses that are identified through the risk assessment and that would not be detected by the general test. A test for pestiviruses is conducted if the source species is susceptible to these.

Bacteria and fungi. Before use, substances are tested for sterility (*2.6.1*), or sterilised to inactivate any bacterial or fungal contaminants.

Mycoplasma. Before use, substances are tested for freedom from mycoplasma (*2.6.7*), or sterilised to inactivate any mycoplasmal contaminants.

5.10. CONTROL OF IMPURITIES IN SUBSTANCES FOR PHARMACEUTICAL USE

5. General texts

5. General texts

5.10. CONTROL OF IMPURITIES IN SUBSTANCES FOR PHARMACEUTICAL USE

Preamble

The monographs of the European Pharmacopoeia on substances for pharmaceutical use are designed to ensure acceptable quality for users. The role of the Pharmacopoeia in public health protection requires that adequate control of impurities be provided by monographs. The quality required is based on scientific, technical and regulatory considerations.

Requirements concerning impurities are given in specific monographs and in the general monograph *Substances for pharmaceutical use (2034)*. Specific monographs and the general monograph are complementary: specific monographs prescribe acceptance criteria for impurities whereas the general monograph deals with the need for qualification, identification and reporting of any organic impurities that occur in *active substances*.

The thresholds for reporting, identification and qualification contained in the general monograph *Substances for pharmaceutical use (2034)* apply to all related substances. However, if a monograph does not contain a related substances test based on a quantitative method, any new impurities occurring above a threshold may be overlooked since the test is not capable to detect those impurities.

The provisions of the Related substances section of the general monograph *Substances for pharmaceutical use (2034)*, notably those concerning thresholds, do not apply to excipients; also excluded from the provisions of this section are: biological and biotechnological products; oligonucleotides; radiopharmaceuticals; fermentation products and semisynthetic products derived therefrom; herbal products and crude products of animal and plant origin. Although the thresholds stated in the general monograph do not apply, the general concepts of reporting, identification (wherever possible) and qualification of impurities are equally valid for these classes.

Basis for the elaboration of monographs of the European Pharmacopoeia

European Pharmacopoeia monographs are elaborated on substances that are present in medicinal products that have been authorised by the competent authorities of Parties to the *European Pharmacopoeia Convention*. Consequently, these monographs do not necessarily cover all sources of substances for pharmaceutical use on the world market.

Organic and inorganic impurities present in those substances that have been evaluated by the competent authorities are qualified with respect to safety at the maximum authorised content (at the maximum daily dose) unless new safety data that become available following evaluation justify lower limits.

European Pharmacopoeia monographs on substances for pharmaceutical use are elaborated by groups of experts and working parties collaborating with national pharmacopoeia authorities, the competent authorities for marketing authorisation, national control laboratories and the European Pharmacopoeia laboratory; they are also assisted by the producers of the substances and/or the pharmaceutical manufacturers that use these substances.

Control of impurities in substances for pharmaceutical use

The quality with respect to impurities is controlled by a set of tests within a monograph. These tests are intended to cover organic and inorganic impurities that are relevant in view of the sources of active substances in authorised medicinal products.

Control of residual solvents is provided by the general monograph *Substances for pharmaceutical use (2034)* and general chapter *5.4. Residual solvents*. The certificate of suitability of a monograph of the European Pharmacopoeia for a given source of a substance indicates the residual solvents that are controlled together with the specified acceptance criteria and the validated control method where this differs from those described in general chapter *2.4.24. Identification and control of residual solvents*.

Monographs on organic chemicals usually have a test entitled "Related substances" that covers relevant organic impurities. This test may be supplemented by specific tests where the general test does not control a given impurity or where there are particular reasons (for example, safety reasons) for requiring special control.

Where a monograph has no Related substances (or equivalent) test but only specific tests, the user of a substance must nevertheless ensure that there is suitable control of organic impurities; those occurring above the identification threshold are to be identified (wherever possible) and, unless justified, those occurring above the qualification threshold are to be qualified (see also under Recommendations to users of monographs of active substances).

Where the monograph covers substances with different impurity profiles, it may have a single related substances test to cover all impurities mentioned in the Impurities section or several tests may be necessary to give control of all known profiles. Compliance may be established by carrying out only the tests relevant to the known impurity profile for the source of the substance.

Instructions for control of impurities may be included in the Production section of a monograph, for example where the only analytical method appropriate for the control of a given impurity is to be performed by the manufacturer since the method is too technically complex for general use or cannot be applied to the final drug substance and/or where validation of the production process (including the purification step) will give sufficient control.

Impurities section in monographs on active substances

The Impurities section in a monograph includes impurities (chemical structure and name wherever possible), which are usually organic, that are known to be detected by the tests prescribed in the monograph. It is based on information available at the time of elaboration or revision of the monograph and is not necessarily exhaustive. The section includes specified impurities and, where so indicated, other detectable impurities.

Specified impurities have an acceptance criterion not greater than that authorised by the competent authorities.

Other detectable impurities are potential impurities with a defined structure but not known to be normally present above the identification threshold in substances used in medicinal products that have been authorised by the competent authorities of Parties to the Convention. They are given in the Impurities section for information.

Where an impurity other than a specified impurity is found in an active substance it is the responsibility of the user of the substance to check whether it has to be identified/qualified, depending on its content, nature, maximum daily dose

5. General texts

and relevant identification/qualification threshold, in accordance with the general monograph on *Substances for pharmaceutical use (2034)*, Related substances section.

It should be noted that specific thresholds are applied to substances exclusively for veterinary use.

Interpretation of the test for related substances in the monographs on active substances

A specific monograph on a substance for pharmaceutical use is to be read and interpreted in conjunction with the general monograph on *Substances for pharmaceutical use (2034)*.

Where a general acceptance criterion for impurities ("any other impurity", "other impurities", "any impurity") equivalent to a nominal content greater than the applicable identification threshold (see the general monograph on *Substances for pharmaceutical use (2034)*) is prescribed, this is valid only for specified impurities mentioned in the Impurities section. The need for identification (wherever possible), reporting, specification and qualification of other impurities that occur must be considered according to the requirements of the general monograph. It is the responsibility of the user of the substance to determine the validity of the acceptance criteria for impurities not mentioned in the Impurities section and for those indicated as other detectable impurities.

Acceptance criteria for the related substances test are presented in different ways in existing monographs; the decision tree (Figure 5.10.-1) may be used as an aid in the interpretation of general acceptance criteria and their relation with the Impurities section of the monograph.

General acceptance criteria for "other" impurities are expressed in various ways in the monographs: "any other impurity", "other impurities", "any impurity", "any spot", "any band", etc. The general acceptance criteria may apply to certain specified impurities only or to unspecified impurities and certain specified impurities, depending on the nature of the active substance and the applicable identification threshold. Pending editorial adaptation of already published monographs using unequivocal terminology, the decision tree (Figure 5.10.-1) may be used to determine the acceptance criterion to be applied.

Recommendations to users of monographs of active substances

Monographs give a specification for suitable quality of substances with impurity profiles corresponding to those taken into account during elaboration and/or revision of the monograph. It is the responsibility of the user of the substance to check that the monograph provides adequate control of impurities for a substance for pharmaceutical use from a given source, notably by using the procedure for certification of suitability of the monographs of the European Pharmacopoeia.

A monograph with a related substances test based on a quantitative method (such as liquid chromatography, gas chromatography and capillary electrophoresis) provides adequate control of impurities for a substance from a given source if impurities present in amounts above the applicable identification threshold are specified impurities mentioned in the Impurities section.

If the substance contains impurities other than those mentioned in the Impurities section, it has to be verified that these impurities are detectable by the method described in the monograph, otherwise a new method must be developed and revision of the monograph must be requested. Depending on the contents found and the limits proposed, the identification and/or the qualification of these impurities must be considered.

Where a single related substances test covers different impurity profiles, only impurities for the known profile from a single source need to be reported in the certificate of analysis unless the marketing authorisation holder uses active substances with different impurity profiles.

Identification of impurities (peak assignment)

Where a monograph has an individual limit for an impurity, it is often necessary to define means of identification, for example using a reference substance, a representative chromatogram or relative retention. The user of the substance may find it necessary to identify impurities other than those for which the monograph provides a means of identification, for example to check the suitability of the specification for a given impurity profile by comparison with the Impurities section. The European Pharmacopoeia does not provide reference substances, representative chromatograms or information on relative retentions for this purpose, unless prescribed in the monograph. Users will therefore have to apply the available scientific techniques for identification.

New impurities/Specified impurities above the specified limit

Where a new manufacturing process or change in an established process leads to the occurrence of a new impurity, it is necessary to apply the provisions of the general monograph on *Substances for pharmaceutical use (2034)* regarding identification and qualification and to verify the suitability of the monograph for control of the impurity. A certificate of suitability is a means for confirming for a substance from a given source that the new impurity is adequately controlled or the certificate contains a method for control with a defined acceptance criterion. In the latter case revision of the monograph will be initiated.

Where a new manufacturing process or change in an established process leads to the occurrence of a specified impurity above the specified limit, it is necessary to apply the provisions of the general monograph on *Substances for pharmaceutical use (2034)* regarding qualification.

Chromatographic methods

General chapter *2.2.46. Chromatographic separation techniques* deals with various aspects of impurities control.

Information is available via the EDQM website on commercial names for columns and other reagents and equipment found suitable during monograph development, where this is considered useful.

GLOSSARY

Disregard limit: in chromatographic tests, the nominal content at or below which peaks/signals are not taken into account for calculating a sum of impurities. The numerical values for the disregard limit and the reporting threshold are usually the same.

Identification threshold: a limit above which an impurity is to be identified.

Identified impurity: an impurity for which structural characterisation has been achieved.

Impurity: any component of a substance for pharmaceutical use that is not the chemical entity defined as the substance.

Nominal concentration: concentration calculated on the basis of the concentration of the prescribed reference and taking account of the prescribed correction factor.

Other detectable impurities: potential impurities with a defined structure that are known to be detected by the tests in a monograph but not known to be normally present above the identification threshold in substances used in medicinal products that have been authorised by the competent authorities of Parties to the Convention. They are unspecified impurities and are thus limited by a general acceptance criterion.

Potential impurity: an impurity that theoretically can arise during manufacture or storage. It may or may not actually appear in the substance. Where a potential impurity is known to be detected by the tests in a monograph but not known to be normally present in substances used in medicinal products that have been authorised by the competent authorities of Parties to the Convention, it will be included in the Impurities section under *Other detectable impurities* for information.

Qualification: the process of acquiring and evaluating data that establishes the biological safety of an individual impurity or a given impurity profile at the level(s) specified.

Qualification threshold: a limit above which an impurity is to be qualified.

Related substances: title used in monographs for general tests for organic impurities.

Reporting threshold: a limit above which an impurity is to be reported. Synonym: reporting level.

Specified impurity: an impurity that is individually listed and limited with a specific acceptance criterion in a monograph. A specified impurity can be either identified or unidentified.

Unidentified impurity: an impurity for which a structural characterisation has not been achieved and that is defined solely by qualitative analytical properties (for example, relative retention).

Unspecified impurity: an impurity that is limited by a general acceptance criterion and not individually listed with its own specific acceptance criterion.

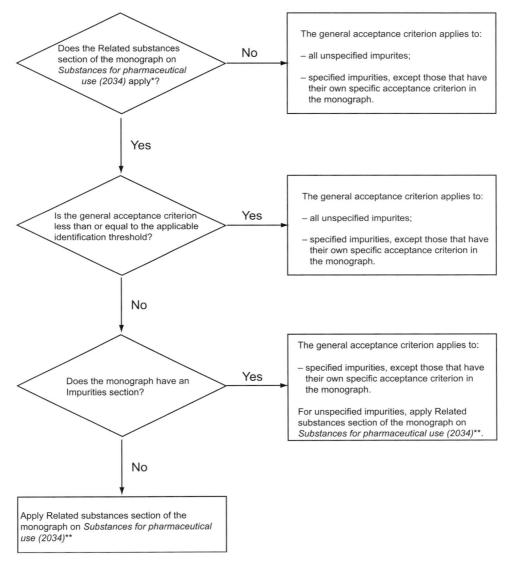

* The requirements of this section apply to active substances, with the exception of: biological and biotechnological products; oligonucleotides; radiopharmaceuticals; products of fermentation and semi-synthetic products derived therefrom; crude products of animal or plant origin; herbal products.

** To apply the Related substances section of the monograph *Substances for pharmaceutical use (2034)*:
— an individual acceptance criterion must be defined for any impurity that may be present above the identification threshold;
— any impurity with an acceptance criterion above the identification threshold must wherever possible be identified;
— any impurity with an acceptance criterion above the qualification threshold must be qualified.

Figure 5.10.-1. − *Decision tree for interpretation of general acceptance criteria for 'other' impurities in monographs*

GENERAL MONOGRAPHS

General
monographs

07/2009:2034

SUBSTANCES FOR PHARMACEUTICAL USE

Corpora ad usum pharmaceuticum

DEFINITION

Substances for pharmaceutical use are any organic or inorganic substances that are used as active substances or excipients for the production of medicinal products for human or veterinary use. They may be obtained from natural sources or produced by extraction from raw materials, fermentation or synthesis.

This general monograph does not apply to herbal drugs, herbal drugs for homoeopathic preparations, herbal drug preparations, extracts, or mother tinctures for homoeopathic preparations, which are the subject of separate general monographs (*Herbal drugs (1433), Herbal drugs for homoeopathic preparations (2045), Herbal drug preparations (1434), Extracts (0765), Mother tinctures for homoeopathic preparations (2029)*). It does not apply to raw materials for homoeopathic preparations, except where there is an individual monograph for the substance in the non-homoeopathic part of the Pharmacopoeia.

Where a substance for pharmaceutical use not described in an individual monograph of the Pharmacopoeia is used in a medicinal product prepared for the special needs of individual patients, the need for compliance with the present general monograph is decided in the light of a risk assessment that takes account of the available quality of the substance and its intended use.

Where medicinal products are manufactured using substances for pharmaceutical use of human or animal origin, the requirements of chapter *5.1.7. Viral safety* apply.

Substances for pharmaceutical use may be used as such or as starting materials for subsequent formulation to prepare medicinal products. Depending on the formulation, certain substances may be used either as active substances or as excipients. Solid substances may be compacted, coated, granulated, powdered to a certain fineness, or processed in other ways. A monograph is applicable to a substance processed with an excipient only where such processing is mentioned in the definition section of the monograph.

Substance for pharmaceutical use of special grade. Unless otherwise indicated or restricted in the individual monographs, a substance for pharmaceutical use is intended for human and veterinary use, and is of appropriate quality for the manufacture of all dosage forms in which it can be used.

Polymorphism. Individual monographs do not usually specify crystalline or amorphous forms, unless bioavailability is affected. All forms of a substance for pharmaceutical use comply with the requirements of the monograph, unless otherwise indicated.

PRODUCTION

Substances for pharmaceutical use are manufactured by procedures that are designed to ensure a consistent quality and comply with the requirements of the individual monograph or approved specification.

The provisions of general chapter *5.10* apply to the control of impurities in substances for pharmaceutical use.

Whether or not it is specifically stated in the individual monograph that the substance for pharmaceutical use:

– is a recombinant protein or another substance obtained as a direct gene product based on genetic modification, where applicable, the substance also complies with the requirements of the general monograph *Products of recombinant DNA technology (0784)*;

– is obtained from animals susceptible to transmissible spongiform encephalopathies other than by experimental challenge, where applicable, the substance also complies with the requirements of the general monograph *Products with risk of transmitting agents of animal spongiform encephalopathies (1483)*;

– is a substance derived from a fermentation process, whether or not the micro-organisms involved are modified by traditional procedures or recombinant DNA (rDNA) technology, where applicable, the substance also complies with the requirements of the general monograph *Products of fermentation (1468)*.

If solvents are used during production, they are of suitable quality. In addition, their toxicity and their residual level are taken into consideration (*5.4*). If water is used during production, it is of suitable quality.

If substances are produced or processed to yield a certain form or grade, that specific form or grade of the substance complies with the requirements of the monograph. Certain functionality-related tests may be described to control properties that may influence the suitability of the substance and subsequently the properties of dosage forms prepared from it.

Powdered substances may be processed to obtain a certain degree of fineness (*2.9.35*).

Compacted substances are processed to increase the particle size or to obtain particles of a specific form and/or to obtain a substance with a higher bulk density.

Coated active substances consist of particles of the active substance coated with one or more suitable excipients.

Granulated active substances are particles of a specified size and/or form produced from the active substance by granulation directly or with one or more suitable excipients.

If substances are processed with excipients, these excipients comply with the requirements of the relevant monograph or, where no such monograph exists, the approved specification.

Where active substances have been processed with excipients to produce, for example, coated or granulated substances, the processing is carried out under conditions of good manufacturing practice and the processed substances are regarded as intermediates in the manufacture of a medicinal product.

CHARACTERS

The statements under the heading Characters (e.g. statements about the solubility or a decomposition point) are not to be interpreted in a strict sense and are not requirements. They are given for information.

Where a substance may show polymorphism, this may be stated under Characters in order to draw this to the attention of the user who may have to take this characteristic into consideration during formulation of a preparation.

IDENTIFICATION

Where under Identification an individual monograph contains subdivisions entitled 'First identification' and 'Second identification', the test or tests that constitute the 'First identification' may be used in all circumstances. The test or tests that constitute the 'Second identification' may be used in pharmacies provided it can be demonstrated that the substance or preparation is fully traceable to a batch certified to comply with all the other requirements of the monograph.

Certain monographs give two or more sets of tests for the purpose of the first identification, which are equivalent and may be used independently. One or more of these sets usually contain a cross-reference to a test prescribed in the Tests section of the monograph. It may be used to simplify the work of the analyst carrying out the identification and the prescribed tests. For example, one identification set cross-refers to a test for enantiomeric purity while the other set gives a test for specific optical rotation: the intended purpose of the two is the same, that is, verification that the correct enantiomer is present.

TESTS

Polymorphism (*5.9*). If the nature of a crystalline or amorphous form imposes restrictions on its use in preparations, the nature of the specific crystalline or amorphous form is identified, its morphology is adequately controlled and its identity is stated on the label.

Related substances. Unless otherwise prescribed or justified and authorised, organic impurities in active substances are to be reported, identified wherever possible, and qualified as indicated in Table 2034.-1 or in Table 2034.-2 for peptides obtained by chemical synthesis.

Table 2034.-1. – *Reporting, identification and qualification of organic impurities in active substances*

Use	Maximum daily dose	Reporting threshold	Identification threshold	Qualification threshold
Human use or human and veterinary use	≤ 2 g/day	> 0.05 per cent	> 0.10 per cent or a daily intake of > 1.0 mg (whichever is the lower)	> 0.15 per cent or a daily intake of > 1.0 mg (whichever is the lower)
Human use or human and veterinary use	> 2 g/day	> 0.03 per cent	> 0.05 per cent	> 0.05 per cent
Veterinary use only	Not applicable	> 0.10 per cent	> 0.20 per cent	> 0.50 per cent

Table 2034.-2. – *Reporting, identification and qualification of organic impurities in peptides obtained by chemical synthesis*

Reporting threshold	Identification threshold	Qualification threshold
> 0.1 per cent	> 0.5 per cent	> 1.0 per cent

Specific thresholds may be applied for impurities known to be unusually potent or to produce toxic or unexpected pharmacological effects.

If the individual monograph does not provide suitable control for a new impurity, a suitable test for control must be developed and included in the specification for the substance.

The requirements above do not apply to biological and biotechnological products, oligonucleotides, radiopharmaceuticals, products of fermentation and semi-synthetic products derived therefrom, to crude products of animal or plant origin or herbal products.

Residual solvents are limited according to the principles defined in chapter *5.4*, using general method *2.4.24* or another suitable method. Where a quantitative determination of a residual solvent is carried out and a test for loss on drying is not carried out, the content of residual solvent is taken into account for calculation of the assay content of the substance, the specific optical rotation and the specific absorbance.

Microbiological quality. Individual monographs give acceptance criteria for microbiological quality wherever such control is necessary. Table 5.1.4.-2. – *Acceptance criteria for microbiological quality of non-sterile substances for pharmaceutical use* in chapter *5.1.4. Microbiological quality of non-sterile pharmaceutical preparations and substances for pharmaceutical use* gives recommendations on microbiological quality that are of general relevance for substances subject to microbial contamination. Depending on the nature of the substance and its intended use, different acceptance criteria may be justified.

Sterility (*2.6.1*). If intended for use in the manufacture of sterile dosage forms without a further appropriate sterilisation procedure, or if offered as sterile grade, the substance for pharmaceutical use complies with the test for sterility.

Bacterial endotoxins (*2.6.14*). If offered as bacterial endotoxin-free grade, the substance for pharmaceutical use complies with the test for bacterial endotoxins. The limit and test method (if not gelation method A) are stated in the individual monograph. The limit is calculated in accordance with *Test for bacterial endotoxins: guidelines* in chapter *2.6.14. Bacterial endotoxins*, unless a lower limit is justified from results from production batches or is required by the competent authority. Where a test for bacterial endotoxins is prescribed, a test for pyrogens is not required.

Pyrogens (*2.6.8*). If the test for pyrogens is justified rather than the test for bacterial endotoxins and if a pyrogen-free grade is offered, the substance for pharmaceutical use complies with the test for pyrogens. The limit and test method are stated in the individual monograph or approved by the competent authority. Based on appropriate test validation for bacterial endotoxins and pyrogens, the test for bacterial endotoxins may replace the test for pyrogens.

Additional properties. Control of additional properties (e.g. physical characteristics, functionality-related characteristics) may be necessary for individual manufacturing processes or formulations. Grades (such as sterile, endotoxin-free, pyrogen-free) may be produced with a view to manufacture of preparations for parenteral administration or other dosage forms and appropriate requirements may be specified in an individual monograph.

ASSAY

Unless justified and authorised, contents of substances for pharmaceutical use are determined. Suitable methods are used.

LABELLING

In general, labelling is subject to supranational and national regulation and to international agreements. The statements under the heading Labelling therefore are not comprehensive and, moreover, for the purposes of the Pharmacopoeia only those statements that are necessary to demonstrate compliance or non-compliance with the monograph are mandatory. Any other labelling statements are included as recommendations. When the term 'label' is used in the Pharmacopoeia, the labelling statements may appear on the container, the package, a leaflet accompanying the package or a certificate of analysis accompanying the article, as decided by the competent authority.

Where appropriate, the label states that the substance is:

— intended for a specific use;

— of a distinct crystalline form;

— of a specific degree of fineness;
— compacted;
— coated;
— granulated;
— sterile;
— free from bacterial endotoxins;

— free from pyrogens;
— containing gliding agents.

Where applicable, the label states:

— the degree of hydration;
— the name and concentration of any excipient.

General monographs

General
monographs

VACCINES FOR VETERINARY USE

Vaccines

Vaccines

See the information section on general monographs (cover pages)

07/2009:2038

INFECTIOUS CHICKEN ANAEMIA VACCINE (LIVE)

Vaccinum anaemiae infectivae pulli vivum

1. DEFINITION

Infectious chicken anaemia vaccine (live) is a preparation of a suitable strain of chicken anaemia virus. This monograph applies to vaccines intended for administration to breeder chickens for active immunisation, to prevent excretion of the virus, to prevent or reduce egg transmission and to protect passively their future progeny.

2. PRODUCTION

2-1. *PREPARATION OF THE VACCINE*

The vaccine virus is grown in embryonated hens' eggs or in cell cultures.

2-2. *SUBSTRATE FOR VIRUS PROPAGATION*

2-2-1. **Embryonated hens' eggs**. If the vaccine virus is grown in embryonated hens' eggs, they are obtained from flocks free from specified pathogens (SPF) (*5.2.2*).

2-2-2. **Cell cultures**. If the vaccine virus is grown in cell cultures, they comply with the requirements for cell cultures for production of veterinary vaccines (*5.2.4*).

2-3. *SEED LOTS*

2-3-1. **Extraneous agents**. The master seed lot complies with the test for extraneous agents in seed lots (*2.6.24*). In these tests on the master seed lot, the organisms used are not more than 5 passages from the master seed lot at the start of the tests.

2-4. *CHOICE OF VACCINE VIRUS*

The vaccine virus is shown to be satisfactory with respect to safety (*5.2.6*) and efficacy (*5.2.7*) for the chickens for which it is intended.

The following tests for safety (section 2-4-1), increase in virulence (section 2-4-2) and immunogenicity (section 2-4-3) may be used during the demonstration of safety and efficacy.

2-4-1. **Safety**. Carry out the test for each route and method of administration to be recommended for vaccination in chickens not older than the minimum age to be recommended for vaccination and from an SPF flock (*5.2.2*). Use vaccine virus at the least attenuated passage level that will be present between the master seed lot and a batch of the vaccine.

2-4-1-1. *General safety*. For each test, use not fewer than 20 chickens not older than the minimum age to be recommended for vaccination and from an SPF flock (*5.2.2*). Administer to each chicken a quantity of the vaccine virus equivalent to not less than 10 times the maximum virus titre likely to be contained in 1 dose of the vaccine. 14 days after vaccination, collect blood samples from half of the chickens and determine the haematocrit value. Euthanise these chickens and carry out post-mortem examination. Note any pathological changes attributable to chicken anaemia virus, such as thymic atrophy and specific bone-marrow lesions. Observe the remaining chickens at least daily for 21 days.

The vaccine virus complies with the test if during the observation period no chicken shows notable signs of chicken anaemia or dies from causes attributable to the vaccine virus.

2-4-1-2. *Safety for young chickens*. Use not fewer than twenty 1-day-old chickens from an SPF flock (*5.2.2*). Administer to each chicken by the oculonasal route a quantity of the vaccine virus equivalent to not less than the maximum titre likely to be contained in 1 dose of the vaccine. Observe the chickens at least daily. Record the incidence of any signs attributable to the vaccine virus, such as depression, and any deaths. 14 days after vaccination, collect blood samples from half of the chickens and determine the haematocrit value. Euthanise these chickens and carry out post-mortem examination. Note any pathological changes attributable to chicken anaemia virus, such as thymic atrophy and specific bone marrow lesions. Observe the remaining chickens at least daily for 21 days. Assess the extent to which the vaccine strain is pathogenic for 1-day-old susceptible chickens from the results of the clinical observations and mortality rates and the proportion of chickens examined at 14 days that show anaemia (haematocrit value less than 27 per cent) and signs of infectious chicken anaemia on post-mortem examination. The results are used to formulate the label statement on safety for young chickens.

2-4-2. **Increase in virulence**. The test for increase in virulence consists of the administration of the vaccine virus at the least attenuated passage level that will be present between the master seed lot and a batch of the vaccine to a group of five 1-day-old chickens from an SPF flock (*5.2.2*), sequential passages, 5 times where possible, to further similar groups of 1-day-old chickens and testing of the final recovered virus for increase in virulence. If the properties of the vaccine virus allow sequential passage to 5 groups via natural spreading, this method may be used, otherwise passage as described below is carried out and the maximally passaged virus that has been recovered is tested for increase in virulence. Care must be taken to avoid contamination by virus from previous passages.

Administer to each animal by the intramuscular route a quantity of the vaccine virus that will allow recovery of virus for the passages described below. Prepare 7 to 9 days after administration a suspension from the liver of each chicken and pool these samples. Depending on the tropism of the virus, other tissues such as spleen or bone marrow may be used. Administer 0.1 ml of the pooled samples by the intramuscular route to each of 5 other chickens of the same age and origin. Carry out this passage operation not fewer than 5 times; verify the presence of the virus at each passage. If the virus is not found at a passage level, carry out a second series of passages.

Carry out the tests for safety (section 2-4-1) using the unpassaged vaccine virus and the maximally passaged vaccine virus that has been recovered.

The vaccine virus complies with the test if no indication of increased virulence of the maximally passaged virus compared with the unpassaged virus is observed. If virus is not recovered at any passage level in the first and second series of passages, the vaccine virus also complies with the test.

2-4-3. **Immunogenicity**. A test is carried out for each route and method of administration to be recommended using chickens not older than the minimum age to be recommended for vaccination and from an SPF flock (*5.2.2*). The test for prevention of virus excretion is intended to demonstrate reduction of egg transmission through viraemia and virus excretion in the faeces. The quantity of the vaccine virus to be administered to each chicken is not greater than the minimum virus titre to be stated on the label and the virus is at the most attenuated passage level that will be present in a batch of vaccine.

2-4-3-1. *Passive immunisation of chickens*. Vaccinate according to the recommended schedule not fewer than 10 breeder chickens not older than the minimum age recommended for vaccination and from an SPF flock (*5.2.2*); keep not fewer than 10 unvaccinated breeder chickens of the same origin and from an SPF flock (5.2.2) as controls. At a suitable time after excretion of vaccine virus has ceased, collect fertilised eggs from each vaccinated and control breeder chicken and incubate them. Challenge at least 3 randomly chosen 1-day-old chickens from each vaccinated and control breeder chicken by intramuscular administration of a sufficient quantity of virulent chicken anaemia virus. Observe the chickens at least daily for 14 days after challenge. Record the deaths and the surviving chickens that show signs of disease. At the end of the observation period determine the haematocrit value of each surviving chicken. Euthanise these chickens and carry out post-mortem examination. Note any pathological signs attributable to chicken anaemia virus, such as thymic atrophy and specific bone-marrow lesions. The test is not valid if:

— during the observation period after challenge fewer than 90 per cent of the chickens of the control breeder chickens die or show severe signs of infectious chicken anaemia, including haematocrit value under 27 per cent, and/or notable macroscopic lesions of the bone marrow and thymus;

— and/or during the period between vaccination and egg collection more than 10 per cent of vaccinated or control breeder chickens show notable signs of disease or die from causes not attributable to the vaccine.

The vaccine complies with the test if during the observation period after challenge not fewer than 90 per cent of the chickens of the vaccinated breeder chickens survive and show no notable signs of disease and/or macroscopic lesions of the bone marrow and thymus.

2-4-3-2. *Prevention of virus excretion.* Vaccinate according to the recommended schedule not fewer than 10 chickens not older than the minimum age recommended for vaccination and from an SPF flock (5.2.2). Maintain separately not fewer than 10 chickens of the same age and origin as controls. At a suitable time after excretion of vaccine virus has ceased, challenge all the chickens by intramuscular administration of a sufficient quantity of virulent chicken anaemia virus. Collect blood samples from the chickens on days 3, 5 and 7 after challenge and faecal samples from the chickens on days 7, 14 and 21 after challenge and carry out a test for presence of virus to determine whether or not the chickens are viraemic and are excreting the virus. The test is not valid if:

— fewer than 70 per cent of the control chickens are viraemic and excrete the virus at one or more times of sampling;

— and/or during the period between vaccination and challenge more than 10 per cent of control or vaccinated chickens show abnormal clinical signs or die from causes not attributable to the vaccine.

The vaccine complies with the test if not fewer than 90 per cent of the vaccinated chickens do not develop viraemia or excrete the virus.

3. BATCH TESTING

3-1. **Identification.** The vaccine, diluted if necessary and mixed with a monospecific chicken anaemia virus antiserum, no longer infects susceptible cell cultures or eggs from an SPF flock (5.2.2) into which it is inoculated.

3-2. **Bacteria and fungi.** Vaccines intended for administration by injection comply with the test for sterility prescribed in the monograph *Vaccines for veterinary use (0062)*.

Vaccines not intended for administration by injection either comply with the test for sterility prescribed in the monograph *Vaccines for veterinary use (0062)* or with the following test: carry out a quantitative test for bacterial and fungal contamination; carry out identification tests for microorganisms detected in the vaccine; the vaccine does

not contain pathogenic microorganisms and contains not more than 1 non-pathogenic microorganism per dose.

Any liquid supplied with the vaccine complies with the test for sterility prescribed in the monograph *Vaccines for veterinary use (0062)*.

3-3. **Mycoplasmas.** The vaccine complies with the test for mycoplasmas (2.6.7).

3-4. **Extraneous agents.** The vaccine complies with the tests for extraneous agents in batches of finished product (2.6.25).

3-5. **Safety.** Use not fewer than 10 chickens not older than the minimum age recommended for vaccination and from an SPF flock (5.2.2). Administer by a recommended route to each chicken 10 doses of the vaccine. Observe the chickens at least daily for 21 days. The test is not valid if more than 20 per cent of the chickens show abnormal signs or die from causes not attributable to the vaccine.

The vaccine complies with the test if no chicken shows notable signs of disease or dies from causes attributable to the vaccine.

3-6. **Virus titre.** Titrate the vaccine virus by inoculation into suitable cell cultures (5.2.4) or eggs from an SPF flock (5.2.2). The vaccine complies with the test if 1 dose contains not less than the minimum virus titre stated on the label.

3-7. **Potency.** The vaccine complies with the requirements of the tests prescribed under Immunogenicity (sections 2-4-3-1 and 2-4-3-2) when administered by a recommended route and method. It is not necessary to carry out the potency test for each batch of the vaccine if it has been carried out on a representative batch using a vaccinating dose containing not more than the minimum virus titre stated on the label.

4. LABELLING

The label states to which extent the vaccine virus causes disease if it spreads to susceptible young chickens.

07/2009:2448

PORCINE ENZOOTIC PNEUMONIA VACCINE (INACTIVATED)

Vaccinum pneumoniae enzooticae suillae inactivatum

1. DEFINITION

Porcine enzootic pneumonia vaccine (inactivated) is a preparation of a suitable strain of *Mycoplasma hyopneumoniae* that has been inactivated while maintaining adequate immunogenic properties. This monograph applies to vaccines intended for the active immunisation of pigs against enzootic pneumonia caused by *M. hyopneumoniae*.

2. PRODUCTION

2-1. *PREPARATION OF THE VACCINE*

Production of the vaccine is based on a seed-lot system. The seed material is cultured in a suitable solid and/or liquid medium to ensure optimal growth under the chosen incubation conditions. The identity of the strain is verified using a suitable method.

During production, various parameters such as growth rate are monitored by suitable methods; the values are within the limits approved for the particular vaccine. Purity of the harvest is verified using a suitable method.

After cultivation, the mycoplasma suspension is collected and inactivated by a suitable method. The vaccine may contain an adjuvant.

2-2. *CHOICE OF VACCINE COMPOSITION*

The vaccine is shown to be satisfactory with respect to safety (*5.2.6*) and efficacy (*5.2.7*) for the pigs for which it is intended.

The following tests for safety (section 2-2-1) and immunogenicity (section 2-2-2) may be used during the demonstration of safety and efficacy.

2-2-1. **Safety**

2-2-1-1. *Laboratory tests*. Carry out the test for each route and method of administration to be recommended for vaccination and in each category of animals for which the vaccine is intended. Use a batch of vaccine containing not less than the maximum potency that may be expected in a batch of vaccine.

2-2-1-1-1. General safety. For each test, use not fewer than 10 pigs that do not have antibodies against *M. hyopneumoniae*. Administer to each pig a double dose of the vaccine, then, where applicable, one dose after the interval to be recommended. Observe the pigs at least daily until 14 days after the last administration for signs of abnormal local or systemic reactions. Record body temperature the day before vaccination, at vaccination, 4 h later and then daily for 4 days; note the maximum temperature increase for each pig.

The vaccine complies with the test if no pig shows notable signs of disease or dies from causes attributable to the vaccine, and, in particular, if the average body temperature increase for all pigs does not exceed 1.5 °C and no pig shows a rise greater than 2 °C.

2-2-1-2. *Field studies*. The animals used for field trials are also used to evaluate safety. Carry out a test in each category of animals for which the vaccine is intended. Use not fewer than 3 groups each of not fewer than 20 animals with corresponding groups of not fewer than 10 controls. Examine the injection site for local reactions after vaccination. Record body temperature the day before vaccination, at vaccination, at the time interval after which a rise in temperature, if any, was seen in test 2-2-1-1, and daily during the 2 days following vaccination; note the maximum temperature increase for each animal.

The vaccine complies with the test if:

— no animal shows notable signs of disease or dies from causes attributable to the vaccine;

— the average body temperature increase for all animals does not exceed 1.5 °C; and

— no animal shows a rise in body temperature greater than 2 °C.

2-2-2. **Immunogenicity**. A test is carried out for each route and method of administration to be recommended using in each case pigs not older than the minimum age to be recommended for vaccination. The vaccine to be administered to each pig is of minimum potency.

Use not fewer than 20 pigs that do not have antibodies against *M. hyopneumoniae* and that are from a herd or herds where there are no signs of enzootic pneumonia and that have not been vaccinated against *M. hyopneumoniae*. Vaccinate not fewer than 12 pigs according to the schedule to be recommended. Maintain not fewer than 8 non-vaccinated pigs as controls. Challenge each pig at least 14 days after the last vaccination by the intranasal or intratracheal route or by aerosol with a sufficient quantity of a virulent strain of *M. hyopneumoniae*. The challenge strain used is different from the vaccine strain. 21-30 days after challenge, euthanise the pigs. Conduct a post-mortem examination on each pig in order to evaluate the extent of lung lesions using a validated

lung lesion scoring system that is adapted to the age of the animals. The following scoring system may be used.

A weighted score is allocated to each of the 7 lobes of the lungs according to the relative weight of the lung lobes.

Lobes	Left	Right
Apical	5	11
Cardiac	6	10
Diaphragmatic	29	34
Intermediate	5	

The vaccine complies with the test if the vaccinated pigs, when compared with controls, show a significant reduction in the lung lesion score.

2-3. *MANUFACTURER'S TESTS*

2-3-1. **Batch potency test**. It is not necessary to carry out the potency test (section 3-5) for each batch of the vaccine if it has been carried out using a batch of vaccine with a minimum potency. Where the test is not carried out, an alternative validated method is used, the criteria for acceptance being set with reference to a batch of vaccine that has given satisfactory results in the test described under Potency. A quantification of the antigen (i.e. an *in vitro* test using a reference vaccine that has given satisfactory results in the test described under Potency) together with a test for adjuvant quantification may be used as an alternative method provided the antigen that is measured has been proven to be protective and/or immunorelevant.

Alternatively, a test measuring induction of antibody response in laboratory animals may be used. The following method is given as an example.

Use at least 5 mice weighing 18-20 g and that do not have antibodies against *M. hyopneumoniae*. Vaccinate each mouse by the subcutaneous route with a suitable dose. Maintain not fewer than 5 mice as controls. Where the recommended schedule requires a booster injection to be given, a booster vaccination may also be given in this test provided it has been demonstrated that this will still provide a suitably sensitive test system. Before the vaccination and at a given interval within the range of 14-21 days after the last injection, collect blood from each mouse and prepare serum samples. Determine individually for each serum the titre of specific antibodies against each antigenic component stated on the label, using a suitable validated test such as enzyme-linked immunosorbent assay (*2.7.1*).

The vaccine complies with the test if the mean antibody levels are not significantly lower than those obtained for a batch that has given satisfactory results in the test described under Potency.

3. BATCH TESTS

3-1. **Identification**. When injected into healthy animals that do not have antibodies against *M. hyopneumoniae*, the vaccine stimulates the production of such antibodies. Suitable molecular methods such as nucleic acid amplification techniques (*2.6.21*) may also serve for identification.

3-2. **Bacteria and fungi**. The vaccine and, where applicable, the liquid supplied with it comply with the test for sterility prescribed in the monograph *Vaccines for veterinary use (0062)*.

3-3. **Safety**. Use 2 pigs of the minimum age recommended for vaccination and that do not have antibodies against *M. hyopneumoniae*. Administer to each pig by a recommended route a double dose of vaccine. Observe the pigs at least daily for 14 days. Record body temperature the day before vaccination, at vaccination, 4 h later and then daily for 2 days.

The vaccine complies with the test if no pig shows notable signs of disease or dies from causes attributable to the vaccine; a transient body temperature increase not exceeding 2 °C may occur.

3-4. **Residual live mycoplasmas**. A test for residual live mycoplasmas is carried out to confirm inactivation of *M. hyopneumoniae*. The vaccine complies with a validated test for residual live *M. hyopneumoniae* carried out by a culture method (see for example *2.6.7*, using media shown to be suitable for *M. hyopneumoniae*).

3-5. **Potency**. The vaccine complies with the requirements of the test mentioned under Immunogenicity (section 2-2-2) when administered by a recommended route and method.

RADIOPHARMACEUTICAL PREPARATIONS

Radiopharmaceutical preparations

See the information section on general monographs (cover pages)

07/2009:2350

MEDRONIC ACID FOR RADIOPHARMACEUTICAL PREPARATIONS

Acidum medronicum ad radiopharmaceutica

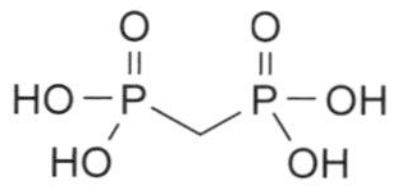

$CH_6O_6P_2$ M_r 176.0
[1984-15-2]

DEFINITION

Methylenediphosphonic acid.

Content: 99.0 per cent to 101.0 per cent (dried substance).

CHARACTERS

Appearance: white or almost white, amorphous or crystalline, hygroscopic powder.

Solubility: very soluble in water, very slightly soluble in anhydrous ethanol, practically insoluble in methylene chloride.

IDENTIFICATION

First identification: A.

Second identification: B.

A. ^{1}H Nuclear magnetic resonance spectrometry (*2.2.33*).

    Preparation: 100 g/l solution in *deuterium oxide R*.

    Comparison: 100 g/l solution of *medronic acid CRS* in *deuterium oxide R*.

B. Infrared absorption spectrophotometry (*2.2.24*).

    Comparison: medronic acid CRS.

TESTS

Impurities A and B. ^{1}H Nuclear magnetic resonance spectrometry (*2.2.33*).

Test solution. To 1.0 g of the substance to be examined add 10 ml of *deuterated chloroform R*. Stir for 1 hour. Pass the resulting solution through a sintered-glass filter to remove the precipitate containing medronic acid. Evaporate the filtrate to about 0.5 ml.

Reference solution (a). Mix 10 µl of *medronic acid impurity A CRS* with 1.0 ml of *deuterated chloroform R*.

Reference solution (b). Mix 10 µl of *medronic acid impurity B CRS* with 1.0 ml of *deuterated chloroform R*.

Reference solution (c). After recording the NMR spectrum of the test solution, add 10 µl of *medronic acid impurity A CRS* and 10 µl of *medronic acid impurity B CRS* to the test solution.

Apparatus: NMR spectrometer operating at minimum 250 MHz.

Record the ^{1}H NMR spectra of the test solution and the reference solutions, if necessary using *tetramethylsilane R* as a chemical shift internal reference compound.

Position of the signals: deuterated chloroform = about 7.3 ppm; impurity A = about 4.4 ppm and 1.3 ppm; impurity B = about 4.7 ppm, 2.4 ppm and 1.3 ppm.

System suitability:

— the positions of the signals due to impurities A and B in the spectrum obtained with reference solution (c) do not differ significantly from those in the spectra obtained with reference solutions (a) and (b).

Limits:

— *integration*: integrate the multiplet at 4.4 ppm due to impurity A and the multiplet at 2.4 ppm due to impurity B in the spectra obtained with the test solution and reference solution (c) to obtain the areas of the peaks used in the comparison of impurity contents;

— *impurities A, B*: for each impurity, not more than 0.5 times the area of the corresponding peak in the spectrum obtained with reference solution (c) (1 per cent).

Phosphates (*2.4.11*): maximum 1.0 per cent.

Dissolve 0.100 g in 10 ml of *water R* and dilute to 100.0 ml with the same solvent. Dilute 1.0 ml of this solution to 100.0 ml with *water R*.

Loss on drying (*2.2.32*): maximum 0.5 per cent, determined on 0.500 g by drying in an oven at 105 °C.

Bacterial endotoxins (*2.6.14*): less than 2.0 IU/mg.

ASSAY

Dissolve 75 mg in *water R* and dilute to 50 ml with the same solvent. Titrate with *0.1 M sodium hydroxide*, using 0.1 ml of *bromocresol green solution R* as indicator.

1 ml of *0.1 M sodium hydroxide* is equivalent to 8.80 mg of $CH_6O_6P_2$.

STORAGE

In an airtight container, protected from light.

LABELLING

The label recommends testing the substance in a production test before its use for the manufacture of radiopharmaceutical preparations. This ensures that, under specified production conditions, the substance yields the radiopharmaceutical preparation in the desired quantity and quality specified.

IMPURITIES

Specified impurities: A, B.

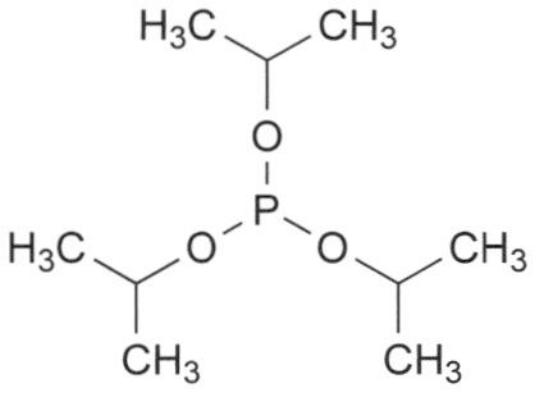

A. tris(1-methylethoxy)phosphane,

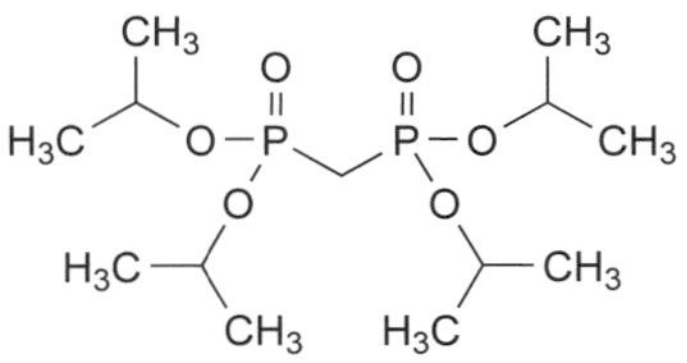

B. tetrakis(1-methylethyl) methylenediphosphonate.

HOMOEOPATHIC PREPARATIONS

Homoeopathic preparations

See the information section on general monographs (cover pages)

07/2009:2045

HERBAL DRUGS FOR HOMOEOPATHIC PREPARATIONS

Plantae medicinales ad praeparationes homoeopathicas

DEFINITION

Herbal drugs for homoeopathic preparations are mainly whole, fragmented or cut plants, parts of plants including algae, fungi or lichens, in an unprocessed state, usually in fresh form. The state, fresh or dried, in which the drug is used, is defined in the individual monograph of the European Pharmacopoeia or, in the absence, in the individual monograph of a national Pharmacopoeia. In the absence of such a monograph, the state in which the herbal drug is used has to be defined. Certain exudates that have not been subjected to a specific treatment are also considered to be herbal drugs for homoeopathic preparations. Herbal drugs for homoeopathic preparations are precisely defined by the botanical scientific name of the source species according to the binomial system (genus, species, variety and author).

PRODUCTION

Herbal drugs for homoeopathic preparations are obtained from cultivated or wild plants. Suitable collection, cultivation, harvesting, sorting, drying, fragmentation and storage conditions are essential to guarantee the quality of herbal drugs for homoeopathic preparations.

Herbal drugs for homoeopathic preparations are, as far as possible, free from impurities such as soil, dust, dirt and other contaminants such as fungal, insect and other animal contaminants. They do not present signs of decay.

If a decontaminating treatment has been used, it is necessary to demonstrate that the constituents of the plant are not affected and that no harmful residues remain. The use of ethylene oxide is prohibited for the decontamination of herbal drugs for homoeopathic preparations.

Fresh herbal drugs are processed as rapidly as possible after harvesting. Where justified and authorised for transportation or storage purposes, fresh plant material may be deep-frozen; it may also be kept in ethanol (96 per cent) or in ethanol of a suitable concentration, provided the whole material including the storage medium is used for processing.

Adequate measures have to be taken in order to ensure that the microbiological quality of homoeopathic preparations containing 1 or more herbal drugs comply with the recommendations given in the text on *5.1.4. Microbiological quality of non-sterile pharmaceutical preparations and substances for pharmaceutical use.*

IDENTIFICATION

Herbal drugs for homoeopathic preparations are identified using their macroscopic and, where necessary, microscopic descriptions and any further tests that may be required (for example, thin-layer chromatography).

TESTS

Foreign matter (*2.8.2*). When a fresh plant is used as a starting material for the manufacture of homoeopathic preparations, the content of foreign matter is as low as possible; if necessary, the maximum content of foreign matter is indicated in the individual monographs. When a dried plant is used as a starting material for the manufacture of homoeopathic preparations, carry out a test for foreign matter, unless otherwise prescribed in the individual monographs. The content of foreign matter is not more than 2 per cent *m/m*, unless otherwise prescribed or justified and authorised.

Adulteration. A specific appropriate test may apply to herbal drugs for homoeopathic preparations liable to be falsified.

Loss on drying (*2.2.32*). Carry out a test for loss on drying on dried herbal drugs for homoeopathic preparations.

Water (*2.2.13*). A determination of water is carried out on herbal drugs for homoeopathic preparations with a high essential oil content. The water content of fresh herbal drugs for homoeopathic preparations may be determined by an appropriate method.

Pesticides (*2.8.13*). Herbal drugs for homoeopathic preparations comply with the requirements for pesticide residues. The requirements take into account the nature of the plant, where necessary the preparation in which the plant might be used, and where available the knowledge of the complete record of treatment of the batch of the plant. The content of pesticide residues may be determined by the method described in the annex to the general method.

If appropriate, the herbal drugs for homoeopathic preparations comply with other tests, such as the following, for example:

Total ash (*2.4.16*).

Bitterness value (*2.8.15*).

Heavy metals. The risk of contamination of herbal drugs for homoeopathic preparations by heavy metals must be considered. If an individual monograph does not prescribe limits for heavy metals or specific elements, such limits may be required if justified.

Aflatoxins (*2.8.18*). Limits for aflatoxins may be required.

Radioactive contamination. In some specific circumstances, the risk of radioactive contamination is to be considered.

ASSAY

Where applicable, herbal drugs for homoeopathic preparations are assayed by an appropriate method.

STORAGE

Store dried herbal drugs protected from light.

Homoeopathic preparations

See the information section on general monographs (cover pages)

A

Monographs
A-C

07/2009:1281

ACECLOFENAC

Aceclofenacum

$C_{16}H_{13}Cl_2NO_4$
[89796-99-6]

M_r 354.2

DEFINITION

[[[2-[(2,6-Dichlorophenyl)amino]phenyl]acetyl]oxy]acetic acid.

Content: 99.0 per cent to 101.0 per cent (dried substance).

CHARACTERS

Appearance: white or almost white, crystalline powder.

Solubility: practically insoluble in water, freely soluble in acetone, soluble in ethanol (96 per cent).

IDENTIFICATION

First identification: B.

Second identification: A, C.

A. Dissolve 50.0 mg in *methanol R* and dilute to 100.0 ml with the same solvent. Dilute 2.0 ml of the solution to 50.0 ml with *methanol R*. Examined between 220 nm and 370 nm (*2.2.25*), the solution shows an absorption maximum at 275 nm. The specific absorbance at the absorption maximum is 320 to 350.

B. Infrared absorption spectrophotometry (*2.2.24*).

   Comparison: Ph. Eur. reference spectrum of aceclofenac.

C. Dissolve about 10 mg in 10 ml of *ethanol (96 per cent) R*. To 1 ml of the solution, add 0.2 ml of a mixture, prepared immediately before use, of equal volumes of a 6 g/l solution of *potassium ferricyanide R* and a 9 g/l solution of *ferric chloride R*. Allow to stand protected from light for 5 min. Add 3 ml of a 10.0 g/l solution of *hydrochloric acid R*. Allow to stand protected from light for 15 min. A blue colour develops and a precipitate is formed.

TESTS

Related substances. Liquid chromatography (*2.2.29*). *Prepare the solutions immediately before use.*

Test solution. Dissolve 50.0 mg of the substance to be examined in a mixture of 30 volumes of mobile phase A and 70 volumes of mobile phase B and dilute to 25.0 ml with the same mixture of solvents.

Reference solution (a). Dissolve 21.6 mg of *diclofenac sodium CRS* (impurity A) in a mixture of 30 volumes of mobile phase A and 70 volumes of mobile phase B and dilute to 50.0 ml with the same mixture of solvents.

Reference solution (b). Dilute 2.0 ml of the test solution to 10.0 ml with a mixture of 30 volumes of mobile phase A and 70 volumes of mobile phase B.

Reference solution (c). Mix 1.0 ml of reference solution (a) and 1.0 ml of reference solution (b) and dilute to 100.0 ml with a mixture of 30 volumes of mobile phase A and 70 volumes of mobile phase B.

Reference solution (d). Dissolve 4.0 mg of *aceclofenac impurity F CRS* and 2.0 mg of *aceclofenac impurity H CRS* in a mixture of 30 volumes of mobile phase A and 70 volumes of mobile phase B then dilute to 10.0 ml with the same mixture of solvents.

Reference solution (e). Mix 1.0 ml of reference solution (b) and 1.0 ml of reference solution (d) and dilute to 100.0 ml with a mixture of 30 volumes of mobile phase A and 70 volumes of mobile phase B.

Reference solution (f). Dissolve the contents of a vial of *diclofenac impurity A CRS* (aceclofenac impurity I) in 1.0 ml of a mixture of 30 volumes of mobile phase A and 70 volumes of mobile phase B, add 1.5 ml of the same mixture of solvents and mix.

Reference solution (g). Dissolve 4 mg of *aceclofenac for peak identification CRS* (containing impurities B, C, D, E and G) in 2.0 ml of a mixture of 30 volumes of mobile phase A and 70 volumes of mobile phase B.

Column:

– *size*: l = 0.25 m, Ø = 4.6 mm;

– *stationary phase*: spherical *end-capped octadecylsilyl silica gel for chromatography R* (5 µm) with a pore size of 10 nm and a carbon loading of 19 per cent;

– *temperature*: 40 °C.

Mobile phase:

– *mobile phase A*: 1.12 g/l solution of *phosphoric acid R* adjusted to pH 7.0 using a 42 g/l solution of *sodium hydroxide R*;

– *mobile phase B*: *water R, acetonitrile R* (1:9 *V/V*);

Time (min)	Mobile phase A (per cent *V/V*)	Mobile phase B (per cent *V/V*)
0 - 25	70 → 50	30 → 50
25 - 30	50 → 20	50 → 80
30 - 50	20	80

Flow rate: 1.0 ml/min.

Detection: spectrophotometer at 275 nm.

Injection: 10 µl of the test solution and reference solutions (c), (e), (f) and (g).

Identification of impurities: use the chromatogram supplied with *aceclofenac for peak identification CRS* and the chromatogram obtained with reference solution (g) to identify the peaks due to impurities B, C, D, E and G.

Relative retention with reference to aceclofenac (retention time = about 11 min): impurity A = about 0.8; impurity G = about 1.3; impurity H = about 1.5; impurity I = about 2.3; impurity D = about 3.1; impurity B = about 3.2; impurity E = about 3.3; impurity C = about 3.5; impurity F = about 3.7.

System suitability: reference solution (c):

– *resolution*: minimum 5.0 between the peaks due to impurity A and aceclofenac.

Limits:

– *impurity A*: not more than the area of the corresponding peak in the chromatogram obtained with reference solution (c) (0.2 per cent);

— *impurities B, C, D, E, G*: for each impurity, not more than the area of the peak due to aceclofenac in the chromatogram obtained with reference solution (e) (0.2 per cent);

— *impurity F*: not more than the area of the corresponding peak in the chromatogram obtained with reference solution (e) (0.2 per cent);

— *impurity H*: not more than the area of the corresponding peak in the chromatogram obtained with reference solution (e) (0.1 per cent);

— *impurity I*: not more than the area of the corresponding peak in the chromatogram obtained with reference solution (f) (0.1 per cent);

— *unspecified impurities*: not more than 0.5 times the area of the peak due to aceclofenac in the chromatogram obtained with reference solution (e) (0.10 per cent);

— *total*: not more than 0.7 per cent;

— *disregard limit*: 0.1 times the area of the peak due to aceclofenac in the chromatogram obtained with reference solution (e) (0.02 per cent).

Heavy metals (*2.4.8*): maximum 10 ppm.

To 2.0 g in a silica crucible, add 2 ml of *sulphuric acid R* to wet the substance. Heat progressively to ignition and continue heating until an almost white or at most a greyish residue is obtained. Carry out the ignition at a temperature not exceeding 800 °C. Allow to cool. Add 3 ml of *hydrochloric acid R* and 1 ml of *nitric acid R*. Heat and evaporate slowly to dryness. Cool and add 1 ml of a 100 g/l solution of *hydrochloric acid R* and 10.0 ml of *distilled water R*. Neutralise with a 1.0 g/l solution of *ammonia R* using 0.1 ml of *phenolphthalein solution R* as indicator. Add 2.0 ml of a 60 g/l solution of *anhydrous acetic acid R* and dilute to 20 ml with *distilled water R*. 12 ml of the solution complies with test A. Prepare the reference solution using *lead standard solution (1 ppm Pb) R*.

Loss on drying (*2.2.32*): maximum 0.5 per cent, determined on 1.000 g by drying in an oven at 105 °C.

Sulphated ash (*2.4.14*): maximum 0.1 per cent, determined on 1.0 g.

ASSAY

Dissolve 0.300 g in 40 ml of *methanol R*. Titrate with *0.1 M sodium hydroxide*, determining the end-point potentiometrically (*2.2.20*).

1 ml of *0.1 M sodium hydroxide* is equivalent to 35.42 mg of $C_{16}H_{13}Cl_2NO_4$.

STORAGE

In an airtight container, protected from light.

IMPURITIES

Specified impurities: A, B, C, D, E, F, G, H, I.

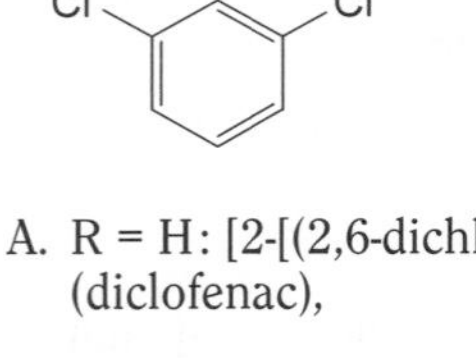

A. R = H: [2-[(2,6-dichlorophenyl)amino]phenyl]acetic acid (diclofenac),

B. R = CH₃: methyl [2-[(2,6-dichlorophenyl)amino]phenyl]-acetate (methyl ester of diclofenac),

C. R = C₂H₅: ethyl [2-[(2,6-dichlorophenyl)amino]phenyl]-acetate (ethyl ester of diclofenac),

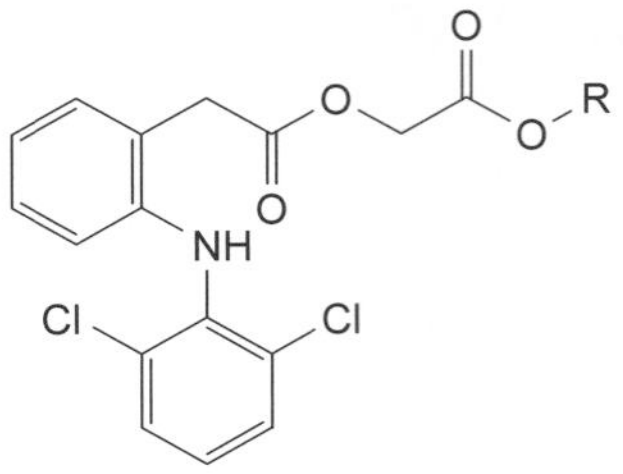

D. R = CH₃: methyl [[[2-[(2,6-dichlorophenyl)-amino]phenyl]acetyl]oxy]acetate (methyl ester of aceclofenac),

E. R = C₂H₅: ethyl [[[2-[(2,6-dichlorophenyl)-amino]phenyl]acetyl]oxy]acetate (ethyl ester of aceclofenac),

F. R = CH₂-C₆H₅: benzyl [[[2-[(2,6-dichlorophenyl)-amino]phenyl]acetyl]oxy]acetate (benzyl ester of aceclofenac),

G. R = CH₂-CO₂H: [[[[2-[(2,6-dichlorophenyl)-amino]phenyl]acetyl]oxy]acetyl]oxy]acetic acid (acetic aceclofenac),

H. R = CH₂-CO-O-CH₂-CO₂H: [[[[[[2-[(2,6-dichlorophenyl)-amino]phenyl]acetyl]oxy]acetyl]oxy]acetyl]oxy]acetic acid (diacetic aceclofenac),

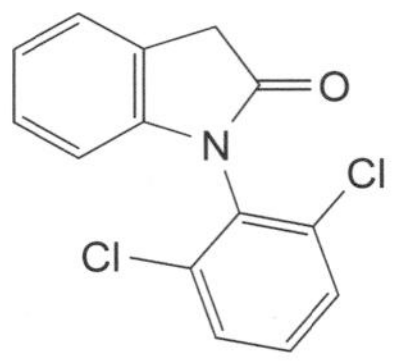

I. 1-(2,6-dichlorophenyl)-1,3-dihydro-2*H*-indol-2-one.

01/2008:0463
corrected 6.5

AMANTADINE HYDROCHLORIDE

Amantadini hydrochloridum

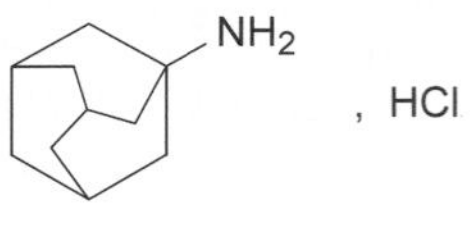

$C_{10}H_{18}ClN$ M_r 187.7
[665-66-7]

DEFINITION

Tricyclo[3.3.1.1³,⁷]decan-1-amine hydrochloride.

Content: 98.5 per cent to 101.0 per cent (anhydrous substance).

CHARACTERS

Appearance: white or almost white, crystalline powder.

Solubility: freely soluble in water and in ethanol (96 per cent).

It sublimes on heating.

IDENTIFICATION

First identification: A, D.

Second identification: B, C, D.

A. Infrared absorption spectrophotometry (*2.2.24*).

Preparation: discs.

Comparison: amantadine hydrochloride CRS.

B. To 0.1 g add 1 ml of *pyridine R*, mix and add 0.1 ml of *acetic anhydride R*. Heat to boiling for about 10 s. Pour the hot solution into 10 ml of *dilute hydrochloric acid R*, cool to 5 °C and filter. The precipitate, washed with *water R* and dried *in vacuo* at 60 °C for 1 h, melts (*2.2.14*) at 147 °C to 151 °C.

C. Dissolve 0.2 g in 1 ml of *0.1 M hydrochloric acid*. Add 1 ml of a 500 g/l solution of *sodium nitrite R*. A white precipitate is formed.

D. 1 ml of solution S (see Tests) gives reaction (a) of chlorides (*2.3.1*).

TESTS

Solution S. Dissolve 2.5 g in *carbon dioxide-free water R* and dilute to 25 ml with the same solvent.

Appearance of solution. Solution S is clear (*2.2.1*) and not more intensely coloured than reference solution Y_7 (*2.2.2, Method II*).

Acidity or alkalinity. Dilute 2 ml of solution S to 10 ml with *carbon dioxide-free water R*. Add 0.1 ml of *methyl red solution R* and 0.2 ml of *0.01 M sodium hydroxide*. The solution is yellow. Add 0.4 ml of *0.01 M hydrochloric acid*. The solution is red.

Related substances. Gas chromatography (*2.2.28*): use the normalisation procedure.

Test solution. Dissolve 0.10 g of the substance to be examined in 2 ml of *water R*. Add 2 ml of a 200 g/l solution of *sodium hydroxide R* and 2 ml of *chloroform R*. Shake for 10 min. Separate the chloroform layer, dry over *anhydrous sodium sulphate R* and filter.

Column:

— *material*: glass;

— *size*: l = 1.8 m, Ø = 2 mm;

— *stationary phase*: mix 19.5 g of *silanised diatomaceous earth for gas chromatography R* with 60 ml of a 3.3 g/l solution of *potassium hydroxide R* in *methanol R* and evaporate the solvent under reduced pressure while rotating the mixture slowly (support); dissolve 0.4 g of *low-vapour-pressure hydrocarbons (type L) R* in 60 ml of *toluene R* (dissolution requires up to 5 h), add this solution to the support and evaporate the solvent under reduced pressure while rotating the mixture slowly.

Carrier gas: *nitrogen for chromatography R*.

Flow rate: 30 ml/min.

Temperature:

	Time (min)	Temperature (°C)
Column	0 - 16.7	100 → 200
Injection port		220
Detector		300

Detection: flame ionisation.

Injection: 1 µl or the chosen volume.

Run time: at least 2.5 times the retention time of amantadine.

Limits:

— *any impurity*: for each impurity, maximum 0.3 per cent;

— *total*: maximum 1 per cent;

— *disregard limit*: disregard the peak due to the solvent.

Heavy metals (*2.4.8*): maximum 20 ppm.

12 ml of solution S complies with test A. Prepare the reference solution using *lead standard solution (2 ppm Pb) R*.

Water (*2.5.12*): maximum 0.5 per cent, determined on 2.000 g.

Sulphated ash (*2.4.14*): maximum 0.1 per cent, determined on 1.0 g.

ASSAY

Dissolve 0.150 g in a mixture of 5.0 ml of *0.01 M hydrochloric acid* and 50 ml of *ethanol (96 per cent) R*. Carry out a potentiometric titration (*2.2.20*), using *0.1 M sodium hydroxide*. Read the volume added between the 2 points of inflexion.

1 ml of *0.1 M sodium hydroxide* is equivalent to 18.77 mg of $C_{10}H_{18}ClN$.

Monographs A-C

See the information section on general monographs (cover pages)

B

Monographs A-C

See the information section on general monographs (cover pages)

07/2009:0256

BENZYL ALCOHOL

Alcohol benzylicus

C_7H_8O M_r 108.1
[100-51-6]

DEFINITION

Phenylmethanol.

Content: 98.0 per cent to 100.5 per cent.

CHARACTERS

Appearance: clear, colourless, oily liquid.

Solubility: soluble in water, miscible with ethanol (96 per cent) and with fatty and essential oils.

Relative density: 1.043 to 1.049.

IDENTIFICATION

Infrared absorption spectrophotometry (*2.2.24*).

Comparison: benzyl alcohol CRS.

TESTS

Appearance of solution. Shake 2.0 ml with 60 ml of *water R*. It dissolves completely. The solution is clear (*2.2.1*) and colourless (*2.2.2, Method II*).

Acidity. To 10 ml add 10 ml of *ethanol (96 per cent) R* and 1 ml of *phenolphthalein solution R*. Not more than 1 ml of *0.1 M sodium hydroxide* is required to change the colour of the indicator to pink.

Refractive index (*2.2.6*): 1.538 to 1.541.

Peroxide value (*2.5.5*): maximum 5.

Related substances. Gas chromatography (*2.2.28*).

Test solution. The substance to be examined.

Standard solution (a). Dissolve 0.100 g of *ethylbenzene R* in the test solution and dilute to 10.0 ml with the same solution. Dilute 2.0 ml of this solution to 20.0 ml with the test solution.

Standard solution (b). Dissolve 2.000 g of *dicyclohexyl R* in the test solution and dilute to 10.0 ml with the same solution. Dilute 2.0 ml of this solution to 20.0 ml with the test solution.

Reference solution (a). Dissolve 0.750 g of *benzaldehyde R* and 0.500 g of *cyclohexylmethanol R* in the test solution and dilute to 25.0 ml with the test solution. Add 1.0 ml of this solution to a mixture of 2.0 ml of standard solution (a) and 3.0 ml of standard solution (b) and dilute to 20.0 ml with the test solution.

Reference solution (b). Dissolve 0.250 g of *benzaldehyde R* and 0.500 g of *cyclohexylmethanol R* in the test solution and dilute to 25.0 ml with the test solution. Add 1.0 ml of this solution to a mixture of 2.0 ml of standard solution (a) and 2.0 ml of standard solution (b) and dilute to 20.0 ml with the test solution.

Column:
– *material*: fused silica;
– *size*: l = 30 m, Ø = 0.32 mm;
– *stationary phase*: *macrogol 20 000 R* (film thickness 0.5 µm).

Carrier gas: *helium for chromatography R*.

Linear velocity: 25 cm/s.

Temperature:

	Time (min)	Temperature (°C)
Column	0 - 34	50 → 220
	34 - 69	220
Injection port		200
Detector		310

Detection: flame ionisation.

Benzyl alcohol not intended for parenteral use

Injection: without air-plug, 0.1 µl of the test solution and reference solution (a).

Relative retention with reference to benzyl alcohol (retention time = about 26 min): ethylbenzene = about 0.28; dicyclohexyl = about 0.59; impurity A = about 0.68; impurity B = about 0.71.

System suitability: reference solution (a):
– *resolution*: minimum 3.0 between the peaks due to impurities A and B.

If any peaks in the chromatogram obtained with the test solution have the same retention time as the peaks due to ethyl benzene or dicyclohexyl, substract the areas of any such peaks from the peak areas at these retention times in the chromatograms obtained with reference solutions (a) or (b) (corrected peak areas of ethyl benzene and dicyclohexyl). Any such peaks in the chromatogram obtained with the test solution are to be included in the assessments for the sum of other peaks.

Limits:
– *impurity A*: not more than the difference between the area of the peak due to impurity A in the chromatogram obtained with reference solution (a) and the area of the peak due to impurity A in the chromatogram obtained with the test solution (0.15 per cent);

– *impurity B*: not more than the difference between the area of the peak due to impurity B in the chromatogram obtained with reference solution (a) and the area of the peak due to impurity B in the chromatogram obtained with the test solution (0.10 per cent);

– *sum of other peaks with a relative retention less than that of benzyl alcohol*: not more than 4 times the area of the peak due to ethylbenzene in the chromatogram obtained with reference solution (a) corrected if necessary as described above (0.04 per cent);

– *sum of peaks with a relative retention greater than that of benzyl alcohol*: not more than the area of the peak due to dicyclohexyl in the chromatogram obtained with reference solution (a) corrected if necessary as described above (0.3 per cent);

– *disregard limit*: 0.01 times the area of the peak due to ethylbenzene in the chromatogram obtained with reference solution (a) corrected if necessary as described above (0.0001 per cent).

Benzyl alcohol intended for parenteral use

Injection: without air-plug, 0.1 µl of the test solution and reference solution (b).

Relative retention with reference to benzyl alcohol (retention time = about 26 min): ethylbenzene = about 0.28; dicyclohexyl = about 0.59; impurity A = about 0.68; impurity B = about 0.71.

System suitability: reference solution (b):

— *resolution*: minimum 3.0 between the peaks due to impurities A and B.

If any peaks in the chromatogram obtained with the test solution have the same retention times as the peaks due to ethyl benzene or dicyclohexyl, substract the areas of any such peaks from the peak areas at these retention times in the chromatograms obtained with reference solutions (a) or (b) (corrected peak areas of ethyl benzene and dicyclohexyl). Any such peaks in the chromatogram obtained with the test solution are to be included in the assessments for the sum of other peaks.

Limits:

— *impurity A*: not more than the difference between the area of the peak due to impurity A in the chromatogram obtained with reference solution (b) and the area of the peak due to impurity A in the chromatogram obtained with the test solution (0.05 per cent);

— *impurity B*: not more than the difference between the area of the peak due to impurity B in the chromatogram obtained with reference solution (b) and the area of the peak due to impurity B in the chromatogram obtained with the test solution (0.10 per cent);

— *sum of other peaks with a relative retention less than that of benzyl alcohol*: not more than twice the area of the peak due to ethylbenzene in the chromatogram obtained with reference solution (b) corrected if necessary as described above (0.02 per cent);

— *sum of peaks with a relative retention greater than that of benzyl alcohol*: not more than the area of the peak due to dicyclohexyl in the chromatogram obtained with reference solution (b) corrected if necessary as described above (0.2 per cent);

— *disregard limit*: 0.01 times the area of the peak due to ethylbenzene in the chromatogram obtained with reference solution (b) corrected if necessary as described above (0.0001 per cent).

Residue on evaporation: maximum 0.05 per cent.

After ensuring that the substance to be examined complies with the test for peroxide value, evaporate 10.0 g to dryness in a tared quartz or porcelain crucible or platinum dish on a hot plate at a temperature not exceeding 200 °C. Ensure that the substance to be examined does not boil during evaporation. Dry the residue on the hot plate for 1 h and allow to cool in a desiccator. The residue weighs a maximum of 5 mg.

ASSAY

To 0.900 g (*m* g) add 15.0 ml of a freshly prepared mixture of 1 volume of *acetic anhydride R* and 7 volumes of *pyridine R* and boil under a reflux condenser on a water-bath for 30 min. Cool and add 25 ml of *water R*. Using 0.25 ml of *phenolphthalein solution R* as indicator, titrate with *1 M sodium hydroxide* (n_1 ml). Carry out a blank titration (n_2 ml).

Calculate the percentage content of C_7H_8O using the following expression:

$$\frac{10.81\left(n_2 - n_1\right)}{m}$$

STORAGE

In an airtight container, under nitrogen, protected from light and at a temperature between 2 °C and 8 °C.

LABELLING

The label states, where applicable, that the substance is suitable for use in the manufacture of parenteral preparations.

IMPURITIES

Specified impurities: A, B.

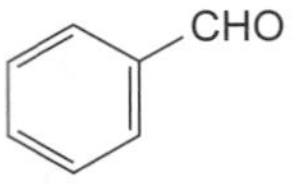

A. benzaldehyde,

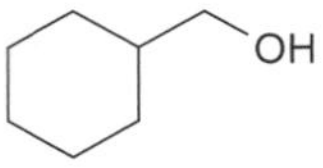

B. cyclohexylmethanol.

01/2008:1395
corrected 6.5

BIFONAZOLE

Bifonazolum

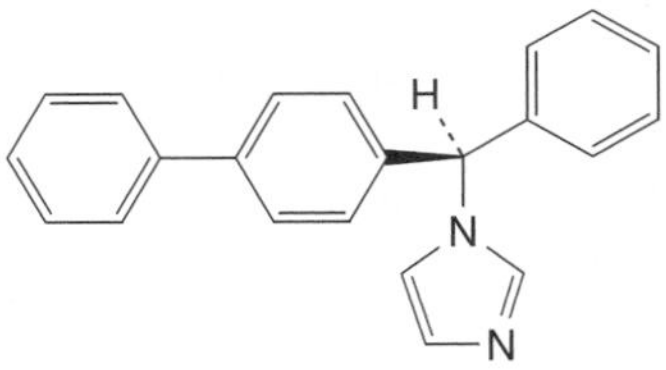

and enantiomer

$C_{22}H_{18}N_2$ [60628-96-8]

M_r 310.4

DEFINITION

1-[(*RS*)-(Biphenyl-4-yl)phenylmethyl]-1*H*-imidazole.

Content: 98.0 per cent to 100.5 per cent (dried substance).

CHARACTERS

Appearance: white or almost white, crystalline powder.

Solubility: practically insoluble in water, sparingly soluble in anhydrous ethanol.

It shows polymorphism (*5.9*).

IDENTIFICATION

Infrared absorption spectrophotometry (*2.2.24*).

Comparison: bifonazole CRS.

If the spectra obtained in the solid state show differences, dissolve the substance to be examined and the reference substance separately in the minimum volume of *2-propanol R*, evaporate to dryness and record new spectra using the residues.

TESTS

Optical rotation (*2.2.7*): − 0.10° to + 0.10°.

Dissolve 0.20 g in 20.0 ml of *methanol R*.

Related substances. Liquid chromatography (*2.2.29*).

Buffer solution pH 3.2. Mix 2.0 ml of *phosphoric acid R* with *water R* and dilute to 1000.0 ml with the same solvent. Adjust to pH 3.2 (*2.2.3*) with *triethylamine R*.

Test solution. Dissolve 50.0 mg of the substance to be examined in 25 ml of *acetonitrile R* and dilute to 50.0 ml with buffer solution pH 3.2.

Reference solution (a). Dilute 0.25 ml of the test solution to 50.0 ml with buffer solution pH 3.2.

Reference solution (b). Dissolve 25.0 mg of *imidazole R* (impurity C) in *acetonitrile R* and dilute to 25.0 ml with the same solvent. Dilute 0.25 ml of this solution to 100.0 ml with buffer solution pH 3.2.

Reference solution (c). Dissolve 5.0 mg of *bifonazole impurity B CRS* in *acetonitrile R* and dilute to 5.0 ml with the same solvent.

Reference solution (d). Mix 0.25 ml of the test solution and 0.25 ml of reference solution (c) and dilute to 50.0 ml with buffer solution pH 3.2.

Column:
— *size*: l = 0.125 m, Ø = 4.6 mm;
— *stationary phase*: *octadecylsilyl silica gel for chromatography R* (5 µm);
— *temperature*: 40 °C.

Mobile phase:
— *mobile phase A*: *acetonitrile R1*, buffer solution pH 3.2 (20:80 *V/V*);
— *mobile phase B*: buffer solution pH 3.2, *acetonitrile R1* (20:80 *V/V*);

Time (min)	Mobile phase A (per cent *V/V*)	Mobile phase B (per cent *V/V*)
0 - 8	60	40
8 - 12	60 → 10	40 → 90
12 - 30	10	90

Flow rate: 1 ml/min.

Detection: spectrophotometer at 210 nm.

Injection: 50 µl of the test solution and reference solutions (a), (b) and (d).

Retention time: impurity B = about 4 min; bifonazole = about 4.5 min.

System suitability: reference solution (d):
— *resolution*: minimum 2.5 between the peaks due to impurity B and bifonazole.

Limits:
— *impurity B*: not more than 3 times the area of the principal peak in the chromatogram obtained with reference solution (a) (1.5 per cent);
— *impurity C*: not more than the area of the corresponding peak in the chromatogram obtained with reference solution (b) (0.25 per cent);
— *impurities A, D*: for each impurity, not more than the area of the principal peak in the chromatogram obtained with reference solution (a) (0.5 per cent);
— *total*: not more than 4 times the area of the principal peak in the chromatogram obtained with reference solution (a) (2 per cent);
— *disregard limit*: 0.1 times the area of the principal peak in the chromatogram obtained with reference solution (a) (0.05 per cent).

Loss on drying (*2.2.32*): maximum 0.5 per cent, determined on 1.000 g by drying in an oven at 105 °C.

Sulphated ash (*2.4.14*): maximum 0.1 per cent, determined on 1.0 g.

ASSAY

Dissolve 0.250 g in 80 ml of *anhydrous acetic acid R*. Titrate with *0.1 M perchloric acid*, determining the end-point potentiometrically (*2.2.20*).

1 ml of *0.1 M perchloric acid* is equivalent to 31.04 mg of $C_{22}H_{18}N_2$.

IMPURITIES

Specified impurities: A, B, C, D.

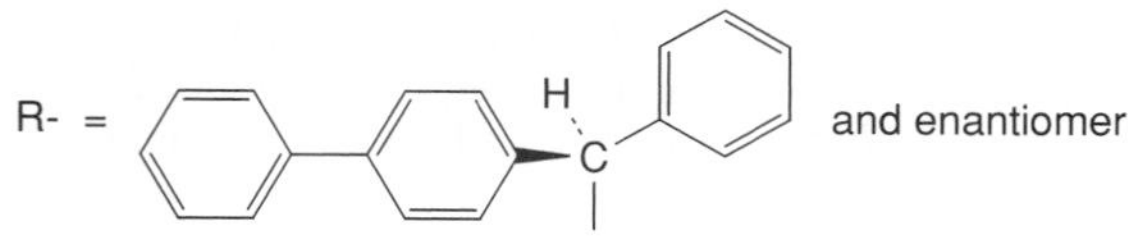

A. R-OH: (*RS*)-(biphenyl-4-yl)phenylmethanol,

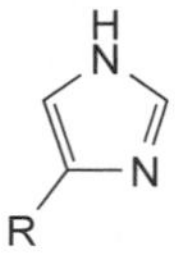

B. 4-[(*RS*)-(biphenyl-4-yl)phenylmethyl]-1*H*-imidazole,

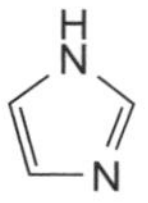

C. 1*H*-imidazole,

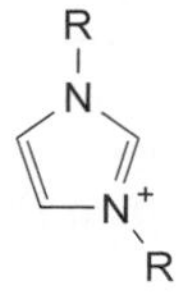

D. 1,3-bis[(biphenyl-4-yl)phenylmethyl]-1*H*-imidazolium ion.

01/2008:1493
corrected 6.5

BISMUTH SUBGALLATE

Bismuthi subgallas

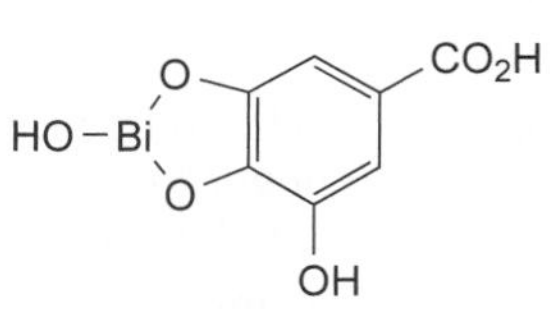

$C_7H_5BiO_6$
[99-26-3]

M_r 394.1

DEFINITION

Complex of bismuth and gallic acid.

Content: 48.0 per cent to 51.0 per cent of Bi (A_r 209.0) (dried substance).

CHARACTERS

Appearance: yellow powder.

Solubility: practically insoluble in water and in ethanol (96 per cent). It dissolves in mineral acids with decomposition and in solutions of alkali hydroxides, producing a reddish-brown liquid.

IDENTIFICATION

A. Mix 0.1 g with 5 ml of *water R* and 0.1 ml of *phosphoric acid R*. Heat to boiling and maintain boiling for 2 min. Cool and filter. To the filtrate, add 1.5 ml of *ferric chloride solution R1*; a blackish-blue colour develops.

B. It gives reaction (b) of bismuth (*2.3.1*).

TESTS

Solution S. In a porcelain or quartz dish, ignite 1.0 g, increasing the temperature very gradually. Heat in a muffle furnace at 600 ± 50 °C for 2 h. Cool and dissolve the residue with warming in 4 ml of a mixture of equal volumes of *lead-free nitric acid R* and *water R* and dilute to 20 ml with *water R*.

Acidity. Shake 1.0 g with 20 ml of *water R* for 1 min and filter. To the filtrate add 0.1 ml of *methyl red solution R*. Not more than 0.15 ml of *0.1 M sodium hydroxide* is required to change the colour of the indicator to yellow.

Chlorides (*2.4.4*): maximum 200 ppm.

To 0.5 g add 10 ml of *dilute nitric acid R*. Heat on a water-bath for 5 min and filter. Dilute 5 ml of the filtrate to 15 ml with *water R*.

Nitrates: maximum 0.2 per cent.

To 1.0 g add 25 ml of *water R* then 25 ml of a mixture of 2 volumes of *sulphuric acid R* and 9 volumes of *water R*. Heat at about 50 °C for 1 min with stirring and filter. To 10 ml of the filtrate, carefully add 30 ml of *sulphuric acid R*. The solution is not more intensely brownish-yellow than a reference solution prepared at the same time as follows: to 0.4 g of *gallic acid R*, add 20 ml of *nitrate standard solution (100 ppm NO₃) R* and 30 ml of a mixture of 2 volumes of *sulphuric acid R* and 9 volumes of *water R*, then filter; to 10 ml of the filtrate, carefully add 30 ml of *sulphuric acid R*.

Copper: maximum 50.0 ppm.

Atomic absorption spectrometry (*2.2.23, Method I*).

Test solution. Solution S.

Reference solutions. Prepare the reference solutions using *copper standard solution (10 ppm Cu) R* and diluting with a 6.5 per cent *V/V* solution of *lead-free nitric acid R*.

Source: copper hollow-cathode lamp.

Wavelength: 324.7 nm.

Atomisation device: air-acetylene flame.

Lead: maximum 20.0 ppm.

Atomic absorption spectrometry (*2.2.23, Method II*).

Test solution. Solution S.

Reference solutions. Prepare the reference solutions using *lead standard solution (10 ppm Pb) R* and diluting with a 6.5 per cent *V/V* solution of *lead-free nitric acid R*.

Source: lead hollow-cathode lamp.

Wavelength: 283.3 nm (depending on the apparatus, the line at 217.0 nm may be used).

Atomisation device: air-acetylene flame.

Silver: maximum 25.0 ppm.

Atomic absorption spectrometry (*2.2.23, Method I*).

Test solution. Solution S.

Reference solutions. Prepare the reference solutions using *silver standard solution (5 ppm Ag) R* and diluting with a 6.5 per cent *V/V* solution of *lead-free nitric acid R*.

Source: silver hollow-cathode lamp.

Wavelength: 328.1 nm.

Atomisation device: air-acetylene flame.

Substances not precipitated by ammonia: maximum 1.0 per cent.

In a porcelain or quartz dish, ignite 2.0 g, increasing the temperature very gradually to 600 ± 50 °C; allow to cool. Moisten the residue with 2 ml of *nitric acid R*, evaporate to dryness on a water-bath and carefully heat and ignite once more at 600 ± 50 °C. After cooling, dissolve the residue in 5 ml of *nitric acid R* and dilute to 20 ml with *water R*. To 10 ml of this solution, add *concentrated ammonia R* until alkaline and filter. Wash the residue with *water R* and evaporate the combined filtrate and washings to dryness on a water-bath. Add 0.3 ml of *dilute sulphuric acid R* and ignite. The residue weighs a maximum of 10 mg.

Loss on drying (*2.2.32*): maximum 7.0 per cent, determined on 1.000 g by drying in an oven at 105 °C for 3 h.

ASSAY

To 0.300 g add 10 ml of a mixture of equal volumes of *nitric acid R* and *water R*, heat to boiling and maintain boiling for 2 min. Add 0.1 g of *potassium chlorate R*, heat to boiling and maintain boiling for 1 min. Add 10 ml of *water R* and heat until the solution becomes colourless. To the hot solution, add 200 ml of *water R* and 50 mg of *xylenol orange triturate R*. Titrate with *0.1 M sodium edetate* until a yellow colour is obtained.

1 ml of *0.1 M sodium edetate* is equivalent to 20.90 mg of Bi.

STORAGE

Protected from light.

07/2009:2380

BITTER-FENNEL HERB OIL

Foeniculi amari herbae aetheroleum

DEFINITION

Essential oil obtained by steam distillation of the aerial parts of *Foeniculum vulgare* Mill. ssp. *vulgare*, var. *vulgare* collected during fruiting.

CHARACTERS

Appearance: clear, pale or intense yellow liquid.

Anise-like odour.

IDENTIFICATION

First identification: B.

Second identification: A.

A. Thin-layer chromatography (*2.2.27*).

  Test solution. Dissolve 0.1 ml of the oil to be examined in 5 ml of *toluene R*.

  Reference solution. Dissolve 10 µl of *fenchone R* and 40 µl of *anethole R* in 5 ml of *toluene R*.

  Plate: TLC silica gel plate R (5-40 µm) [or *TLC silica gel plate R* (2-10 µm)].

  Mobile phase: ethyl acetate R, toluene R (5:95 *V/V*).

  Application: 10 µl [or 3 µl] as bands of 10 mm [or 8 mm].

  Development: over a path of 8 cm [or 6 cm].

  Drying: in air.

  Detection: spray with a freshly prepared 200 g/l solution of *phosphomolybdic acid R* in *ethanol (96 per cent) R* and heat at 150 °C for 15 min; examine in daylight.

See the information section on general monographs (cover pages)

Results: see below the sequence of zones present in the chromatograms obtained with the reference solution and the test solution. Furthermore, other faint zones may be present in the chromatogram obtained with the test solution.

Top of the plate	
Anethole: a dark blue or dark violet zone	A dark blue or dark violet zone (anethole)
_____	_____
Fenchone: a blue or bluish-grey zone	A sometimes faint blue or bluish-grey zone (fenchone)
_____	
Reference solution	**Test solution**

B. Examine the chromatograms obtained in the test for chromatographic profile.

Results:

— *Spanish type*: the characteristic peaks due to α-pinene, β-pinene, β-myrcene, α-phellandrene, limonene, fenchone, estragole and *trans*-anethole in the chromatogram obtained with the test solution are similar in retention time to those in the chromatogram obtained with reference solution (a);

— *Tasmanian type*: the characteristic peaks due to α-pinene, α-phellandrene, limonene, fenchone, estragole and *trans*-anethole in the chromatogram obtained with the test solution are similar in retention time to those in the chromatogram obtained with reference solution (a).

TESTS

Relative density (*2.2.5*):

— *Spanish type*: 0.877 to 0.921;

— *Tasmanian type*: 0.940 to 0.973.

Refractive index (*2.2.6*):

— *Spanish type*: 1.487 to 1.501;

— *Tasmanian type*: 1.512 to 1.538.

Optical rotation (*2.2.7*):

— *Spanish type*: + 42° to + 68°;

— *Tasmanian type*: + 11° to + 35°.

Solubility in alcohol (*2.8.10*):

— *Spanish type*: 1 volume is soluble in 2 volumes and more of *ethanol (90 per cent V/V) R*;

— *Tasmanian type*: 1 volume is soluble in 10 volumes and more of *ethanol (85 per cent V/V) R*.

Chromatographic profile. Gas chromatography (*2.2.28*): use the normalisation procedure.

Test solution. Dissolve 0.20 ml of the oil to be examined in *acetone R* and dilute to 10.0 ml with the same solvent.

Reference solution (a). Dissolve 20 µl of *α-pinene R*, 10 µl of *β-pinene R*, 20 µl of *β-myrcene R*, 20 µl of *α-phellandrene R*, 20 µl of *limonene R*, 40 µl of *fenchone R*, 10 µl of *estragole R*, 40 µl of *anethole R*, 10 µl of *anisaldehyde R* and 10 µl of *anise ketone R* in *acetone R* and dilute to 10.0 ml with the same solvent.

Reference solution (b). Dissolve 5 µl of *anethole R* in 25.0 ml of *acetone R*. Dilute 0.5 ml of this solution to 20.0 ml with *acetone R*.

Column:

— *material*: fused silica;

— *size*: l = 60 m, Ø = 0.25 mm;

— *stationary phase*: macrogol 20 000 R (film thickness 0.25 µm).

Carrier gas: helium for chromatography R.

Flow rate: 1 ml/min.

Split ratio: 1:50.

Temperature:

	Time (min)	Temperature (°C)
Column	0 - 35	70 → 210
	35 - 42	210
Injection port		250
Detector		270

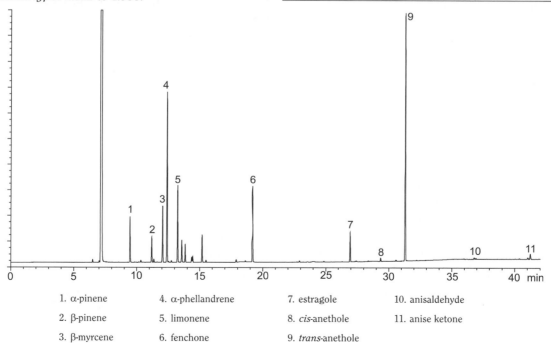

1. α-pinene
2. β-pinene
3. β-myrcene
4. α-phellandrene
5. limonene
6. fenchone
7. estragole
8. *cis*-anethole
9. *trans*-anethole
10. anisaldehyde
11. anise ketone

Figure 2380.-1. – *Chromatogram for the test for chromatographic profile of Spanish-type bitter-fennel herb oil*

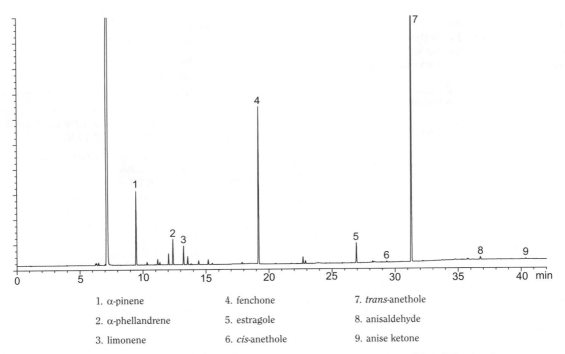

Figure 2380.-2. – *Chromatogram for the test for chromatographic profile of Tasmanian-type bitter-fennel herb oil*

1. α-pinene   4. fenchone   7. *trans*-anethole
2. α-phellandrene   5. estragole   8. anisaldehyde
3. limonene   6. *cis*-anethole   9. anise ketone

Detection: flame ionisation.

Injection: 1 μl.

Elution order: order indicated in the composition of the reference solution; record the retention times of these substances.

System suitability: reference solution (a):

— *resolution*: minimum 1.5 between the peaks due to β-myrcene and α-phellandrene.

Using the chromatogram obtained with the reference solution, locate the relevant components for the type of the essential oil to be examined in the chromatogram obtained with the test solution, and locate *cis*-anethole using Figures 2380.-1 and 2380.-2.

Determine the percentage content of each of these components.

For Spanish-type bitter-fennel herb oil, the percentages are within the following ranges:

— *α-pinene*: 2.0 to 8.0 per cent;
— *β-pinene*: 1.0 to 4.0 per cent;
— *β-myrcene*: 1.0 to 12.0 per cent;
— *α-phellandrene*: 1.0 to 25.0 per cent;
— *limonene*: 8.0 to 30.0 per cent;
— *fenchone*: 7.0 to 16.0 per cent;
— *estragole*: 2.0 to 7.0 per cent;
— *cis-anethole*: less than 0.5 per cent;
— *trans-anethole*: 15.0 to 40.0 per cent;
— *anisaldehyde*: less than 1.0 per cent;
— *anise ketone*: less than 0.05 per cent;
— *disregard limit*: the area of the principal peak in the chromatogram obtained with reference solution (b) (0.025 per cent).

For Tasmanian-type bitter-fennel herb oil, the percentages are within the following ranges:

— *α-pinene*: 2.0 to 11.0 per cent;
— *α-phellandrene*: 1.0 to 8.5 per cent;
— *limonene*: 1.0 to 6.0 per cent;
— *fenchone*: 10.0 to 25.0 per cent;

— *estragole*: 1.5 to 6.0 per cent;
— *cis-anethole*: less than 0.5 per cent;
— *trans-anethole*: 45.0 to 78.0 per cent;
— *anisaldehyde*: less than 1.0 per cent;
— *anise ketone*: less than 0.05 per cent;
— *disregard limit*: the area of the principal peak in the chromatogram obtained with reference solution (b) (0.025 per cent).

STORAGE

At a temperature not exceeding 25 °C.

LABELLING

The label states that the content is Spanish-type or Tasmanian-type.

07/2009:1180

BUPRENORPHINE

Buprenorphinum

$C_{29}H_{41}NO_4$
[52485-79-7]

M_r 467.6

DEFINITION

(2S)-2-[17-(Cyclopropylmethyl)-4,5α-epoxy-3-hydroxy-6-methoxy-6α,14-ethano-14α-morphinan-7α-yl]-3,3-dimethylbutan-2-ol.

Content: 98.5 per cent to 101.5 per cent (dried substance).

CHARACTERS

Appearance: white or almost white, crystalline powder.

Solubility: very slightly soluble in water, freely soluble in acetone, soluble in methanol, slightly soluble in cyclohexane. It dissolves in dilute solutions of acids.

mp: about 217 °C.

IDENTIFICATION

Infrared absorption spectrophotometry (*2.2.24*).

Comparison: buprenorphine CRS.

TESTS

Solution S. Dissolve 0.250 g in *ethanol 96 per cent R* and dilute to 25.0 ml with the same solvent.

Appearance of solution. Solution S is clear (*2.2.1*) and colourless (*2.2.2, Method II*).

Specific optical rotation (*2.2.7*): − 103 to − 107 (dried substance), determined on solution S.

Related substances. Liquid chromatography (*2.2.29*).

Test solution. Dissolve 50.0 mg of the substance to be examined in *methanol R* and dilute to 10.0 ml with the same solvent.

Reference solution (a). Dilute 1.0 ml of the test solution to 100.0 ml with *methanol R*. Dilute 1.0 ml of this solution to 10.0 ml with *methanol R*.

Reference solution (b). Dissolve 5 mg of *buprenorphine for system suitability CRS* (containing impurities A, B, F, G, H and J) in 1.0 ml of *methanol R*.

Column:

– *size*: *l* = 0.05 m, Ø = 4,6 mm;
– *stationary phase*: *end-capped octadecylsilyl silica gel for chromatography R* (3.5 μm);
– *temperature*: 30 °C.

Mobile phase:

– *mobile phase A*: dissolve 5.44 g of *potassium dihydrogen phosphate R* in 900 ml of *water R*, adjust to pH 4.5 with a 5 per cent *V/V* solution of *phosphoric acid R* and dilute to 1000 ml with *water R*; mix 90 volumes of this solution and 10 volumes of *acetonitrile R*;
– *mobile phase B*: *acetonitrile R*;

Time (min)	Mobile phase A (per cent *V/V*)	Mobile phase B (per cent *V/V*)
0 - 2	89	11
2 - 12	89 → 64	11 → 36
12 - 15	64 → 41	36 → 59
15 - 20	41 → 39	59 → 61

Flow rate: 1.3 ml/min.

Detection: spectrophotometer at 240 nm.

Injection: 5 μl.

Identification of impurities: use the chromatogram supplied with *buprenorphine for system suitability CRS* and the chromatogram obtained with reference solution (b) to identify the peaks due to impurities A, B, F, G, H and J.

Relative retention with reference to buprenorphine (retention time = about 8.5 min): impurity B = about 0.4; impurity J = about 1.1; impurity F = about 1.27; impurity H = about 1.33; impurity A = about 1.40; impurity G = about 1.8.

System suitability: reference solution (b):

– *resolution*: minimum 2.0 between the peaks due to buprenorphine and impurity J.

Limits:

– *correction factor*: for the calculation of content, multiply the peak area of impurity G by 0.3;
– *impurity H*: not more than 2.5 times the area of the principal peak in the chromatogram obtained with reference solution (a) (0.25 per cent);
– *impurities A, B, F, J*: for each impurity, not more than twice the area of the principal peak in the chromatogram obtained with reference solution (a) (0.2 per cent);
– *impurity G*: not more than 1.5 times the area of the principal peak in the chromatogram obtained with reference solution (a) (0.15 per cent);
– *unspecified impurities*: for each impurity, not more than the area of the principal peak in the chromatogram obtained with reference solution (a) (0.10 per cent);
– *total*: not more than 7 times the area of the principal peak in the chromatogram obtained with reference solution (a) (0.7 per cent);
– *disregard limit*: 0.5 times the area of the principal peak in the chromatogram obtained with reference solution (a) (0.05 per cent).

Loss on drying (*2.2.32*): maximum 1.0 per cent, determined on 1.000 g by drying in an oven at 105 °C.

ASSAY

Dissolve 0.400 g in 40 ml of *anhydrous acetic acid R*. Titrate with *0.1 M perchloric acid*, determining the end-point potentiometrically (*2.2.20*).

1 ml of *0.1 M perchloric acid* is equivalent to 46.76 mg of $C_{29}H_{41}NO_4$.

STORAGE

Protected from light.

IMPURITIES

Specified impurities: A, B, F, G, H, J.

Other detectable impurities (the following substances would, if present at a sufficient level, be detected by one or other of the tests in the monograph. They are limited by the general acceptance criterion for other/unspecified impurities and/or by the general monograph *Substances for pharmaceutical use (2034)*. It is therefore not necessary to identify these impurities for demonstration of compliance. See also *5.10. Control of impurities in substances for pharmaceutical use*): C, D, E, I.

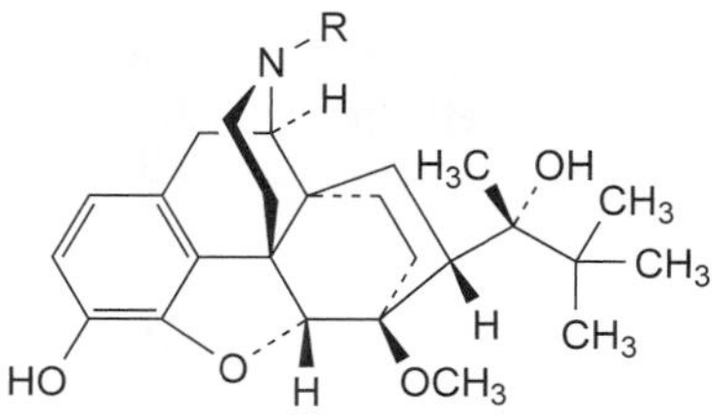

A. R = CH₂-CH₂-CH=CH₂: (2S)-2-[17-(but-3-enyl)-4,5α-epoxy-3-hydroxy-6-methoxy-6α,14-ethano-14α-morphinan-7α-yl]-3,3-dimethylbutan-2-ol,

B. R = H: (2S)-2-(4,5α-epoxy-3-hydroxy-6-methoxy-6α,14-ethano-14α-morphinan-7α-yl)-3,3-dimethylbutan-2-ol (norbuprenorphine),

H. R = CH₂-CH₂-CH₂-CH₃: (2S)-2-[17-butyl-4,5α-epoxy-3-hydroxy-6-methoxy-6α,14-ethano-14α-morphinan-7α-yl]-3,3-dimethylbutan-2-ol,

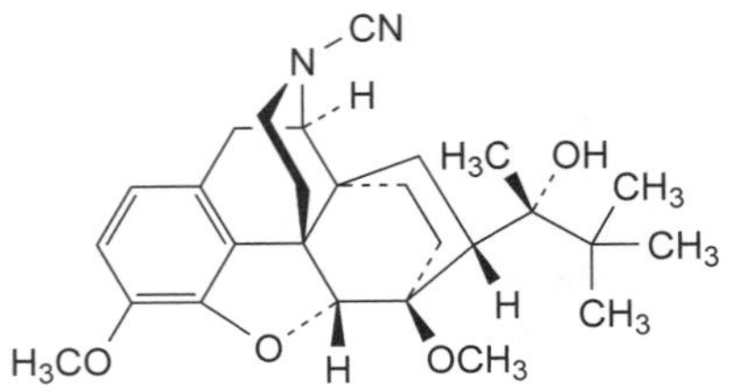

C. 4,5α-epoxy-7α-[(1S)-1-hydroxy-1,2,2-trimethylpropyl]-3,6-dimethoxy-6α,14-ethano-14α-morphinan-17-carbonitrile,

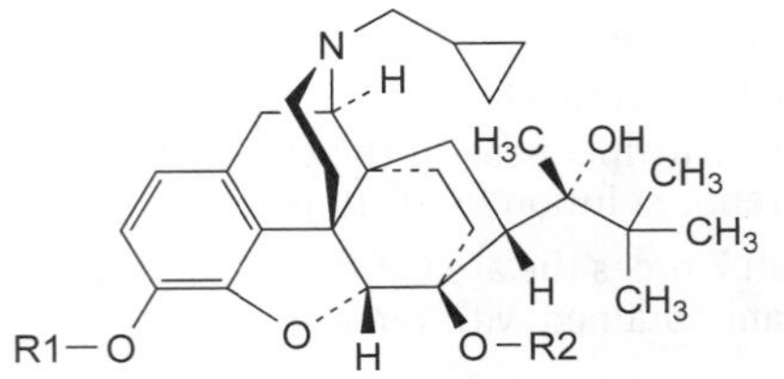

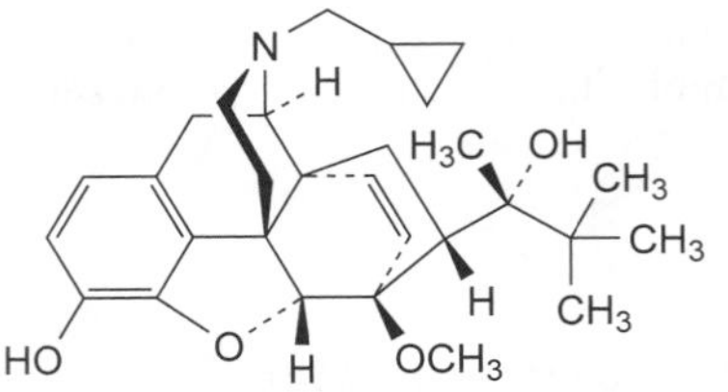

J. (2S)-2-[17-(cyclopropylmethyl)-4,5α-epoxy-3-hydroxy-6-methoxy-6α,14-etheno-14α-morphinan-7α-yl]-3,3-dimethylbutan-2-ol.

D. R1 = R2 = CH₃: (2S)-2-[17-(cyclopropylmethyl)-4,5α-epoxy-3,6-dimethoxy-6α,14-ethano-14α-morphinan-7α-yl]-3,3-dimethylbutan-2-ol (3-O-methylbuprenorphine),

E. R1 = R2 = H: (2S)-2-[17-(cyclopropylmethyl)-4,5α-epoxy-3,6-dihydroxy-6α,14-ethano-14α-morphinan-7α-yl]-3,3-dimethylbutan-2-ol (6-O-desmethylbuprenorphine),

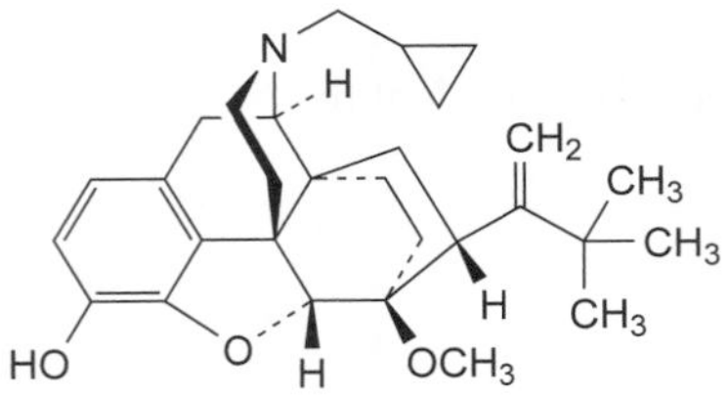

F. 17-(cyclopropylmethyl)-4,5α-epoxy-6-methoxy-7α-[1-(1,1-dimethylethyl)ethenyl]-6α,14-ethano-14α-morphinan-3-ol,

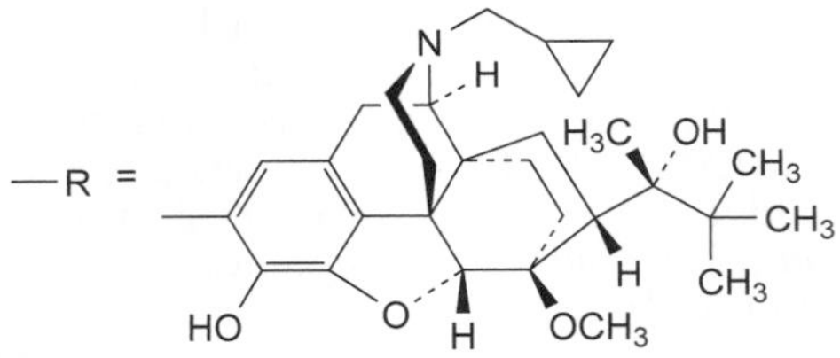

G. R-R: 17,17'-di(cyclopropylmethyl)-4,5α;4',5α'-diepoxy-7α,7α'-di[(1S)-1-hydroxy-1,2,2-trimethylpropyl]-6,6'-dimethoxy-2,2'-bi(6α,14-ethano-14α-morphinan)-3,3'-diol (2,2'-bibuprenorphine),

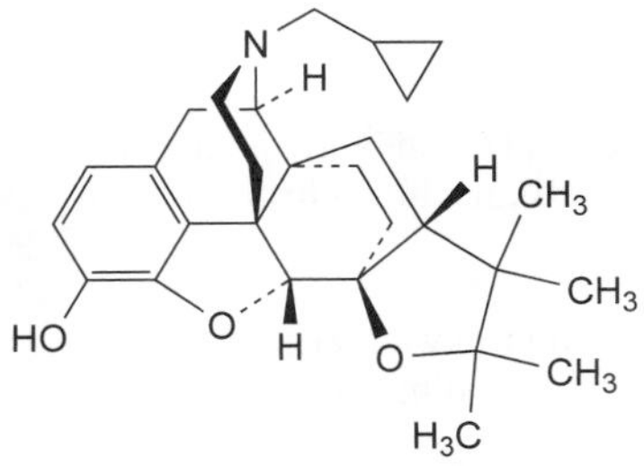

I. 17-(cyclopropylmethyl)-4'',4'',5'',5''-tetramethyl-4'',5''-dihydro-(7βH)-6α,14-ethano-(5βH)-difurano-[2',3',4',5':4,12,13,5;2'',3'':6,7]-14α-morphinan-3-ol,

---

07/2009:1181

BUPRENORPHINE HYDROCHLORIDE

Buprenorphini hydrochloridum

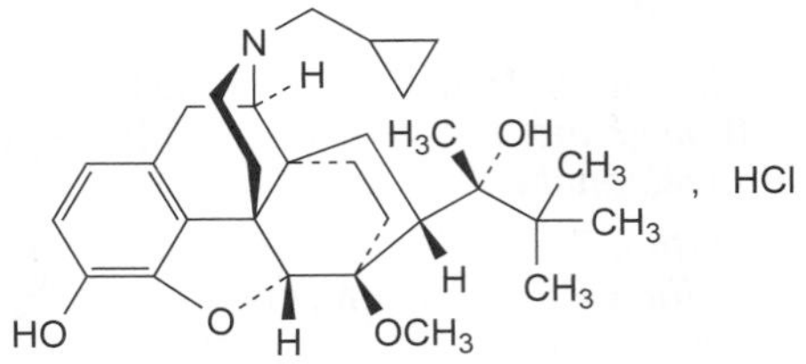

$C_{29}H_{42}ClNO_4$ M_r 504.1
[53152-21-9]

DEFINITION

(2S)-2-[17-(Cyclopropylmethyl)-4,5α-epoxy-3-hydroxy-6-methoxy-6α,14-ethano-14α-morphinan-7α-yl]-3,3-dimethylbutan-2-ol hydrochloride.

Content: 98.5 per cent to 101.5 per cent (dried substance).

CHARACTERS

Appearance: white or almost white, crystalline powder.

Solubility: sparingly soluble in water, freely soluble in methanol, soluble in ethanol (96 per cent), practically insoluble in cyclohexane.

IDENTIFICATION

A. Infrared absorption spectrophotometry (*2.2.24*).

    Comparison: buprenorphine hydrochloride CRS.

B. 3 ml of solution S (see Tests) gives reaction (a) of chlorides (*2.3.1*).

TESTS

Solution S. Dissolve 0.250 g in 5.0 ml of *methanol R* and, while stirring, dilute to 25.0 ml with *carbon dioxide-free water R*.

Appearance of solution. Solution S is clear (*2.2.1*) and colourless (*2.2.2, Method II*).

Acidity or alkalinity. To 10.0 ml of solution S add 0.05 ml of *methyl red solution R*. Not more than 0.2 ml of *0.02 M sodium hydroxide* or *0.02 M hydrochloric acid* is required to change the colour of the indicator.

Specific optical rotation (*2.2.7*): − 92 to − 98 (dried substance).

Dissolve 0.200 g in *methanol R* and dilute to 20.0 ml with the same solvent.

Related substances. Liquid chromatography (*2.2.29*).

Test solution. Dissolve 50.0 mg of the substance to be examined in *methanol R* and dilute to 10.0 ml with the same solvent.

Reference solution (a). Dilute 1.0 ml of the test solution to 100.0 ml with *methanol R*. Dilute 1.0 ml of this solution to 10.0 ml with *methanol R*.

Reference solution (b). Dissolve 5 mg of *buprenorphine for system suitability CRS* (containing impurities A, B, F, G, H and J) in 1.0 ml of *methanol R*.

Column:

— *size*: l = 0.05 m, Ø = 4,6 mm;

— *stationary phase*: *end-capped octadecylsilyl silica gel for chromatography R* (3.5 μm);

— *temperature*: 30 °C.

Mobile phase:

— *mobile phase A*: dissolve 5.44 g of *potassium dihydrogen phosphate R* in 900 ml of *water R*, adjust to pH 4.5 with a 5 per cent *V/V* solution of *phosphoric acid R* and dilute to 1000 ml with *water R*; mix 90 volumes of this solution and 10 volumes of *acetonitrile R*;

— *mobile phase B*: *acetonitrile R*;

Time (min)	Mobile phase A (per cent *V/V*)	Mobile phase B (per cent *V/V*)
0 - 2	89	11
2 - 12	89 → 64	11 → 36
12 - 15	64 → 41	36 → 59
15 - 20	41 → 39	59 → 61

Flow rate: 1.3 ml/min.

Detection: spectrophotometer at 240 nm.

Injection: 5 μl.

Identification of impurities: use the chromatogram supplied with *buprenorphine for system suitability CRS* and the chromatogram obtained with reference solution (b) to identify the peaks due to impurities A, B, F, G, H and J.

Relative retention with reference to buprenorphine (retention time = about 8.5 min): impurity B = about 0.4; impurity J = about 1.1; impurity F = about 1.27; impurity H = about 1.33; impurity A = about 1.40; impurity G = about 1.8.

System suitability: reference solution (b):

— *resolution*: minimum 2.0 between the peaks due to buprenorphine and impurity J.

Limits:

— *correction factor*: for the calculation of content, multiply the peak area of impurity G by 0.3;

— *impurity H*: not more than 2.5 times the area of the principal peak in the chromatogram obtained with reference solution (a) (0.25 per cent);

— *impurities A, B, F, J*: for each impurity, not more than twice the area of the principal peak in the chromatogram obtained with reference solution (a) (0.2 per cent);

— *impurity G*: not more than 1.5 times the area of the principal peak in the chromatogram obtained with reference solution (a) (0.15 per cent);

— *unspecified impurities*: for each impurity, not more than the area of the principal peak in the chromatogram obtained with reference solution (a) (0.10 per cent);

— *total*: not more than 7 times the area of the principal peak in the chromatogram obtained with reference solution (a) (0.7 per cent);

— *disregard limit*: 0.5 times the area of the principal peak in the chromatogram obtained with reference solution (a) (0.05 per cent).

Loss on drying (2.2.32): maximum 1.0 per cent, determined on 1.000 g by heating in an oven at 115-120 °C.

ASSAY

Dissolve 0.400 g in a mixture of 5 ml of *0.01 M hydrochloric acid* and 50 ml of *ethanol (96 per cent) R*. Carry out a potentiometric titration (2.2.20), using *0.1 M sodium hydroxide*. Read the volume added between the 2 points of inflexion. Carry out a blank titration.

1 ml of *0.1 M sodium hydroxide* is equivalent to 50.41 mg of $C_{29}H_{42}ClNO_4$.

STORAGE

Protected from light.

IMPURITIES

Specified impurities: A, B, F, G, H, J.

Other detectable impurities (the following substances would, if present at a sufficient level, be detected by one or other of the tests in the monograph. They are limited by the general acceptance criterion for other/unspecified impurities and/or by the general monograph *Substances for pharmaceutical use (2034)*. It is therefore not necessary to identify these impurities for demonstration of compliance. See also 5.10. *Control of impurities in substances for pharmaceutical use*): C, D, E, I.

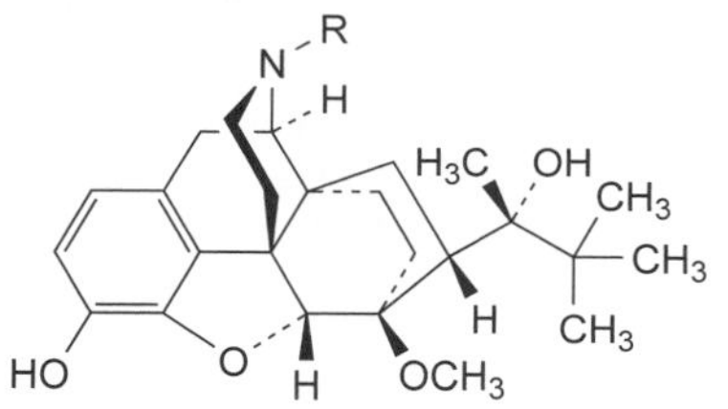

A. R = CH_2-CH_2-CH=CH_2: (2S)-2-[17-(but-3-enyl)-4,5α-epoxy-3-hydroxy-6-methoxy-6α,14-ethano-14α-morphinan-7α-yl]-3,3-dimethylbutan-2-ol,

B. R = H: (2S)-2-(4,5α-epoxy-3-hydroxy-6-methoxy-6α,14-ethano-14α-morphinan-7α-yl)-3,3-dimethylbutan-2-ol (norbuprenorphine),

H. R = CH_2-CH_2-CH_2-CH_3: (2S)-2-[17-butyl-4,5α-epoxy-3-hydroxy-6-methoxy-6α,14-ethano-14α-morphinan-7α-yl]-3,3-dimethylbutan-2-ol,

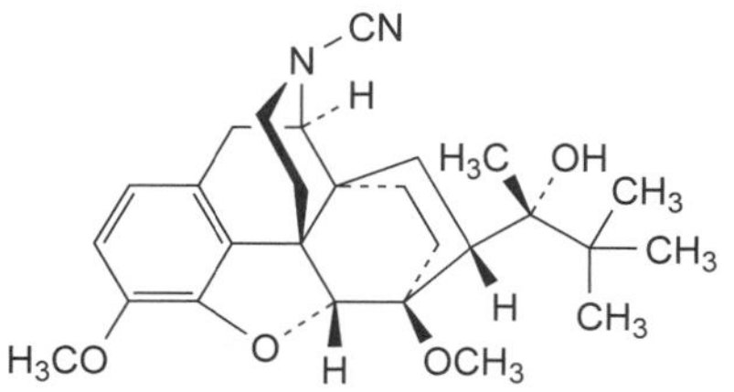

C. 4,5α-epoxy-7α-[(1S)-1-hydroxy-1,2,2-trimethylpropyl]-3,6-dimethoxy-6α,14-ethano-14α-morphinan-17-carbonitrile,

D. R1 = R2 = CH$_3$: (2S)-2-[17-(cyclopropylmethyl)-4,5α-epoxy-3,6-dimethoxy-6α,14-ethano-14α-morphinan-7α-yl]-3,3-dimethylbutan-2-ol (3-O-methylbuprenorphine),

E. R1 = R2 = H: (2S)-2-[17-(cyclopropylmethyl)-4,5α-epoxy-3,6-dihydroxy-6α,14-ethano-14α-morphinan-7α-yl]-3,3-dimethylbutan-2-ol (6-O-desmethylbuprenorphine),

F. 17-(cyclopropylmethyl)-4,5α-epoxy-6-methoxy-7α-[1-(1,1-dimethylethyl)ethenyl]-6α,14-ethano-14α-morphinan-3-ol,

G. R-R: 17,17'-di(cyclopropylmethyl)-4,5α;4',5α'-diepoxy-7α,7α'-di[(1S)-1-hydroxy-1,2,2-trimethylpropyl]-6,6'-dimethoxy-2,2'-bi(6α,14-ethano-14α-morphinan)-3,3'-diol (2,2'-bibuprenorphine),

I. 17-(cyclopropylmethyl)-4″,4″,5″,5″-tetramethyl-4″,5″-dihydro-(7βH)-6α,14-ethano-(5βH)-difurano-[2′,3′,4′,5′:4,12,13,5;2″,3″:6,7]-14α-morphinan-3-ol,

J. (2S)-2-[17-(cyclopropylmethyl)-4,5α-epoxy-3-hydroxy-6-methoxy-6α,14-etheno-14α-morphinan-7α-yl]-3,3-dimethylbutan-2-ol.

C

Monographs
A-C

See the information section on general monographs (cover pages)

07/2009:0268

CAFFEINE MONOHYDRATE

Coffeinum monohydricum

, H₂O

$C_8H_{10}N_4O_2, H_2O$　　　　　　　　　　　　M_r 212.2
[5743-12-4]

DEFINITION

1,3,7-Trimethyl-3,7-dihydro-1*H*-purine-2,6-dione monohydrate.

Content: 98.5 per cent to 101.5 per cent (dried substance).

CHARACTERS

Appearance: white or almost white, crystalline powder or silky, white or almost white crystals.

Solubility: sparingly soluble in water, freely soluble in boiling water, slightly soluble in ethanol (96 per cent). It dissolves in concentrated solutions of alkali benzoates or salicylates.

It sublimes readily.

IDENTIFICATION

First identification: A, B, E.

Second identification: A, C, D, E, F.

A. Melting point (*2.2.14*): 234 °C to 239 °C, determined after drying at 100-105 °C.

B. Infrared absorption spectrophotometry (*2.2.24*).

　　Preparation: dry the substance to be examined at 100-105 °C before use.

　　Comparison: *caffeine CRS*.

C. To 2 ml of a saturated solution add 0.05 ml of *iodinated potassium iodide solution R*; the solution remains clear. Add 0.1 ml of *dilute hydrochloric acid R*; a brown precipitate is formed. Neutralise with *dilute sodium hydroxide solution R*; the precipitate dissolves.

D. In a glass-stoppered tube, dissolve about 10 mg in 0.25 ml of a mixture of 0.5 ml of *acetylacetone R* and 5 ml of *dilute sodium hydroxide solution R*. Heat in a water-bath at 80 °C for 7 min. Cool and add 0.5 ml of *dimethylaminobenzaldehyde solution R2*. Heat again in a water-bath at 80 °C for 7 min. Allow to cool and add 10 ml of *water R*; an intense blue colour develops.

E. Loss on drying (see Tests).

F. It gives the reaction of xanthines (*2.3.1*).

TESTS

Solution S. Dissolve 0.5 g with heating in 50 ml of *carbon dioxide-free water R* prepared from *distilled water R*, cool, and dilute to 50 ml with the same solvent.

Appearance of solution. Solution S is clear (*2.2.1*) and colourless (*2.2.2, Method II*).

Acidity. To 10 ml of solution S add 0.05 ml of *bromothymol blue solution R1*; the solution is green or yellow. Not more than 0.2 ml of *0.01 M sodium hydroxide* is required to change the colour of the indicator to blue.

Related substances. Liquid chromatography (*2.2.29*).

Test solution. Dissolve 0.110 g of the substance to be examined in the mobile phase and dilute to 50.0 ml with the mobile phase. Dilute 1.0 ml of this solution to 10.0 ml with the mobile phase.

Reference solution (a). Dilute 2.0 ml of the test solution to 100.0 ml with the mobile phase. Dilute 1.0 ml of this solution to 10.0 ml with the mobile phase.

Reference solution (b). Dissolve 5 mg of *caffeine for system suitability CRS* (containing impurities A, C, D and F) in the mobile phase and dilute to 5.0 ml with the mobile phase. Dilute 2.0 ml of this solution to 10.0 ml with the mobile phase.

Column:
- *size*: *l* = 0.15 m, Ø = 4.6 mm;
- *stationary phase*: base-deactivated end-capped octadecylsilyl silica gel for chromatography R (5 µm).

Mobile phase. Mix 20 volumes of *tetrahydrofuran R*, 25 volumes of *acetonitrile R* and 955 volumes of a solution containing 0.82 g/l of *anhydrous sodium acetate R* previously adjusted to pH 4.5 with *glacial acetic acid R*.

Flow rate: 1.0 ml/min.

Detection: spectrophotometer at 275 nm.

Injection: 10 µl.

Run time: 1.5 times the retention time of caffeine.

Identification of impurities: use the chromatogram supplied with *caffeine for system suitability CRS* and the chromatogram obtained with reference solution (b) to identify the peaks due to impurities A, C, D and F.

Retention time: caffeine = about 8 min.

System suitability: reference solution (b):
- *resolution*: minimum 2.5 between the peaks due to impurities C and D; minimum 2.5 between the peaks due to impurities F and A.

Limits:
- *unspecified impurities*: for each impurity, not more than 0.5 times the area of the principal peak in the chromatogram obtained with reference solution (a) (0.10 per cent);
- *total*: not more than 0.5 times the area of the principal peak in the chromatogram obtained with reference solution (a) (0.1 per cent);
- *disregard limit*: 0.25 times the area of the principal peak in the chromatogram obtained with reference solution (a) (0.05 per cent).

Sulphates (*2.4.13*): maximum 500 ppm, determined on 15 ml of solution S.

Prepare the standard using a mixture of 7.5 ml of *sulphate standard solution (10 ppm SO₄) R* and 7.5 ml of *distilled water R*.

Heavy metals (*2.4.8*): maximum 20 ppm.

1.0 g complies with test C. Prepare the reference solution using 2 ml of *lead standard solution (10 ppm Pb) R*.

Loss on drying (*2.2.32*): 5.0 per cent to 9.0 per cent, determined on 1.000 g by drying in an oven at 105 °C for 1 h.

Sulphated ash (*2.4.14*): maximum 0.1 per cent, determined on 1.0 g.

ASSAY

Dissolve 0.170 g, previously dried at 100-105 °C, with heating in 5 ml of *anhydrous acetic acid R*. Allow to cool, and add 10 ml of *acetic anhydride R* and 20 ml of *toluene R*. Titrate with *0.1 M perchloric acid*, determining the end-point potentiometrically (*2.2.20*).

1 ml of *0.1 M perchloric acid* is equivalent to 19.42 mg of $C_8H_{10}N_4O_2$.

IMPURITIES

Other detectable impurities (the following substances would, if present at a sufficient level, be detected by one or other of the tests in the monograph. They are limited by the general acceptance criterion for other/unspecified impurities and/or by the general monograph *Substances for pharmaceutical use (2034)*. It is therefore not necessary to identify these impurities for demonstration of compliance. See also *5.10. Control of impurities in substances for pharmaceutical use*): A, B, C, D, E, F.

A. theophylline,

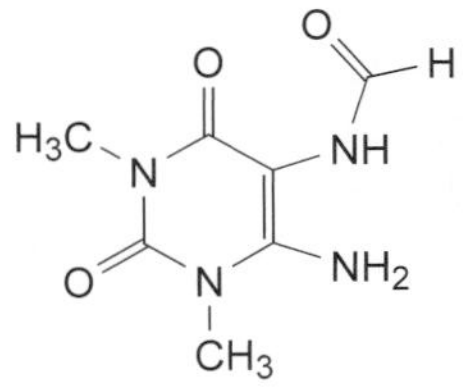

B. *N*-(6-amino-1,3-dimethyl-2,4-dioxo-1,2,3,4-tetrahydropyrimidin-5-yl)formamide,

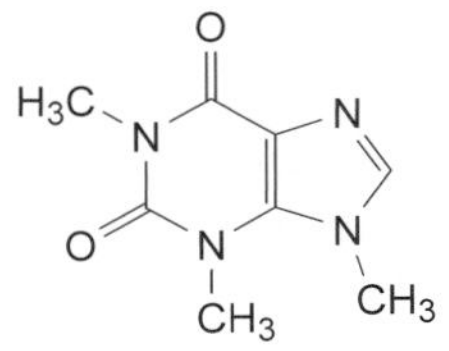

C. 1,3,9-trimethyl-3,9-dihydro-1*H*-purine-2,6-dione (isocaffeine),

D. theobromine,

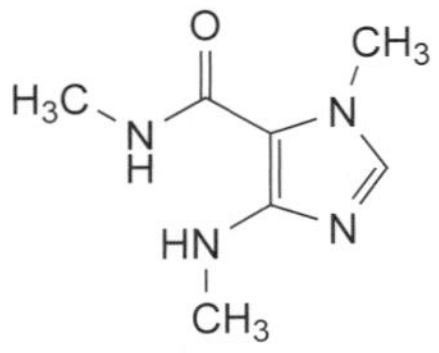

E. *N*,1-dimethyl-4-(methylamino)-1*H*-imidazole-5-carboxamide (caffeidine),

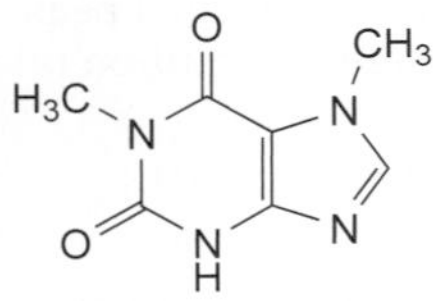

F. 1,7-dimethyl-3,7-dihydro-1*H*-purine-2,6-dione.

07/2009:1081

CARBOPLATIN

Carboplatinum

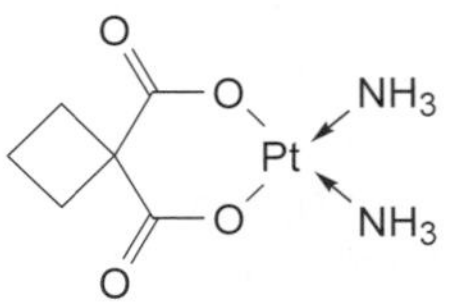

$C_6H_{12}N_2O_4Pt$
[41575-94-4]

M_r 371.3

DEFINITION

(*SP*-4-2)-Diammine[cyclobutan-1,1-dicarboxylato(2-)-*O,O'*]-platin.

Content: 98.0 per cent to 102.0 per cent (dried substance).

CHARACTERS

Appearance: colourless, crystalline powder.

Solubility: sparingly soluble in water, very slightly soluble in acetone and in ethanol (96 per cent).

mp: about 200 °C, with decomposition.

IDENTIFICATION

Infrared absorption spectrophotometry (*2.2.24*).

Comparison: Ph. Eur. reference spectrum of carboplatin.

TESTS

Solution S. Dissolve 0.25 g in *carbon dioxide-free water R* and dilute to 25 ml with the same solvent.

Appearance of solution. Solution S is clear (*2.2.1*) and colourless (*2.2.2, Method II*).

Impurity B and acidity: maximum 0.5 per cent, calculated as impurity B.

To 10 ml of solution S add 0.1 ml of *phenolphthalein solution R1*. The solution is colourless. Not more than 0.7 ml of *0.01 M sodium hydroxide* is required to change the colour of the indicator to pink.

Related substances. Liquid chromatography (*2.2.29*).

Test solution. Dissolve 20.0 mg of the substance to be examined in a mixture of equal volumes of *acetonitrile R* and *water R* and dilute to 20.0 ml with the same mixture of solvents.

Reference solution. Dilute 0.5 ml of the test solution to 200.0 ml with the mobile phase.

Column:
— *size*: *l* = 0.25 m, Ø = 4.6 mm;
— *stationary phase*: *aminopropylsilyl silica gel for chromatography R* (5 µm).

Mobile phase: *water R*, *acetonitrile R* (13:87 *V/V*).

Flow rate: 2 ml/min.

Detection: spectrophotometer at 230 nm.

Injection: 10 µl.

Run time: 2.5 times the retention time of carboplatin.

System suitability: test solution:
— *number of theoretical plates*: minimum 5000; if necessary, adjust the concentration of acetonitrile in the mobile phase;
— *mass distribution ratio*: minimum 4.0; if necessary, adjust the concentration of acetonitrile in the mobile phase;
— *symmetry factor*: maximum 2.0; if necessary, adjust the concentration of acetonitrile in the mobile phase.

Limits:
— *impurity A*: not more than the area of the principal peak in the chromatogram obtained with the reference solution (0.25 per cent);
— *total*: not more than twice the area of the principal peak in the chromatogram obtained with the reference solution (0.5 per cent);
— *disregard limit*: 0.2 times the area of the principal peak in the chromatogram obtained with the reference solution (0.05 per cent).

Chlorides (*2.4.4*): maximum 100 ppm.

Dissolve 0.5 g in *water R*, heating slightly if necessary, and dilute to 20 ml with the same solvent. Filter if necessary. Dilute 10 ml of this solution to 15 ml with *water R*. Prepare the standard using 5 ml of *chloride standard solution (5 ppm Cl) R*.

Ammonium (*2.4.1, Method B*): maximum 100 ppm, determined on 0.20 g.

Prepare the standard using 0.2 ml of *ammonium standard solution (100 ppm NH₄) R*.

Silver: maximum 10.0 ppm.

Atomic emission spectrometry (*2.2.22, Method I*).

Test solution. Dissolve 0.50 g in a 1 per cent *V/V* solution of *nitric acid R* and dilute to 50.0 ml with the same solution.

Reference solutions. Prepare the reference solutions using *silver standard solution (5 ppm Ag) R*, diluting with a 1 per cent *V/V* solution of *nitric acid R*.

Wavelength: 328.1 nm.

Soluble barium: maximum 10.0 ppm.

Atomic emission spectrometry (*2.2.22, Method I*).

Test solution. Use the solution described in the test for silver.

Reference solutions. Prepare the reference solutions using *barium standard solution (50 ppm Ba) R*, diluting with a 1 per cent *V/V* solution of *nitric acid R*.

Wavelength: 455.4 nm.

Loss on drying (*2.2.32*): maximum 0.5 per cent, determined on 1.000 g by drying in an oven at 105 °C.

ASSAY

Use the residue obtained in the test for loss on drying. Ignite 0.200 g of the residue to constant mass at 800 ± 50 °C.

1 mg of the residue is equivalent to 1.903 mg of $C_6H_{12}N_2O_4Pt$.

STORAGE

Protected from light.

IMPURITIES

Specified impurities: A, B.

A. cisplatin,

B. cyclobutane-1,1-dicarboxylic acid.

01/2008:0986
corrected 6.5

CEFACLOR

Cefaclorum

, H_2O

$C_{15}H_{14}ClN_3O_4S,H_2O$ M_r 385.8
[70356-03-5]

DEFINITION

(6*R*,7*R*)-7-[[(2*R*)-2-Amino-2-phenylacetyl]amino]-3-chloro-8-oxo-5-thia-1-azabicyclo[4.2.0]oct-2-ene-2-carboxylic acid monohydrate.

Semi-synthetic product derived from a fermentation product.

Content: 96.0 per cent to 102.0 per cent of $C_{15}H_{14}ClN_3O_4S$ (anhydrous substance).

CHARACTERS

Appearance: white or slightly yellow powder.

Solubility: slightly soluble in water, practically insoluble in methanol and in methylene chloride.

IDENTIFICATION

Infrared absorption spectrophotometry (*2.2.24*).

Comparison: cefaclor CRS.

TESTS

pH (*2.2.3*): 3.0 to 4.5.

Suspend 0.250 g in *carbon dioxide-free water R* and dilute to 10 ml with the same solvent.

Specific optical rotation (*2.2.7*): + 101 to + 111 (anhydrous substance).

Dissolve 0.250 g in a 10 g/l solution of *hydrochloric acid R* and dilute to 25.0 ml with the same solution.

Related substances. Liquid chromatography (*2.2.29*).

Test solution. Dissolve 50.0 mg of the substance to be examined in 10.0 ml of a 2.7 g/l solution of *sodium dihydrogen phosphate R* adjusted to pH 2.5 with *phosphoric acid R*.

Reference solution (a). Dissolve 2.5 mg of cefaclor CRS and 5.0 mg of *delta-3-cefaclor CRS* (impurity D) in 100.0 ml of a 2.7 g/l solution of *sodium dihydrogen phosphate R* adjusted to pH 2.5 with *phosphoric acid R*.

Reference solution (b). Dilute 1.0 ml of the test solution to 100.0 ml with a 2.7 g/l solution of *sodium dihydrogen phosphate R* adjusted to pH 2.5 with *phosphoric acid R*.

Column:
— *size*: *l* = 0.25 m, Ø = 4.6 mm;
— *stationary phase*: *end-capped octadecylsilyl silica gel for chromatography R* (5 μm).

Mobile phase:
— *mobile phase A*: 7.8 g/l solution of *sodium dihydrogen phosphate R* adjusted to pH 4.0 with *phosphoric acid R*;
— *mobile phase B*: mix 450 ml of *acetonitrile R* with 550 ml of mobile phase A;

Time (min)	Mobile phase A (per cent *V/V*)	Mobile phase B (per cent *V/V*)
0 - 30	95 → 75	5 → 25
30 - 45	75 → 0	25 → 100
45 - 55	0	100

Flow rate: 1.0 ml/min.

Detection: spectrophotometer at 220 nm.

Injection: 20 μl.

System suitability: reference solution (a):
— *resolution*: minimum 2 between the peaks due to cefaclor and impurity D; if necessary, adjust the acetonitrile content in the mobile phase;
— *symmetry factor*: maximum 1.2 for the peak due to cefaclor; if necessary, adjust the acetonitrile content in the mobile phase.

Limits:
- *any impurity*: for each impurity, not more than 0.5 times the area of the principal peak in the chromatogram obtained with reference solution (b) (0.5 per cent);
- *total*: not more than twice the area of the principal peak in the chromatogram obtained with reference solution (b) (2 per cent);
- *disregard limit*: 0.1 times the area of the principal peak in the chromatogram obtained with reference solution (b) (0.1 per cent).

Heavy metals (*2.4.8*): maximum 30 ppm.

1.0 g complies with test C. Prepare the reference solution using 3 ml of *lead standard solution (10 ppm Pb) R*.

Water (*2.5.12*): 3.0 per cent to 6.5 per cent, determined on 0.200 g.

ASSAY

Liquid chromatography (*2.2.29*).

Test solution. Dissolve 15.0 mg of the substance to be examined in the mobile phase and dilute to 50.0 ml with the mobile phase.

Reference solution (a). Dissolve 15.0 mg of *cefaclor CRS* in the mobile phase and dilute to 50.0 ml with the mobile phase.

Reference solution (b). Dissolve 3.0 mg of *cefaclor CRS* and 3.0 mg of *delta-3-cefaclor CRS* (impurity D) in the mobile phase and dilute to 10.0 ml with the mobile phase.

Column:
- *size*: l = 0.25 m, Ø = 4.6 mm;
- *stationary phase*: *octadecylsilyl silica gel for chromatography R* (5 µm).

Mobile phase: add 220 ml of *methanol R* to a mixture of 780 ml of *water R*, 10 ml of *triethylamine R* and 1 g of *sodium pentanesulphonate R*, then adjust to pH 2.5 with *phosphoric acid R*.

Flow rate: 1.5 ml/min.

Detection: spectrophotometer at 265 nm.

Injection: 20 µl.

System suitability:
- *resolution*: minimum 2.5 between the peaks due to cefaclor and impurity D in the chromatogram obtained with reference solution (b); if necessary, adjust the concentration of methanol in the mobile phase;
- *symmetry factor*: maximum 1.5 for the peak due to cefaclor in the chromatogram obtained with reference solution (b);
- *repeatability*: maximum relative standard deviation of 1.0 per cent after 6 injections of reference solution (a).

IMPURITIES

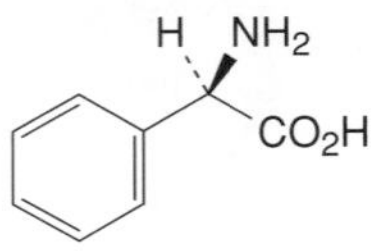

A. (2R)-2-amino-2-phenylacetic acid (phenylglycine),

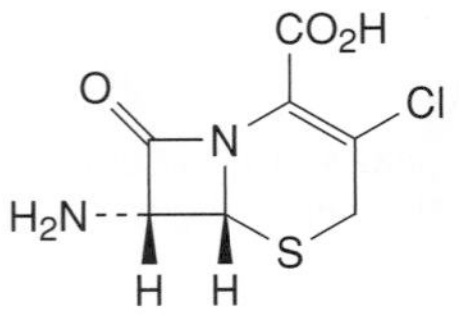

B. (6R,7R)-7-amino-3-chloro-8-oxo-5-thia-1-azabicyclo-[4.2.0]oct-2-ene-2-carboxylic acid,

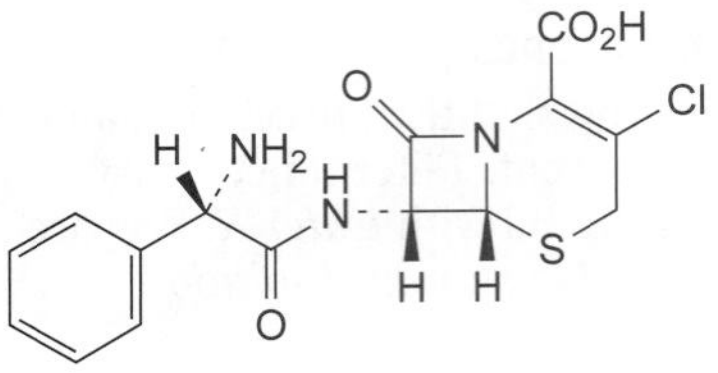

C. (6R,7R)-7-[[(2S)-2-amino-2-phenylacetyl]amino]-3-chloro-8-oxo-5-thia-1-azabicyclo[4.2.0]oct-2-ene-2-carboxylic acid,

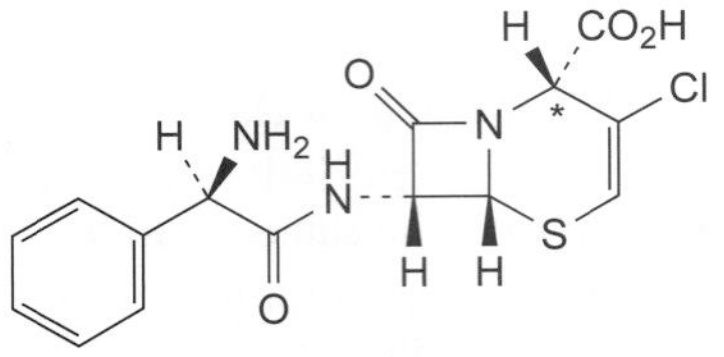

and epimer at C*

D. (2R,6R,7R)- and (2S,6R,7R)-7-[[(2R)-2-amino-2-phenylacetyl]amino]-3-chloro-8-oxo-5-thia-1-azabicyclo[4.2.0]oct-3-ene-2-carboxylic acid (delta-3-cefaclor),

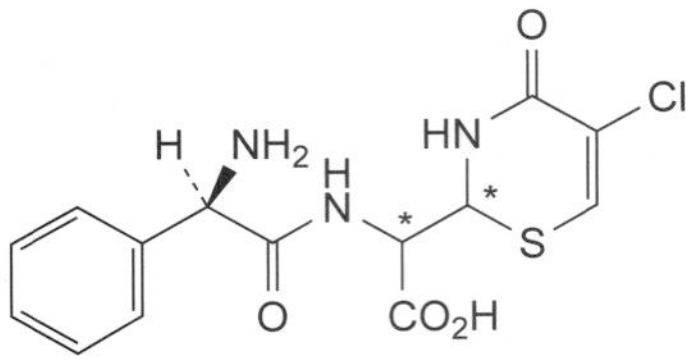

E. 2-[[(2R)-2-amino-2-phenylacetyl]amino]-2-(5-chloro-4-oxo-3,4-dihydro-2H-1,3-thiazin-2-yl)acetic acid,

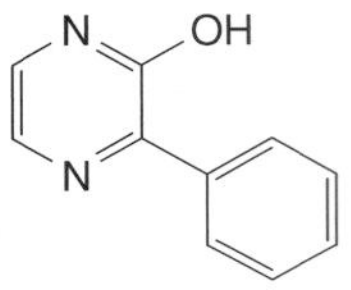

F. 3-phenylpyrazin-2-ol,

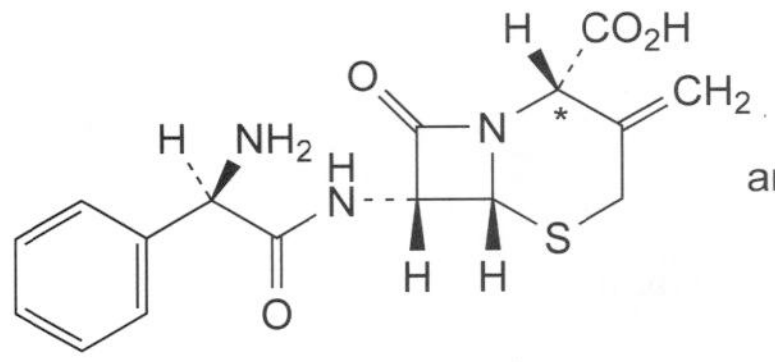

and epimer at C*

G. (2R,6R,7R)- and (2S,6R,7R)-7-[[(2R)-2-amino-2-phenylacetyl]amino]-3-methylene-8-oxo-5-thia-1-azabicyclo[4.2.0]octane-2-carboxylic acid (isocefalexine),

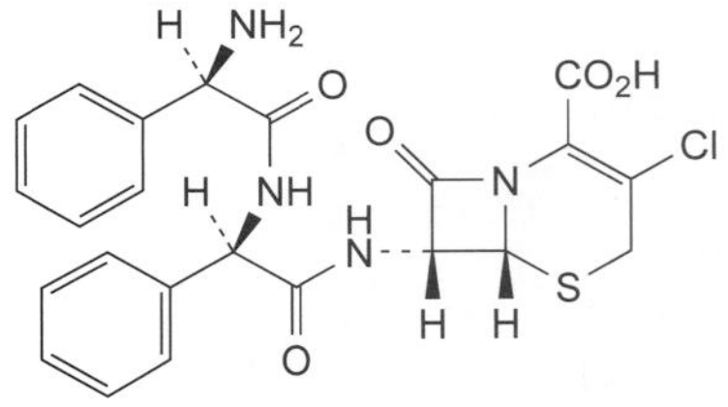

H. (6R,7R)-7-[[(2R)-2-[[(2R)-2-amino-2-phenylacetyl]amino]-2-phenylacetyl]amino]-3-chloro-8-oxo-5-thia-1-azabicyclo[4.2.0]oct-2-ene-2-carboxylic acid (N-phenylglycyl cefaclor).

04/2008:0813
corrected 6.5

CEFADROXIL MONOHYDRATE

Cefadroxilum monohydricum

$C_{16}H_{17}N_3O_5S,H_2O$ M_r 381.4

[66592-87-8]

DEFINITION

(6R,7R)-7-[[(2R)-2-Amino-2-(4-hydroxyphenyl)acetyl]amino]-3-methyl-8-oxo-5-thia-1-azabicyclo[4.2.0]oct-2-ene-2-carboxylic acid monohydrate.

Semi-synthetic product derived from a fermentation product.

Content: 95.0 per cent to 102.0 per cent (anhydrous substance).

CHARACTERS

Appearance: white or almost white powder.

Solubility: slightly soluble in water, very slightly soluble in ethanol (96 per cent).

IDENTIFICATION

Infrared absorption spectrophotometry (*2.2.24*).

Comparison: cefadroxil CRS.

TESTS

pH (*2.2.3*): 4.0 to 6.0.

Suspend 1.0 g in *carbon dioxide-free water R* and dilute to 20 ml with the same solvent.

Specific optical rotation (*2.2.7*): + 165 to + 178 (anhydrous substance).

Dissolve 0.500 g in *water R* and dilute to 50.0 ml with the same solvent.

Related substances. Liquid chromatography (*2.2.29*).

Test solution. Dissolve 50.0 mg of the substance to be examined in mobile phase A and dilute to 50.0 ml with mobile phase A.

Reference solution (a). Dissolve 10.0 mg of D-α-(4-hydroxyphenyl)glycine CRS (impurity A) in mobile phase A and dilute to 10.0 ml with mobile phase A.

Reference solution (b). Dissolve 10.0 mg of 7-aminodesacetoxycephalosporanic acid CRS (impurity B) in *phosphate buffer solution pH 7.0 R5* and dilute to 10.0 ml with the same buffer solution.

Reference solution (c). Dilute 1.0 ml of reference solution (a) and 1.0 ml of reference solution (b) to 100.0 ml with mobile phase A.

Reference solution (d). Dissolve 10 mg of *dimethylformamide R* and 10 mg of *dimethylacetamide R* in mobile phase A and dilute to 10.0 ml with mobile phase A. Dilute 1.0 ml of this solution to 100.0 ml with mobile phase A.

Reference solution (e). Dilute 1.0 ml of reference solution (c) to 25.0 ml with mobile phase A.

Column:
— *size*: l = 0.10 m, Ø = 4.6 mm,

— *stationary phase*: spherical *octadecylsilyl silica gel for chromatography R* (5 μm).

Mobile phase:
— *mobile phase A*: phosphate buffer solution pH 5.0 R,
— *mobile phase B*: methanol R2,

Time (min)	Mobile phase A (per cent V/V)	Mobile phase B (per cent V/V)
0 - 1	98	2
1 - 20	98 → 70	2 → 30
20 - 23	70 → 98	30 → 2
23 - 30	98	2

Flow rate: 1.5 ml/min.

Detection: spectrophotometer at 220 nm.

Injection: 20 μl of the test solution and reference solutions (c), (d) and (e).

Relative retention with reference to cefadroxil (retention time = about 6 min): dimethylformamide = about 0.4; dimethylacetamide = about 0.75.

System suitability:
— *resolution*: minimum 5.0 between the peaks due to impurities A and B in the chromatogram obtained with reference solution (c),
— *signal-to-noise ratio*: minimum 10 for the 2nd peak in the chromatogram obtained with reference solution (e).

Limits:
— *impurity A*: not more than the area of the 1st peak in the chromatogram obtained with reference solution (c) (1.0 per cent),
— *any other impurity*: for each impurity, not more than the area of the 2nd peak in the chromatogram obtained with reference solution (c) (1.0 per cent),
— *total*: not more than 3 times the area of the 2nd peak in the chromatogram obtained with reference solution (c) (3.0 per cent),
— *disregard limit*: 0.05 times the area of the 2nd peak in the chromatogram obtained with reference solution (c) (0.05 per cent); disregard the peaks due to dimethylformamide and dimethylacetamide.

N,N-Dimethylaniline (*2.4.26, Method B*): maximum 20 ppm.

Water (*2.5.12*): 4.0 per cent to 6.0 per cent, determined on 0.200 g.

Sulphated ash (*2.4.14*): maximum 0.5 per cent, determined on 1.0 g.

ASSAY

Liquid chromatography (*2.2.29*).

Test solution. Dissolve 50.0 mg of the substance to be examined in the mobile phase and dilute to 100.0 ml with the mobile phase.

Reference solution (a). Dissolve 50.0 mg of *cefadroxil CRS* in the mobile phase and dilute to 100.0 ml with the mobile phase.

Reference solution (b). Dissolve 5 mg of *cefadroxil CRS* and 50 mg of *amoxicillin trihydrate CRS* in the mobile phase and dilute to 100 ml with the mobile phase.

Column:
— *size*: l = 0.25 m, Ø = 4.6 mm,
— *stationary phase*: octadecylsilyl silica gel for chromatography R (5 μm).

Mobile phase: acetonitrile R, a 2.72 g/l solution of potassium dihydrogen phosphate R (4:96 V/V).

Flow rate: 1 ml/min.

Detection: spectrophotometer at 254 nm.

Injection: 20 µl.

System suitability: reference solution (b):

— *resolution*: minimum 5.0 between the peaks due to cefadroxil and to amoxicillin.

Calculate the percentage content of cefadroxil.

STORAGE

Protected from light.

IMPURITIES

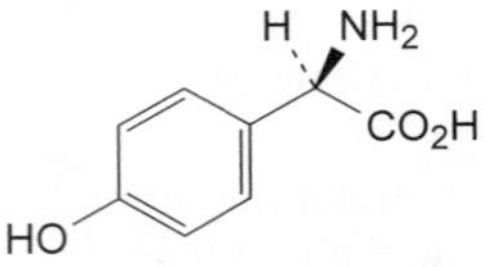

A. (2R)-2-amino-2-(4-hydroxyphenyl)acetic acid,

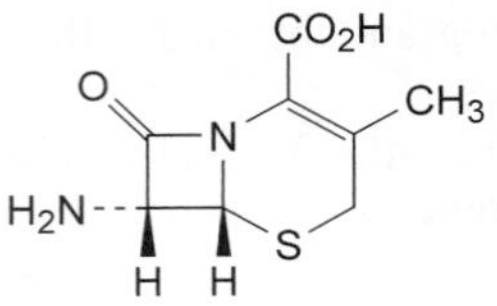

B. (6R,7R)-7-amino-3-methyl-8-oxo-5-thia-1-azabicyclo-[4.2.0]oct-2-ene-2-carboxylic acid (7-ADCA),

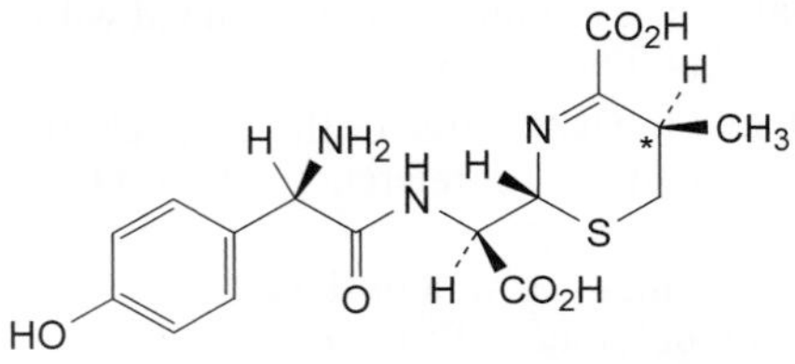

C. (2R,5RS)-2-[(R)-[[(2R)-2-amino-2-(4-hydroxyphenyl)-acetyl]amino]carboxymethyl]-5-methyl-5,6-dihydro-2H-1,3-thiazine-4-carboxylic acid,

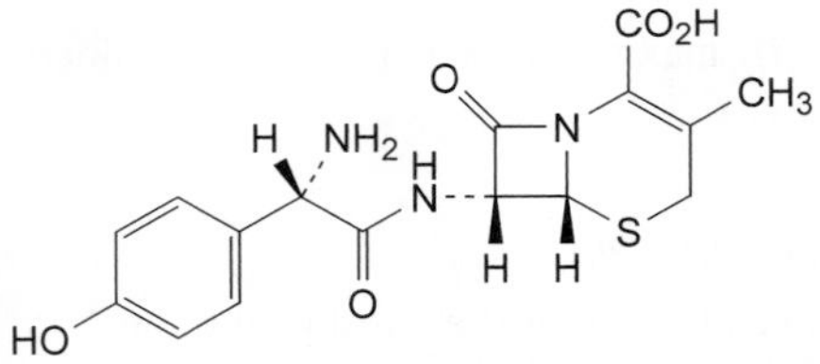

D. (6R,7R)-7-[[(2S)-2-amino-2-(4-hydroxyphenyl)-acetyl]amino]-3-methyl-8-oxo-5-thia-1-azabicyclo-[4.2.0]oct-2-ene-2-carboxylic acid (L-cefadroxil),

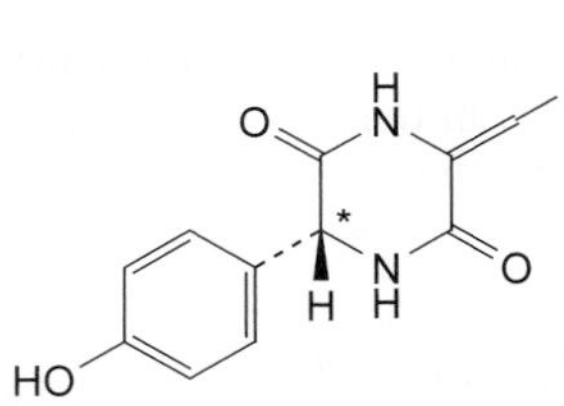

E. (6RS)-3-(aminomethylene)-6-(4-hydroxyphenyl)piperazine-2,5-dione,

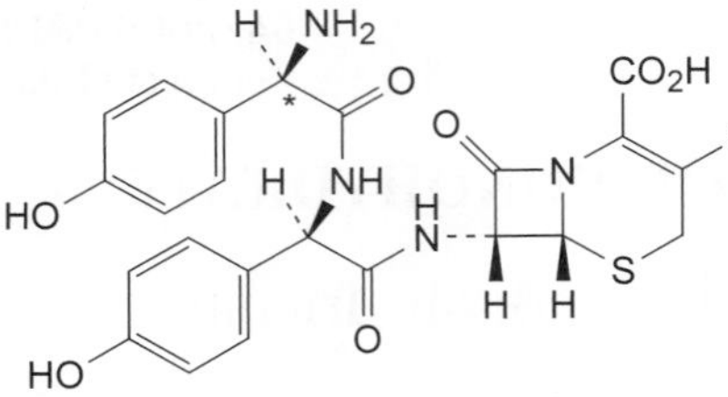

F. (6R,7R)-7-[[(2R)-2-[[(2RS)-2-amino-2-(4-hydroxyphenyl)-acetyl]amino]-2-(4-hydroxyphenyl)acetyl]amino]-3-methyl-8-oxo-5-thia-1-azabicyclo[4.2.0]oct-2-ene-2-carboxylic acid,

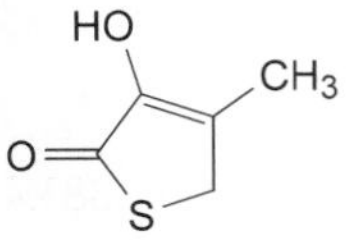

G. 3-hydroxy-4-methylthiophen-2(5H)-one,

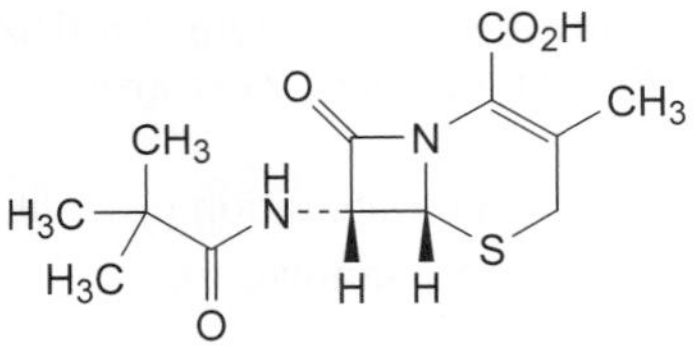

H. (6R,7R)-7-[(2,2-dimethylpropanoyl)amino]-3-methyl-8-oxo-5-thia-1-azabicyclo[4.2.0]oct-2-ene-2-carboxylic acid (7-ADCA pivalamide).

07/2009:1405

CEFTAZIDIME PENTAHYDRATE

Ceftazidimum pentahydricum

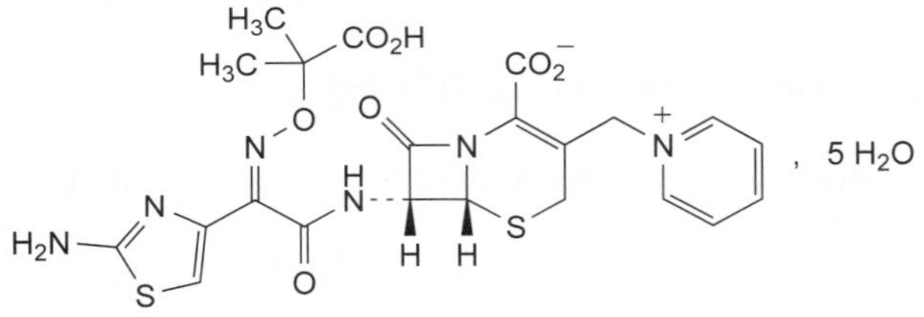

, 5 H$_2$O

$C_{22}H_{22}N_6O_7S_2,5H_2O$ M_r 637
[78439-06-2]

DEFINITION

(6R,7R)-7-[[(2Z)-2-(2-Aminothiazol-4-yl)-2-[(1-carboxy-1-methylethoxy)imino]acetyl]amino]-8-oxo-3-[(1-pyridinio)methyl]-5-thia-1-azabicyclo[4.2.0]oct-2-ene-2-carboxylate pentahydrate.

Semi-synthetic product derived from a fermentation product.

Content: 95.0 per cent to 102.0 per cent (anhydrous substance).

CHARACTERS

Appearance: white or almost white, crystalline powder.

Solubility: slightly soluble in water and in methanol, practically insoluble in acetone and in ethanol (96 per cent). It dissolves in acid and alkali solutions.

IDENTIFICATION

Infrared absorption spectrophotometry (*2.2.24*).

Comparison: ceftazidime CRS.

TESTS

Solution S. Dissolve 0.25 g in *carbon dioxide-free water R* and dilute to 50 ml with the same solvent.

Appearance of solution. Solution S is clear (*2.2.1*) and colourless (*2.2.2, Method II*).

pH (*2.2.3*): 3.0 to 4.0 for solution S.

Related substances. Liquid chromatography (*2.2.29*).

Test solution. Suspend 0.150 g of the substance to be examined in 5 ml of *acetonitrile R*, dissolve by adding *water R* and dilute to 100 ml with the same solvent.

Reference solution (a). To 1.0 ml of the test solution add 5.0 ml of *acetonitrile R* and dilute to 100.0 ml with *water R*. Dilute 1.0 ml of this solution to 5.0 ml with *water R*.

Reference solution (b). Suspend 3 mg of *ceftazidime impurity A CRS* and 3 mg of *ceftazidime CRS* in 5 ml of *acetonitrile R*, dissolve by adding *water R* and dilute to 20 ml with the same solvent. Dilute 1 ml of this solution to 20 ml with *water R*.

Reference solution (c). Suspend 3 mg of *ceftazidime for peak identification CRS* (containing impurities A, B and G) in 0.5 ml of *acetonitrile R*, dissolve by adding *water R* and dilute to 2 ml with the same solvent.

Column:
— *size*: l = 0.25 m, Ø = 4.6 mm;
— *stationary phase*: octadecylsilyl silica gel for chromatography R (5 µm);
— *temperature*: 40 °C.

Mobile phase:
— *mobile phase A*: solution containing 3.6 g of *disodium hydrogen phosphate R* and 1.4 g of *potassium dihydrogen phosphate R* in 1 litre of *water R*, adjusted to pH 3.4 with a 10 per cent *V/V* solution of *phosphoric acid R*;
— *mobile phase B*: acetonitrile for chromatography R;

Time (min)	Mobile phase A (per cent *V/V*)	Mobile phase B (per cent *V/V*)
0 - 4	96 → 89	4 → 11
4 - 5	89	11
5 - 8	89 → 84	11 → 16
8 - 11	84 → 80	16 → 20
11 - 15	80 → 50	20 → 50
15 - 18	50 → 20	50 → 80
18 - 22	20	80

Flow rate: 1.3 ml/min.

Detection: spectrophotometer at 254 nm.

Injection: 10 µl.

Relative retention with reference to ceftazidime (retention time = about 8 min): impurity F = about 0.4; impurity G = about 0.8; impurity A = about 0.9; impurity B = about 1.4.

Identification of impurities: use the chromatogram supplied with *ceftazidime for peak identification CRS* and the chromatogram obtained with reference solution (c) to identify the peaks due to impurities A, B and G.

System suitability: reference solution (b):
— *resolution*: minimum 4.0 between the peaks due to impurity A and ceftazidime.

Limits:
— *correction factor*: for the calculation of content, multiply the peak area of impurity G by 3.0;

— *impurities A, B, G*: for each impurity, not more than the area of the principal peak in the chromatogram obtained with reference solution (a) (0.2 per cent);
— *unspecified impurities*: for each impurity, not more than 0.5 times the area of the principal peak in the chromatogram obtained with reference solution (a) (0.10 per cent);
— *total*: not more than 5 times the area of the principal peak in the chromatogram obtained with reference solution (a) (1.0 per cent);
— *disregard limit*: 0.25 times the area of the principal peak in the chromatogram obtained with reference solution (a) (0.05 per cent); disregard the peak due to impurity F.

Impurity F. Liquid chromatography (*2.2.29*). *Prepare the solutions immediately before use.*

Test solution. Dissolve 0.500 g of the substance to be examined in a 10 per cent *V/V* solution of *phosphate buffer solution pH 7.0 R4* and dilute to 100.0 ml with the same solvent.

Reference solution (a). Dissolve 1.00 g of *pyridine R* in *water R* and dilute to 100.0 ml with the same solvent. Dilute 5.0 ml of this solution to 200.0 ml with *water R*. To 1.0 ml of this solution, add 10 ml of *phosphate buffer solution pH 7.0 R4* and dilute to 100.0 ml with *water R*.

Reference solution (b). Dilute 1 ml of the test solution to 200 ml with a 10 per cent *V/V* solution of *phosphate buffer solution pH 7.0 R4*. To 1 ml of this solution add 20 ml of reference solution (a) and dilute to 200 ml with a 10 per cent *V/V* solution of *phosphate buffer solution pH 7.0 R4*.

Column:
— *size*: l = 0.25 m, Ø = 4.6 mm;
— *stationary phase*: octadecylsilyl silica gel for chromatography R (5 µm).

Mobile phase: mix 8 volumes of a 28.8 g/l solution of *ammonium dihydrogen phosphate R* previously adjusted to pH 7.0 with *ammonia R*, 24 volumes of *acetonitrile R* and 68 volumes of *water R*.

Flow rate: 1.0 ml/min.

Detection: spectrophotometer at 255 nm.

Injection: 20 µl.

Run time: 10 min.

System suitability: reference solution (b):
— *resolution*: minimum 7.0 between the peaks due to ceftazidime and impurity F.

Limit:
— *impurity F*: not more than the area of the principal peak in the chromatogram obtained with reference solution (a) (500 ppm).

Heavy metals (*2.4.8*): maximum 20 ppm.

1.0 g complies with test F. Prepare the reference solution using 2.0 ml of *lead standard solution (10 ppm Pb) R*.

Water (*2.5.12*): 13.0 per cent to 15.0 per cent, determined on 0.100 g.

Bacterial endotoxins (*2.6.14*): less than 0.10 IU/mg, if intended for use in the manufacture of parenteral preparations without a further appropriate procedure for the removal of bacterial endotoxins.

ASSAY

Liquid chromatography (*2.2.29*).

Test solution. Dissolve 25.0 mg of the substance to be examined in the mobile phase and dilute to 25.0 ml with mobile phase.

Reference solution (a). Dissolve 25.0 mg of *ceftazidime CRS* in the mobile phase and dilute to 25.0 ml with the mobile phase.

Reference solution (b). Dissolve 5.0 mg of *ceftazidime impurity A CRS* in 5.0 ml of reference solution (a).

Column:
- *size*: l = 0.15 m, Ø = 4.6 mm;
- *stationary phase*: *hexylsilyl silica gel for chromatography R* (5 µm).

Mobile phase: dissolve 4.3 g of *disodium hydrogen phosphate R* and 2.7 g of *potassium dihydrogen phosphate R* in 980 ml of *water R*, then add 20 ml of *acetonitrile R*.

Flow rate: 2 ml/min.

Detection: spectrophotometer at 245 nm.

Injection: 20 µl.

Run time: 6 min.

Relative retention with reference to ceftazidime (retention time = about 4.5 min): impurity A = about 0.7.

System suitability: reference solution (b):
- *resolution*: minimum 1.5 between the peaks due to impurity A and ceftazidime.

Calculate the content of ceftazidime ($C_{22}H_{22}N_6O_7S_2$) from the declared content of $C_{22}H_{22}N_6O_7S_2$ in *ceftazidime CRS*.

STORAGE

In an airtight container. If the substance is sterile, store in a sterile, airtight, tamper-proof container.

IMPURITIES

Specified impurities: A, B, F, G.

Other detectable impurities (the following substances would, if present at a sufficient level, be detected by one or other of the tests in the monograph. They are limited by the general acceptance criterion for other/unspecified impurities and/or by the general monograph *Substances for pharmaceutical use (2034)*. It is therefore not necessary to identify these impurities for demonstration of compliance. See also *5.10. Control of impurities in substances for pharmaceutical use*): *C, E, H.*

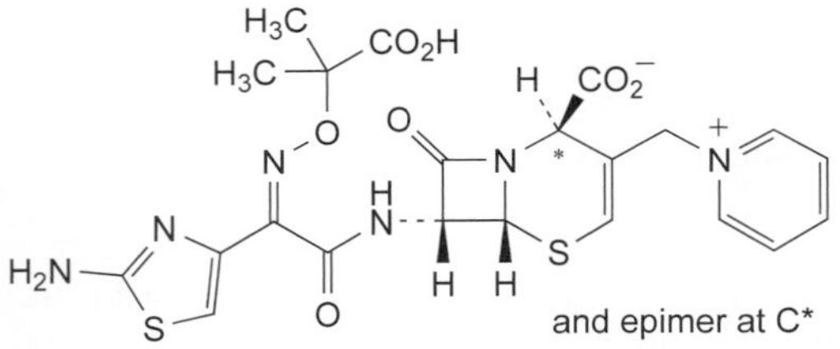

A. (2RS,6R,7R)-7-[[(2Z)-2-(2-aminothiazol-4-yl)-2-[(1-carboxy-1-methylethoxy)imino]acetyl]amino]-8-oxo-3-[(1-pyridinio)methyl]-5-thia-1-azabicyclo[4.2.0]oct-3-ene-2-carboxylate (Δ-2-ceftazidime),

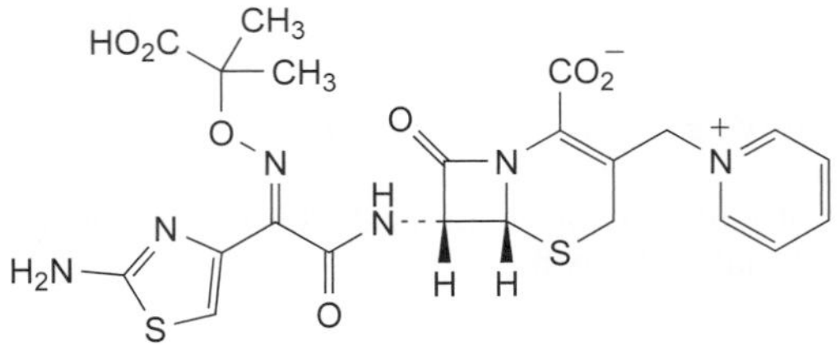

B. (6R,7R)-7-[[(2E)-2-(2-aminothiazol-4-yl)-2-[(1-carboxy-1-methylethoxy)imino]acetyl]amino]-8-oxo-3-[(1-pyridinio)methyl]-5-thia-1-azabicyclo[4.2.0]oct-2-ene-2-carboxylate,

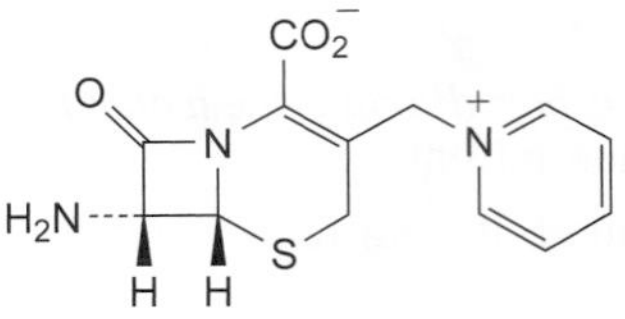

C. (6R,7R)-7-amino-8-oxo-3-[(1-pyridinio)methyl]-5-thia-1-azabicyclo[4.2.0]oct-2-ene-2-carboxylate,

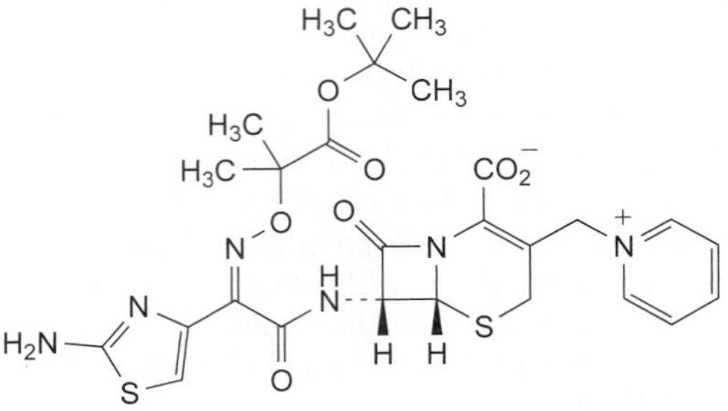

E. (6R,7R)-7-[[(2Z)-2-(2-aminothiazol-4-yl)-2-[[2-(1,1-dimethylethoxy)-1,1-dimethyl-2-oxoethoxy]imino]acetyl]amino]-8-oxo-3-[(1-pyridinio)methyl]-5-thia-1-azabicyclo[4.2.0]oct-2-ene-2-carboxylate,

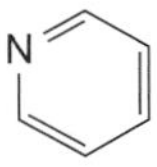

F. pyridine,

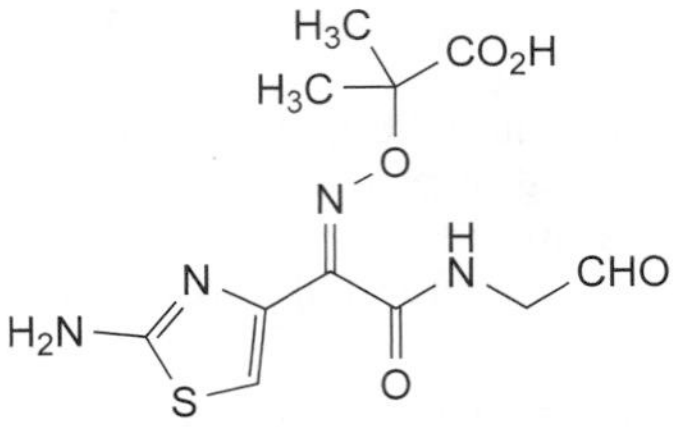

G. 2-[[[(1Z)-1-(2-aminothiazol-4-yl)-2-[(oxoethyl)amino]-2-oxoethylidene]amino]oxy]-2-methylpropanoic acid,

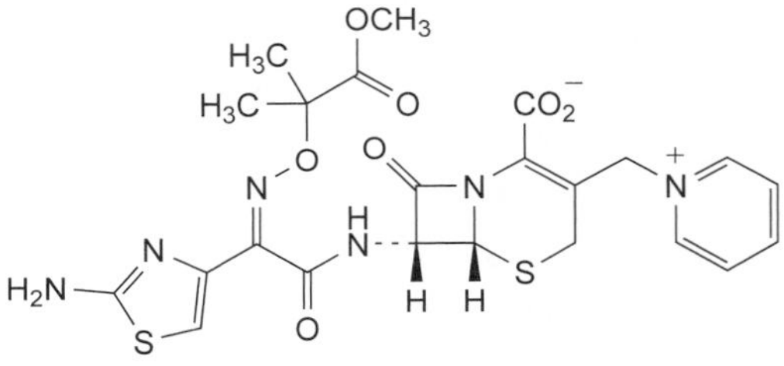

H. (6R,7R)-7-[[(2Z)-2-(2-aminothiazol-4-yl)-2-[(2-methoxy-1,1-dimethyl-2-oxoethoxy)imino]acetyl]amino]-8-oxo-3-[(1-pyridinio)methyl]-5-thia-1-azabicyclo[4.2.0]oct-2-ene-2-carboxylate.

07/2009:2344

CEFTAZIDIME PENTAHYDRATE WITH SODIUM CARBONATE FOR INJECTION

Ceftazidimum pentahydricum et natrii carbonas ad iniectabile

DEFINITION

Sterile mixture of *Ceftazidime pentahydrate (1405)* and *Anhydrous sodium carbonate (0773)*.

Ceftazidime pentahydrate is a semi-synthetic product derived from a fermentation product.

Content:

— *ceftazidime*: 93.0 per cent to 105.0 per cent (dried and carbonate-free substance);

— *sodium carbonate*: 8.0 per cent to 10.0 per cent.

CHARACTERS

Appearance: white or pale yellow powder.

Solubility: freely soluble in water and in methanol, practically insoluble in acetone.

IDENTIFICATION

A. Examine the chromatograms obtained in the assay.

Results: the principal peak in the chromatogram obtained with the test solution is similar in retention time to the principal peak in the chromatogram obtained with reference solution (a).

B. It gives the reaction of carbonates (*2.3.1*).

TESTS

Solution S. Dissolve 2.60 g in *carbon dioxide-free water R* and dilute to 20.0 ml with the same solvent.

Appearance of solution. Solution S is clear (*2.2.1*) and its absorbance (*2.2.25*) at 425 nm is not greater than 0.50.

pH (*2.2.3*): 5.0 to 7.5 for solution S.

Related substances. Liquid chromatography (*2.2.29*).

Test solution. Suspend 0.150 g of the substance to be examined in 5 ml of *acetonitrile R*, dissolve by adding *water R* and dilute to 100 ml with the same solvent.

Reference solution (a). To 1.0 ml of the test solution add 5.0 ml of *acetonitrile R* and dilute to 100.0 ml with *water R*. Dilute 1.0 ml of this solution to 5.0 ml with *water R*.

Reference solution (b). Suspend 3 mg of *ceftazidime CRS* and 3 mg of *ceftazidime impurity A CRS* in 5 ml of *acetonitrile R*, dissolve by adding *water R* and dilute to 20 ml with the same solvent. Dilute 1 ml of this solution to 20 ml with *water R*.

Reference solution (c). Suspend 3 mg of *ceftazidime for peak identification CRS* (containing impurities A, B and G) in 0.5 ml of *acetonitrile R*, dissolve by adding *water R* and dilute to 2 ml with the same solvent.

Column:

— *size*: l = 0.25 m, Ø = 4.6 mm;

— *stationary phase*: *octadecylsilyl silica gel for chromatography R* (5 µm);

— *temperature*: 40 °C.

Mobile phase:

— *mobile phase A*: solution containing 3.6 g of *disodium hydrogen phosphate R* and 1.4 g of *potassium dihydrogen phosphate R* in 1 litre of *water R*, adjusted to pH 3.4 with a 10 per cent *V/V* solution of *phosphoric acid R*;

— *mobile phase B*: *acetonitrile for chromatography R*;

Time (min)	Mobile phase A (per cent *V/V*)	Mobile phase B (per cent *V/V*)
0 - 4	96 → 89	4 → 11
4 - 5	89	11
5 - 8	89 → 84	11 → 16
8 - 11	84 → 80	16 → 20
11 - 15	80 → 50	20 → 50
15 - 18	50 → 20	50 → 80
18 - 22	20	80

Flow rate: 1.3 ml/min.

Detection: spectrophotometer at 254 nm.

Injection: 10 µl.

Relative retention with reference to ceftazidime (retention time = about 8 min): impurity F = about 0.4; impurity G = about 0.8; impurity A = about 0.9; impurity B = about 1.4.

Identification of impurities: use the chromatogram supplied with *ceftazidime for peak identification CRS* and the chromatogram obtained with reference solution (c) to identify the peaks due to impurities A, B and G.

System suitability: reference solution (b):

— *resolution*: minimum 4.0 between the peaks due to impurity A and ceftazidime.

Limits:

— *correction factor*: for the calculation of content, multiply the peak area of impurity G by 3.0;

— *impurities A, B, G*: for each impurity, not more than the area of the principal peak in the chromatogram obtained with reference solution (a) (0.2 per cent);

— *unspecified impurities*: for each impurity, not more than 0.5 times the area of the principal peak in the chromatogram obtained with reference solution (a) (0.10 per cent);

— *total*: not more than 5 times the area of the principal peak in the chromatogram obtained with reference solution (a) (1.0 per cent);

— *disregard limit*: 0.25 times the area of the principal peak in the chromatogram obtained with reference solution (a) (0.05 per cent); disregard the peak due to impurity F.

Impurity F. Liquid chromatography (*2.2.29*). *Prepare the solutions immediately before use.*

Test solution. Dissolve 0.500 g of the substance to be examined in a 10 per cent *V/V* phosphate buffer solution pH 7.0 R4 and dilute to 100.0 ml with the same buffer solution.

Reference solution (a). Dissolve 1.00 g of *pyridine R* in *water R* and dilute to 100.0 ml with the same solvent. Dilute 5.0 ml of this solution to 200.0 ml with *water R*. To 1.0 ml of this solution add 10.0 ml of *phosphate buffer solution pH 7.0 R4* and dilute to 100.0 ml with *water R*.

Reference solution (b). Dilute 1.0 ml of the test solution to 200.0 ml with a 10 per cent *V/V* phosphate buffer solution pH 7.0 R4. To 1.0 ml of this solution add 20.0 ml of reference solution (a) and dilute to 200.0 ml with a 10 per cent *V/V* phosphate buffer solution pH 7.0 R4.

Column:

— *size*: l = 0.25 m, Ø = 4.6 mm;

— *stationary phase*: *octadecylsilyl silica gel for chromatography R* (5 µm).

Mobile phase: mix 8 volumes of a 28.8 g/l solution of *ammonium dihydrogen phosphate R* previously adjusted to pH 7.0 with *ammonia R*, 24 volumes of *acetonitrile R* and 68 volumes of *water R*.

Flow rate: 1.0 ml/min.

Detection: spectrophotometer at 255 nm.

Injection: 20 µl.

Run time: 10 min.

System suitability: reference solution (b):

— *resolution*: minimum 7.0 between the peaks due to ceftazidime and impurity F.

Limit:

— *impurity F*: not more than 6 times the area of the principal peak in the chromatogram obtained with reference solution (a) (0.3 per cent).

Loss on drying (*2.2.32*): maximum 13.5 per cent, determined on 0.300 g. Dry *in vacuo* at 25 °C at a pressure not exceeding 0.67 kPa for 4 h then heat the residue *in vacuo* at 100 °C at a pressure not exceeding 0.67 kPa for 3 h.

Bacterial endotoxins (*2.6.14*): less than 0.10 IU/mg, if intended for use in the manufacture of parenteral preparations without a further appropriate procedure for the removal of bacterial endotoxins.

ASSAY

Ceftazidime. Liquid chromatography (*2.2.29*).

Test solution. Dissolve 25.0 mg of the substance to be examined in the mobile phase and dilute to 25.0 ml with the mobile phase.

Reference solution (a). Dissolve 25.0 mg of *ceftazidime CRS* in the mobile phase and dilute to 25.0 ml with the mobile phase.

Reference solution (b). Dissolve 5.0 mg of *ceftazidime impurity A CRS* in 5.0 ml of reference solution (a).

Column:

— *size*: l = 0.15 m, Ø = 4.6 mm;

— *stationary phase*: *hexylsilyl silica gel for chromatography R* (5 μm).

Mobile phase: dissolve 4.3 g of *disodium hydrogen phosphate R* and 2.7 g of *potassium dihydrogen phosphate R* in 980 ml of *water R*, then add 20 ml of *acetonitrile R*.

Flow rate: 2 ml/min.

Detection: spectrophotometer at 245 nm.

Injection: 20 μl.

Run time: 6 min.

Relative retention with reference to ceftazidime (retention time = about 4.5 min): impurity A = about 0.7.

System suitability: reference solution (b):

— *resolution*: minimum 1.5 between the peaks due to impurity A and ceftazidime.

Calculate the content of ceftazidime ($C_{22}H_{22}N_6O_7S_2$) from the declared content of $C_{22}H_{22}N_6O_7S_2$ in *ceftazidime CRS*.

Sodium carbonate. Atomic absorption spectrometry (*2.2.23, Method I*).

Caesium chloride buffer solution. To 12.7 g of *caesium chloride R* add 500 ml of *water R* and 86 ml of *hydrochloric acid R* and dilute to 1000.0 ml with *water R*.

Sodium standard solution (1000 mg/l). Dissolve 3.70 g of *sodium nitrate R* in *water R* and dilute to 500 ml with the same solvent, add 48.5 g of *nitric acid R* and dilute to 1000 ml with *water R*.

Test solution. Dissolve 650.0 mg of the substance to be examined in *water R* and dilute to 100.0 ml with the same solvent. To 10.0 ml of this solution add 5.0 ml of caesium chloride buffer solution and dilute to 50.0 ml with *water R*.

Reference solution. Into 4 identical flasks, each containing 20.0 ml of caesium chloride buffer solution, introduce respectively 0 ml, 5.00 ml, 10.00 ml and 15.00 ml of sodium standard solution (1000 mg/l) and dilute to 200.0 ml with *water R*.

Source: sodium hollow-cathode lamp.

Wavelength: 330.2 nm to 330.3 nm.

Atomisation device: air-acetylene flame.

Calculate the percentage content of sodium carbonate.

STORAGE

In a sterile, airtight, tamper-proof container, protected from light and humidity.

LABELLING

The label states the percentage content *m/m* of ceftazidime.

IMPURITIES

Specified impurities: A, B, F, G.

Other detectable impurities (the following substances would, if present at a sufficient level, be detected by one or other of the tests in the monograph. They are limited by the general acceptance criterion for other/unspecified impurities and/or by the general monograph *Substances for pharmaceutical use (2034)*. It is therefore not necessary to identify these impurities for demonstration of compliance. See also *5.10. Control of impurities in substances for pharmaceutical use*): *C, E, H*.

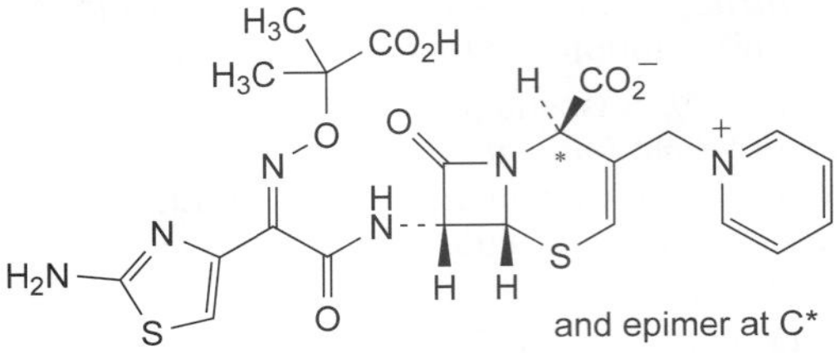

A. (2RS,6R,7R)-7-[[(2Z)-2-(2-aminothiazol-4-yl)-2-[(1-carboxy-1-methylethoxy)imino]acetyl]amino]-8-oxo-3-[(1-pyridinio)methyl]-5-thia-1-azabicyclo[4.2.0]oct-3-ene-2-carboxylate (Δ-2-ceftazidime),

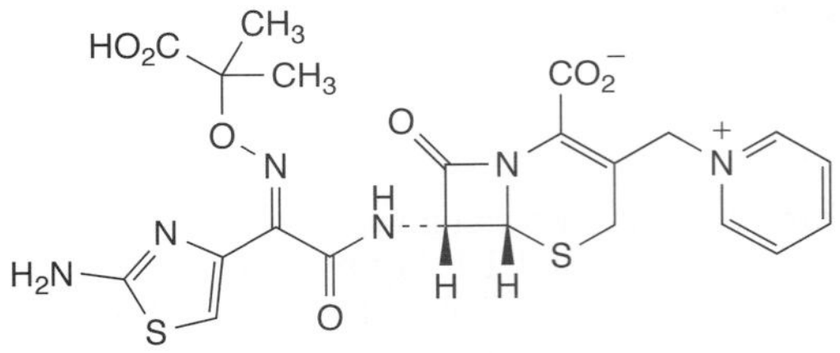

B. (6R,7R)-7-[[(2E)-2-(2-aminothiazol-4-yl)-2-[(1-carboxy-1-methylethoxy)imino]acetyl]amino]-8-oxo-3-[(1-pyridinio)methyl]-5-thia-1-azabicyclo[4.2.0]oct-2-ene-2-carboxylate,

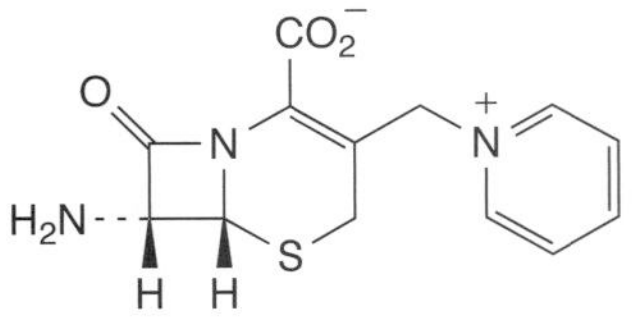

C. (6R,7R)-7-amino-8-oxo-3-[(1-pyridinio)methyl]-5-thia-1-azabicyclo[4.2.0]oct-2-ene-2-carboxylate,

Monographs
A-C

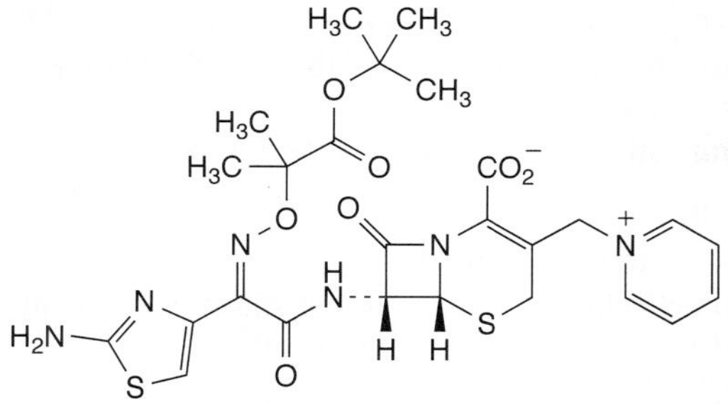

E. (6R,7R)-7-[[(2Z)-2-(2-aminothiazol-4-yl)-2-[[2-(1,1-dimethylethoxy)-1,1-dimethyl-2-oxoethoxy]imino]acetyl]-amino]-8-oxo-3-[(1-pyridinio)methyl]-5-thia-1-azabicyclo[4.2.0]oct-2-ene-2-carboxylate,

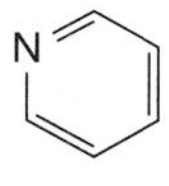

F. pyridine,

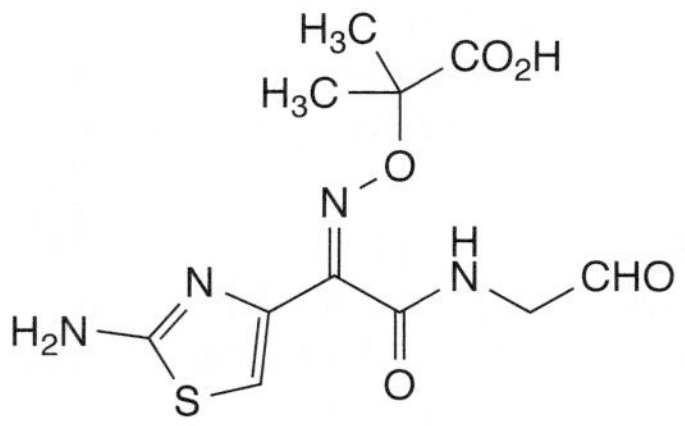

G. 2-[[[(1Z)-1-(2-aminothiazol-4-yl)-2-[(oxoethyl)amino]-2-oxoethylidene]amino]oxy]-2-methylpropanoic acid,

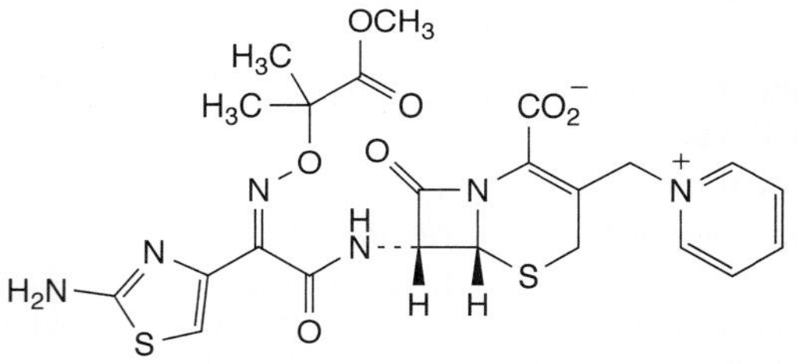

H. (6R,7R)-7-[[(2Z)-2-(2-aminothiazol-4-yl)-2-[(2-methoxy-1,1-dimethyl-2-oxoethoxy)imino]acetyl]amino]-8-oxo-3-[(1-pyridinio)methyl]-5-thia-1-azabicyclo[4.2.0]oct-2-ene-2-carboxylate.

01/2008:1774
corrected 6.5

CHITOSAN HYDROCHLORIDE

Chitosani hydrochloridum

DEFINITION

Chitosan hydrochloride is the chloride salt of an unbranched binary heteropolysaccharide consisting of the two units N-acetyl-D-glucosamine and D-glucosamine, obtained by partial deacetylation of chitin normally leading to a degree of deacetylation of 70.0 per cent to 95.0 per cent. Chitin is extracted from the shells of shrimp and crab.

PRODUCTION

The animals from which chitosan hydrochloride is derived must fulfil the requirements for the health of animals suitable for human consumption to the satisfaction of the competent authority. It must have been shown to what extent the method of production allows inactivation or removal of any contamination by viruses or other infectious agents.

CHARACTERS

Appearance: white or almost white, fine powder.

Solubility: sparingly soluble in water, practically insoluble in anhydrous ethanol.

IDENTIFICATION

A. Infrared absorption spectrophotometry (2.2.24).

Preparation: discs.

Comparison: chitosan hydrochloride CRS.

B. It gives reaction (a) of chlorides (2.3.1).

C. Dilute 50 ml of solution S (see Tests) to 250 ml with a 25 per cent V/V solution of *ammonia R*. A voluminous gelatinous mass is formed.

D. To 10 ml of solution S add 90 ml of *acetone R*. A voluminous gelatinous mass is formed.

TESTS

Solution S. Dissolve 1.0 g in 100 ml of *water R* and stir vigorously for 20 min with a mechanical stirrer.

Appearance of solution. Solution S is not more opalescent than reference suspension II (2.2.1) and not more intensely coloured than reference solution BY_5 (2.2.2, Method II).

Matter insoluble in water: maximum 0.5 per cent.

Add 2.00 g to 400.0 ml of *water R* while stirring until no further dissolution takes place. Transfer the solution to a 2 litre beaker, and add 200 ml of *water R*. Boil the solution gently for 2 h, covering the beaker during the operation. Filter through a sintered-glass filter (40) (2.1.2), wash the residue with water and dry to constant weight in an oven at 100-105 °C. The residue weighs a maximum of 10 mg.

pH (2.2.3): 4.0 to 6.0 for solution S.

Viscosity (2.2.10): 80 per cent to 120 per cent of the value stated on the label, determined on solution S.

Determine the viscosity using a rotating viscometer at 20 °C with a spindle rotating at 20 r/min, using a suitable spindle for the range of the expected viscosity.

Degree of deacetylation

Test solution. Dissolve 0.250 g in *water R* and dilute to 50.0 ml with the same solvent, stirring vigorously. Dilute 1.0 ml of this solution to 100.0 ml with *water R*. Measure the absorbance (2.2.25) from 200 nm to 205 nm as the first derivative of the absorbance curve. Determine the pH of the solution.

Reference solutions. Prepare solutions of 1.0 µg/ml, 5.0 µg/ml, 15.0 µg/ml and 35.0 µg/ml of *N-acetylglucosamine R* in *water R*. Measure the absorbance (2.2.25) from 200 nm to 205 nm of each solution as the first derivative of the absorption curve. Make a standard curve by plotting the first derivative at 202 nm as a function of the concentration of N-acetylglucosamine, and calculate the slope of the curve by least squares linear regression. Use the standard curve to determine the equivalent amount of N-acetylglucosamine for the substance to be examined.

Calculate the degree of deacetylation (molar) using the following expression:

$$\frac{100 \times M_1 \times (C_1 - C_2)}{(M_1 \times C_1) - [(M_1 - M_3) \times C_2]}$$

C_1 = concentration of chitosan hydrochloride in the test solution in micrograms per millilitre;

C_2 = concentration of N-acetylglucosamine in the test solution, as determined from the standard curve prepared using the reference solution in micrograms per millilitre;

M_1 = 203 (relative molecular mass of N-acetylglucosamine unit ($C_8H_{13}NO_5$) in polymer);

M_3 = relative molecular mass of chitosan hydrochloride.

M_3 is calculated from the pH in solution, assuming a pKa value of 6.8, using the following equations:

$$M_3 = f \times M_2 + (1 - f) \times (M_2 + 36.5)$$

$$f = \frac{p}{1 + p}$$

$$p = 10^{(pH - pKa)}$$

M_2 = 161 (relative molecular mass of deacetylated unit (glucosamine) ($C_6H_{11}NO_4$) in polymer).

Chlorides: 10.0 per cent to 20.0 per cent.

Introduce 0.200 g into a 250 ml borosilicate flask fitted with a reflux condenser. Add 40 ml of a mixture of 1 volume of *nitric acid R* and 2 volumes of *water R*. Boil gently under a reflux condenser for 5 min. Cool and add 25 ml of *water R* through the condenser. Add 16.0 ml of *0.1 M silver nitrate*, shake vigorously and titrate with *0.1 M ammonium thiocyanate*, using 1 ml of *ferric ammonium sulphate solution R2* as indicator, and shaking vigorously towards the end-point. Carry out a blank titration.

1 ml of *0.1 M silver nitrate* is equivalent to 3.55 mg of Cl.

Heavy metals (*2.4.8*): maximum 40 ppm.

1.0 g complies with test F. Prepare the reference solution using 4 ml of *lead standard solution (10 ppm Pb) R*.

Loss on drying (*2.2.32*): maximum 10 per cent, determined on 1.000 g by drying in an oven at 105 °C.

Sulphated ash (*2.4.14*): maximum 1.0 per cent, determined on 1.0 g.

STORAGE

At a temperature of 2-8 °C, protected from moisture and light.

LABELLING

The label states the nominal viscosity in millipascal seconds for a 10 g/l solution in *water R*.

01/2008:0575
corrected 6.5

CHOLECALCIFEROL CONCENTRATE (OILY FORM)

Cholecalciferolum densatum oleosum

DEFINITION

Solution of *Cholecalciferol (0072)* in a suitable vegetable fatty oil, authorised by the competent authority.

Content: 90.0 per cent to 110.0 per cent of the cholecalciferol content stated on the label, which is not less than 500 000 IU/g.

It may contain suitable stabilisers such as antioxidants.

CHARACTERS

Appearance: clear, yellow liquid.

Solubility: practically insoluble in water, slightly soluble in anhydrous ethanol, miscible with solvents of fats.

Partial solidification may occur, depending on the temperature.

IDENTIFICATION

First identification: A, C.

Second identification: A, B.

A. Thin-layer chromatography (*2.2.27*). *Prepare the solutions immediately before use.*

Test solution. Dissolve an amount of the preparation to be examined corresponding to 400 000 IU in *ethylene chloride R* containing 10 g/l of *squalane R* and 0.1 g/l of *butylhydroxytoluene R* and dilute to 4 ml with the same solution.

Reference solution (a). Dissolve 10 mg of *cholecalciferol CRS* in *ethylene chloride R* containing 10 g/l of *squalane R* and 0.1 g/l of *butylhydroxytoluene R* and dilute to 4 ml with the same solution.

Reference solution (b). Dissolve 10 mg of *ergocalciferol CRS* in *ethylene chloride R* containing 10 g/l of *squalane R* and 0.1 g/l of *butylhydroxytoluene R* and dilute to 4 ml with the same solution.

Plate: *TLC silica gel G plate R.*

Mobile phase: a 0.1 g/l solution of *butylhydroxytoluene R* in a mixture of equal volumes of *cyclohexane R* and *peroxide-free ether R*.

Application: 20 µl.

Development: immediately, protected from light, over a path of 15 cm.

Drying: in air.

Detection: spray with *sulphuric acid R*.

Results: the chromatogram obtained with the test solution shows immediately a bright yellow principal spot which rapidly becomes orange-brown, then gradually greenish-grey, remaining so for 10 min. This spot is similar in position, colour and size to the spot in the chromatogram obtained with reference solution (a). The chromatogram obtained with reference solution (b) shows immediately at the same level an orange principal spot which gradually becomes reddish-brown and remains so for 10 min.

B. Ultraviolet and visible absorption spectrophotometry (*2.2.25*).

Test solution. Prepare a solution in *cyclohexane R* containing the equivalent of about 400 IU/ml.

Spectral range: 250-300 nm.

Absorption maximum: at 267 nm.

C. Examine the chromatograms obtained in the assay.

Results: the principal peak in the chromatogram obtained with the test solution is similar in retention time to the principal peak in the chromatogram obtained with reference solution (a).

TESTS

Acid value (*2.5.1*): maximum 2.0.

Dissolve 5.0 g in 25 ml of the prescribed mixture of solvents.

Peroxide value (*2.5.5, Method A*): maximum 20.

Related substances

The thresholds indicated under Related substances (Table 2034.-1) in the general monograph *Substances for pharmaceutical use (2034)* do not apply.

ASSAY

Carry out the assay as rapidly as possible, avoiding exposure to actinic light and air.

Liquid chromatography (*2.2.29*).

Test solution. Dissolve a quantity of the preparation to be examined, weighed with an accuracy of 0.1 per cent, equivalent to about 400 000 IU, in 10.0 ml of *toluene R* and dilute to 100.0 ml with the mobile phase.

Reference solution (a). Dissolve 10.0 mg of *cholecalciferol CRS* without heating in 10.0 ml of *toluene R* and dilute to 100.0 ml with the mobile phase.

Reference solution (b). Dilute 1.0 ml of *cholecalciferol for system suitability CRS* to 5.0 ml with the mobile phase. Heat in a water-bath at 90 °C under a reflux condenser for 45 min and cool.

Reference solution (c). Dissolve 0.10 g of *cholecalciferol CRS* without heating in *toluene R* and dilute to 100.0 ml with the same solvent.

Reference solution (d). Dilute 5.0 ml of reference solution (c) to 50.0 ml with the mobile phase. Keep the solution in iced water.

Reference solution (e). Place 5.0 ml of reference solution (c) in a volumetric flask, add about 10 mg of *butylhydroxytoluene R* and displace air from the flask with *nitrogen R*. Heat in a water-bath at 90 °C under a reflux condenser protected from light and under *nitrogen R* for 45 min. Cool and dilute to 50.0 ml with the mobile phase.

Column:

— *size*: l = 0.25 m, Ø = 4.6 mm;

— *stationary phase*: *silica gel for chromatography R* (5 μm).

Mobile phase: *pentanol R*, *hexane R* (3:997 *V/V*).

Flow rate: 2 ml/min.

Detection: spectrophotometer at 254 nm.

Injection: the chosen volume of each solution (the same volume for reference solution (a) and for the test solution); automatic injection device or sample loop recommended.

Relative retention with reference to cholecalciferol: pre-cholecalciferol = about 0.4; *trans*-cholecalciferol = about 0.5.

System suitability: reference solution (b):

— *resolution*: minimum 1.0 between the peaks due to pre-cholecalciferol and *trans*-cholecalciferol; if necessary adjust the proportions of the constituents and the flow rate of the mobile phase to obtain this resolution;

— *repeatability*: maximum relative standard deviation of 1.0 per cent for the peak due to cholecalciferol after 6 injections.

Calculate the conversion factor (*f*) using the following expression:

$$\frac{K - L}{M}$$

K = area (or height) of the peak due to cholecalciferol in the chromatogram obtained with reference solution (d);

L = area (or height) of the peak due to cholecalciferol in the chromatogram obtained with reference solution (e);

M = area (or height) of the peak due to pre-cholecalciferol in the chromatogram obtained with reference solution (e).

The value of *f* determined in duplicate on different days may be used during the entire procedure.

Calculate the content of cholecalciferol in International Units per gram using the following expression:

$$\frac{m'}{V'} \times \frac{V}{m} \times \frac{S_D + (f \times S_p)}{S'_D} \times 40\,000 \times 1000$$

m = mass of the preparation to be examined in the test solution, in milligrams;

m' = mass of *cholecalciferol CRS* in reference solution (a), in milligrams;

V = volume of the test solution (100 ml);

V' = volume of reference solution (a) (100 ml);

S_D = area (or height) of the peak due to cholecalciferol in the chromatogram obtained with the test solution;

S'_D = area (or height) of the peak due to cholecalciferol in the chromatogram obtained with reference solution (a);

S_p = area (or height) of the peak due to pre-cholecalciferol in the chromatogram obtained with the test solution;

f = conversion factor.

STORAGE

In an airtight, well-filled container, protected from light. The contents of an opened container are to be used as soon as possible; any unused part is to be protected by an atmosphere of nitrogen.

LABELLING

The label states:

— the number of International Units per gram;

— the method of restoring the solution if partial solidification occurs.

01/2008:0574
corrected 6.5

CHOLECALCIFEROL CONCENTRATE (POWDER FORM)

Cholecalciferoli pulvis

DEFINITION

Powder concentrate obtained by dispersing an oily solution of *Cholecalciferol (0072)* in an appropriate matrix, which is usually based on a combination of gelatin and carbohydrates of suitable quality, authorised by the competent authority.

Content: 90.0 per cent to 110.0 per cent of the cholecalciferol content stated on the label, which is not less than 100 000 IU/g.

It may contain suitable stabilisers such as antioxidants.

CHARACTERS

Appearance: white or yellowish-white, small particles.

Solubility: practically insoluble, swells, or forms a dispersion in water, depending on the formulation.

IDENTIFICATION

First identification: A, C.

Second identification: A, B.

A. Thin-layer chromatography (*2.2.27*). *Prepare the solutions immediately before use.*

Test solution. Place 10.0 ml of the test solution prepared for the assay in a suitable flask and evaporate to dryness under reduced pressure by swirling in a water-bath at 40 °C. Cool under running water and restore atmospheric pressure with *nitrogen R*. Dissolve the residue immediately in 0.4 ml of *ethylene chloride R* containing 10 g/l of *squalane R* and 0.1 g/l of *butylhydroxytoluene R*.

Reference solution (a). Dissolve 10 mg of *cholecalciferol CRS* in *ethylene chloride R* containing 10 g/l of *squalane R* and 0.1 g/l of *butylhydroxytoluene R* and dilute to 4 ml with the same solution.

Reference solution (b). Dissolve 10 mg of *ergocalciferol CRS* in *ethylene chloride R* containing 10 g/l of *squalane R* and 0.1 g/l of *butylhydroxytoluene R* and dilute to 4 ml with the same solution.

Plate: TLC silica gel G plate R.

Mobile phase: a 0.1 g/l solution of *butylhydroxytoluene R* in a mixture of equal volumes of *cyclohexane R* and *peroxide-free ether R*.

Application: 20 µl.

Development: immediately, protected from light, over a path of 15 cm.

Drying: in air.

Detection: spray with *sulphuric acid R*.

Results: the chromatogram obtained with the test solution shows immediately a bright yellow principal spot, which rapidly becomes orange-brown, then gradually greenish-grey, remaining so for 10 min. This spot is similar in position, colour and size to the spot in the chromatogram obtained with reference solution (a). The chromatogram obtained with reference solution (b) shows immediately at the same level an orange principal spot, which gradually becomes reddish-brown and remains so for 10 min.

B. Ultraviolet and visible absorption spectrophotometry (*2.2.25*).

Test solution. Place 5.0 ml of the test solution prepared for the assay in a suitable flask and evaporate to dryness under reduced pressure by swirling in a water-bath at 40 °C. Cool under running water and restore atmospheric pressure with *nitrogen R*. Dissolve the residue immediately in 50.0 ml of *cyclohexane R*.

Spectral range: 250-300 nm.

Absorption maximum: at 265 nm.

C. Examine the chromatograms obtained in the assay.

Results: the principal peak in the chromatogram obtained with the test solution is similar in retention time to the principal peak in the chromatogram obtained with reference solution (a).

TESTS

Related substances

The thresholds indicated under Related substances (Table 2034.-1) in the general monograph *Substances for pharmaceutical use (2034)* do not apply.

ASSAY

Carry out the assay as rapidly as possible, avoiding exposure to actinic light and air.

Liquid chromatography (*2.2.29*).

Test solution. Introduce into a saponification flask a quantity of the preparation to be examined, weighed with an accuracy of 0.1 per cent, equivalent to about 100 000 IU. Add 5 ml of *water R*, 20 ml of *anhydrous ethanol R*, 1 ml of *sodium ascorbate solution R* and 3 ml of a freshly prepared 50 per cent *m/m* solution of *potassium hydroxide R*. Heat in a water-bath under a reflux condenser for 30 min. Cool rapidly under running water. Transfer the liquid to a separating funnel with the aid of 2 quantities, each of 15 ml, of *water R*, 1 quantity of 10 ml of *ethanol (96 per cent) R* and 2 quantities, each of 50 ml, of *pentane R*. Shake vigorously for 30 s. Allow to stand until the 2 layers are clear. Transfer the lower aqueous-alcoholic layer to a 2nd separating funnel and shake with a mixture of 10 ml of *ethanol (96 per cent) R* and 50 ml of *pentane R*. After separation, transfer the aqueous-alcoholic layer to a 3rd separating funnel and the pentane layer to the 1st separating funnel, washing the 2nd separating funnel with 2 quantities, each of 10 ml, of *pentane R* and adding the washings to the 1st separating funnel. Shake the aqueous-alcoholic layer with 50 ml of *pentane R* and add the pentane layer to the 1st funnel. Wash the pentane layer with 2 quantities, each of 50 ml, of a freshly prepared 30 g/l solution of *potassium hydroxide R* in *ethanol (10 per cent V/V) R*, shaking vigorously, then wash with successive quantities, each of 50 ml, of *water R* until the washings are neutral to phenolphthalein. Transfer the washed pentane extract to a ground-glass-stoppered flask. Evaporate the contents of the flask to dryness under reduced pressure by swirling in a water-bath at 40 °C. Cool under running water and restore atmospheric pressure with *nitrogen R*. Dissolve the residue immediately in 5.0 ml of *toluene R* and add 20.0 ml of the mobile phase to obtain a solution containing about 4000 IU/ml.

Reference solution (a). Dissolve 10.0 mg of *cholecalciferol CRS*, without heating, in 10.0 ml of *toluene R* and dilute to 100.0 ml with the mobile phase.

Reference solution (b). Dilute 1.0 ml of *cholecalciferol for system suitability CRS* to 5.0 ml with the mobile phase. Heat in a water-bath at 90 °C under a reflux condenser for 45 min and cool.

Reference solution (c). Dissolve 0.10 g of *cholecalciferol CRS*, without heating, in *toluene R* and dilute to 100.0 ml with the same solvent.

Reference solution (d). Dilute 5.0 ml of reference solution (c) to 50.0 ml with the mobile phase. Keep the solution in iced water.

Reference solution (e). Place 5.0 ml of reference solution (c) in a volumetric flask, add about 10 mg of *butylhydroxytoluene R* and displace the air from the flask with *nitrogen R*. Heat in a water-bath at 90 °C under a reflux condenser, protected from light and under *nitrogen R*, for 45 min. Cool and dilute to 50.0 ml with the mobile phase.

Column:
— *size*: l = 0.25 m, Ø = 4.6 mm;
— *stationary phase*: *silica gel for chromatography R* (5 µm).

Mobile phase: pentanol R, hexane R (3:997 V/V).

Flow rate: 2 ml/min.

Detection: spectrophotometer at 254 nm.

Injection: the chosen volume of each solution (the same volume for reference solution (a) and for the test solution); automatic injection device or sample loop recommended.

Relative retention with reference to cholecalciferol: pre-cholecalciferol = about 0.4; *trans*-cholecalciferol = about 0.5.

System suitability: reference solution (b):

— *resolution*: minimum 1.0 between the peaks due to pre-cholecalciferol and *trans*-cholecalciferol; if necessary, adjust the proportions of the constituents and the flow rate of the mobile phase to obtain this resolution;

— *repeatability*: maximum relative standard deviation of 1.0 per cent for the peak due to cholecalciferol after 6 injections.

Calculate the conversion factor (*f*) using the following expression:

$$\frac{K - L}{M}$$

K = area (or height) of the peak due to cholecalciferol in the chromatogram obtained with reference solution (d);

L = area (or height) of the peak due to cholecalciferol in the chromatogram obtained with reference solution (e);

M = area (or height) of the peak due to pre-cholecalciferol in the chromatogram obtained with reference solution (e).

The value of *f* determined in duplicate on different days may be used during the entire procedure.

Calculate the content of cholecalciferol in International Units per gram using the following expression:

$$\frac{m'}{V'} \times \frac{V}{m} \times \frac{S_D + (f \times S_p)}{S'_D} \times 40\ 000 \times 1000$$

m = mass of the preparation to be examined in the test solution, in milligrams;

m' = mass of *cholecalciferol CRS* in reference solution (a), in milligrams;

V = volume of the test solution (25 ml);

V' = volume of reference solution (a) (100 ml);

S_D = area (or height) of the peak due to cholecalciferol in the chromatogram obtained with the test solution;

S'_D = area (or height) of the peak due to cholecalciferol in the chromatogram obtained with reference solution (a);

S_p = area (or height) of the peak due to pre-cholecalciferol in the chromatogram obtained with the test solution;

f = conversion factor.

STORAGE

In an airtight, well-filled container, protected from light. The contents of an opened container are to be used as soon as possible; any unused part is to be protected by an atmosphere of nitrogen.

LABELLING

The label states the number of International Units per gram.

01/2008:0598
corrected 6.5

CHOLECALCIFEROL CONCENTRATE (WATER-DISPERSIBLE FORM)

Cholecalciferolum in aqua dispergibile

DEFINITION

Solution of *Cholecalciferol (0072)* in a suitable vegetable fatty oil, authorised by the competent authority, to which suitable solubilisers have been added.

Content: 90.0 per cent to 115.0 per cent of the cholecalciferol content stated on the label, which is not less than 100 000 IU/g.

It may contain suitable stabilisers such as antioxidants.

CHARACTERS

Appearance: slightly yellowish liquid of variable opalescence and viscosity.

Highly concentrated solutions may become cloudy at low temperatures or form a gel at room temperature.

IDENTIFICATION

First identification: A, C, D.

Second identification: A, B, D.

A. Thin-layer chromatography (*2.2.27*). *Prepare the solutions immediately before use.*

Test solution. Place 10.0 ml of the test solution prepared for the assay in a suitable flask and evaporate to dryness under reduced pressure by swirling in a water-bath at 40 °C. Cool under running water and restore atmospheric pressure with *nitrogen R*. Dissolve the residue immediately in 0.4 ml of *ethylene chloride R* containing 10 g/l of *squalane R* and 0.1 g/l of *butylhydroxytoluene R*.

Reference solution (a). Dissolve 10 mg of *cholecalciferol CRS* in *ethylene chloride R* containing 10 g/l of *squalane R* and 0.1 g/l of *butylhydroxytoluene R* and dilute to 4 ml with the same solution.

Reference solution (b). Dissolve 10 mg of *ergocalciferol CRS* in *ethylene chloride R* containing 10 g/l of *squalane R* and 0.1 g/l of *butylhydroxytoluene R* and dilute to 4 ml with the same solution.

Plate: TLC silica gel G plate R.

Mobile phase: a 0.1 g/l solution of *butylhydroxytoluene R* in a mixture of equal volumes of *cyclohexane R* and *peroxide-free ether R*.

Application: 20 µl.

Development: immediately, protected from light, over a path of 15 cm.

Drying: in air.

Detection: spray with *sulphuric acid R*.

Results: the chromatogram obtained with the test solution shows immediately a bright yellow principal spot, which rapidly becomes orange-brown, then gradually greenish-grey, remaining so for 10 min. This spot is similar in position, colour and size to the principal spot in the chromatogram obtained with reference solution (a). The chromatogram obtained with reference solution (b) shows immediately at the same level an orange principal spot, which gradually becomes reddish-brown and remains so for 10 min.

B. Ultraviolet and visible absorption spectrophotometry (*2.2.25*).

Test solution. Place 5.0 ml of the test solution prepared for the assay in a suitable flask and evaporate to dryness under reduced pressure by swirling in a water-bath at 40 °C. Cool under running water and restore atmospheric pressure with *nitrogen R*. Dissolve the residue immediately in 50.0 ml of *cyclohexane R*.

Spectral range: 250-300 nm.

Absorption maximum: at 265 nm.

C. Examine the chromatograms obtained in the assay.

Results: the principal peak in the chromatogram obtained with the test solution is similar in retention time to the principal peak in the chromatogram obtained with reference solution (a).

D. Mix about 1 g with 10 ml of *water R* previously warmed to 50 °C, and cool to 20 °C. Immediately after cooling, a uniform, slightly opalescent and slightly yellow dispersion is obtained.

TESTS

Related substances

The thresholds indicated under Related substances (Table 2034.-1) in the general monograph *Substances for pharmaceutical use (2034)* do not apply.

ASSAY

Carry out the assay as rapidly as possible, avoiding exposure to actinic light and air.

Liquid chromatography (*2.2.29*).

Test solution. Introduce into a saponification flask a quantity of the preparation to be examined, weighed with an accuracy of 0.1 per cent, equivalent to about 100 000 IU. Add 5 ml of *water R*, 20 ml of *anhydrous ethanol R*, 1 ml of *sodium ascorbate solution R* and 3 ml of a freshly prepared 50 per cent *m/m* solution of *potassium hydroxide R*. Heat in a water-bath under a reflux condenser for 30 min. Cool rapidly under running water. Transfer the liquid to a separating funnel with the aid of 2 quantities, each of 15 ml, of *water R*, 1 quantity of 10 ml of *ethanol (96 per cent) R* and 2 quantities, each of 50 ml, of *pentane R*. Shake vigorously for 30 s. Allow to stand until the 2 layers are clear. Transfer the aqueous-alcoholic layer to a 2nd separating funnel and shake with a mixture of 10 ml of *ethanol (96 per cent) R* and 50 ml of *pentane R*. After separation, transfer the aqueous-alcoholic layer to a 3rd separating funnel and the pentane layer to the 1st separating funnel, washing the 2nd separating funnel with 2 quantities, each of 10 ml, of *pentane R* and adding the washings to the 1st separating funnel. Shake the aqueous-alcoholic layer with 50 ml of *pentane R* and add the pentane layer to the 1st funnel. Wash the pentane layer with 2 quantities, each of 50 ml, of a freshly prepared 30 g/l solution of *potassium hydroxide R* in *ethanol (10 per cent V/V) R*, shaking vigorously, and then wash with successive quantities, each of 50 ml, of *water R* until the washings are neutral to phenolphthalein. Transfer the washed pentane extract to a ground-glass-stoppered flask. Evaporate the contents of the flask to dryness under reduced pressure by swirling in a water-bath at 40 °C. Cool under running water and restore atmospheric pressure with *nitrogen R*. Dissolve the residue immediately in 5.0 ml of *toluene R* and add 20.0 ml of the mobile phase to obtain a solution containing about 4000 IU/ml.

Reference solution (a). Dissolve 10.0 mg of *cholecalciferol CRS*, without heating, in 10.0 ml of *toluene R* and dilute to 100.0 ml with the mobile phase.

Reference solution (b). Dilute 1.0 ml of *cholecalciferol for system suitability CRS* to 5.0 ml with the mobile phase. Heat in a water-bath at 90 °C under a reflux condenser for 45 min and cool.

Reference solution (c). Dissolve 0.10 g of *cholecalciferol CRS*, without heating, in *toluene R* and dilute to 100.0 ml with the same solvent.

Reference solution (d). Dilute 5.0 ml of reference solution (c) to 50.0 ml with the mobile phase. Keep the solution in iced water.

Reference solution (e). Place 5.0 ml of reference solution (c) in a volumetric flask, add about 10 mg of *butylhydroxytoluene R* and displace the air from the flask with *nitrogen R*. Heat in a water-bath at 90 °C under a reflux condenser, protected from light and under *nitrogen R*, for 45 min. Cool and dilute to 50.0 ml with the mobile phase.

Column:
— *size*: l = 0.25 m, $\varnothing$ = 4.6 mm;
— *stationary phase*: *silica gel for chromatography R* (5 μm).

Mobile phase: pentanol R, hexane R (3:997 *V/V*).

Flow rate: 2 ml/min.

Detection: spectrophotometer at 254 nm.

Injection: the chosen volume of each solution (the same volume for reference solution (a) and for the test solution); automatic injection device or sample loop recommended.

Relative retention with reference to cholecalciferol: pre-cholecalciferol = about 0.4; *trans*-cholecalciferol = about 0.5.

System suitability: reference solution (b):
— *resolution*: minimum 1.0 between the peaks due to pre-cholecalciferol and *trans*-cholecalciferol; if necessary, adjust the proportions of the constituents and the flow rate of the mobile phase to obtain this resolution;
— *repeatability*: maximum relative standard deviation of 1.0 per cent for the peak due to cholecalciferol after 6 injections.

Calculate the conversion factor (*f*) using the following expression:

$$\frac{K - L}{M}$$

K = area (or height) of the peak due to cholecalciferol in the chromatogram obtained with reference solution (d);

L = area (or height) of the peak due to cholecalciferol in the chromatogram obtained with reference solution (e);

M = area (or height) of the peak due to pre-cholecalciferol in the chromatogram obtained with reference solution (e).

The value of *f* determined in duplicate on different days may be used during the entire procedure.

Calculate the content of cholecalciferol in International Units per gram using the following expression:

$$\frac{m'}{V'} \times \frac{V}{m} \times \frac{S_D + (f \times S_P)}{S'_D} \times 40\,000 \times 1000$$

m = mass of the preparation to be examined in the test solution, in milligrams;

m' = mass of *cholecalciferol CRS* in reference solution (a), in milligrams;

V = volume of the test solution (25 ml);

V' = volume of reference solution (a) (100 ml);

S_D = area (or height) of the peak due to cholecalciferol in the chromatogram obtained with the test solution;

S'_D = area (or height) of the peak due to cholecalciferol in the chromatogram obtained with reference solution (a);

S_p = area (or height) of the peak due to pre-cholecalciferol in the chromatogram obtained with the test solution;

f = conversion factor.

STORAGE

In an airtight, well-filled container, protected from light, at the temperature stated on the label.

The contents of an opened container are to be used as soon as possible; any unused part is to be protected by an atmosphere of inert gas.

LABELLING

The label states:

– the number of International Units per gram;

– the storage temperature.

01/2009:0985
corrected 6.5

CROSCARMELLOSE SODIUM

Carmellosum natricum conexum

DEFINITION

Cross-linked sodium carboxymethylcellulose.

Sodium salt of a cross-linked, partly O-carboxymethylated cellulose.

CHARACTERS

Appeareance: white or greyish-white powder.

Solubility: practically insoluble in acetone, in anhydrous ethanol and in toluene.

IDENTIFICATION

A. Mix 1 g with 100 ml of a solution containing 4 ppm of *methylene blue R*, stir the mixture and allow it to settle. The substance to be examined absorbs the methylene blue and settles as a blue, fibrous mass.

B. Mix 1 g with 50 ml of *water R*. Transfer 1 ml of the mixture to a small test-tube and add 1 ml of *water R* and 0.05 ml of a freshly prepared 40 g/l solution of *α-naphthol R* in *methanol R*. Incline the test-tube and carefully add 2 ml of *sulphuric acid R* down the side so that it forms a lower layer. A reddish-violet colour develops at the interface.

C. The solution prepared from the sulphated ash in the test for heavy metals (see Tests) gives reaction (a) of sodium (*2.3.1*).

TESTS

pH (*2.2.3*): 5.0 to 7.0 for the suspension.

Shake 1 g with 100 ml of *carbon dioxide-free water R* for 5 min.

Sodium chloride and sodium glycollate: maximum 0.5 per cent (dried substance) for the sum of the percentage contents of sodium chloride and sodium glycollate.

Sodium chloride. Place 5.00 g in a 250 ml conical flask, add 50 ml of *water R* and 5 ml of *strong hydrogen peroxide*

solution R and heat on a water-bath for 20 min, stirring occasionally to ensure total hydration. Cool, add 100 ml of *water R* and 10 ml of *nitric acid R*. Titrate with *0.05 M silver nitrate*, determining the end-point potentiometrically (*2.2.20*) using a silver indicator electrode and a double-junction reference electrode containing a 100 g/l solution of *potassium nitrate R* in the outer jacket and a standard filling solution in the inner jacket, and stirring constantly.

1 ml of *0.05 M silver nitrate* is equivalent to 2.922 mg of NaCl.

Sodium glycollate. Place a quantity of the substance to be examined equivalent to 0.500 g of the dried substance in a 100 ml beaker. Add 5 ml of *glacial acetic acid R* and 5 ml of *water R* and stir to ensure total hydration (about 15 min). Add 50 ml of *acetone R* and 1 g of *sodium chloride R*. Stir for several minutes to ensure complete precipitation of the carboxymethylcellulose. Filter through a fast filter paper impregnated with *acetone R* into a volumetric flask, rinse the beaker and the filter with 30 ml of *acetone R* and dilute the filtrate to 100.0 ml with the same solvent. Allow to stand for 24 h without shaking. Use the clear supernatant to prepare the test solution.

Prepare the reference solutions as follows: in a 100 ml volumetric flask, dissolve 0.100 g of *glycollic acid R*, previously dried *in vacuo* over *diphosphorus pentoxide R* at room temperature overnight, in *water R* and dilute to 100.0 ml with the same solvent; use the solution within 30 days; transfer 1.0 ml, 2.0 ml, 3.0 ml and 4.0 ml of the solution to separate volumetric flasks, dilute the contents of each flask to 5.0 ml with *water R*, add 5 ml of *glacial acetic acid R*, dilute to 100.0 ml with *acetone R* and mix.

Transfer 2.0 ml of the test solution and 2.0 ml of each of the reference solutions to separate 25 ml volumetric flasks. Heat the uncovered flasks for 20 min on a water-bath to eliminate acetone. Allow to cool and add 5.0 ml of *2,7-dihydroxynaphthalene solution R* to each flask. Mix, add a further 15.0 ml of *2,7-dihydroxynaphthalene solution R* and mix again. Close the flasks with aluminium foil and heat on a water-bath for 20 min. Cool and dilute to 25.0 ml with *sulphuric acid R*.

Measure the absorbance (*2.2.25*) of each solution at 540 nm. Prepare a blank using 2.0 ml of a solution containing 5 per cent *V/V* each of *glacial acetic acid R* and *water R* in *acetone R*. Prepare a standard curve using the absorbances obtained with the reference solutions. From the standard curve and the absorbance of the test solution, determine the mass (*a*) of glycollic acid in the substance to be examined, in milligrams, and calculate the content of sodium glycollate using the following expression:

$$\frac{10 \times 1.29 \times a}{(100 - b)\, m}$$

1.29 = the factor converting glycollic acid to sodium glycollate;

b = loss on drying as a percentage;

m = mass of the substance to be examined, in grams.

Water-soluble substances: maximum 10.0 per cent.

Disperse 10.00 g in 800.0 ml of *water R* and stir for 1 min every 10 min during the first 30 min. Allow to stand for 1 h and centrifuge if necessary. Decant 200.0 ml of the supernatant liquid onto a fast filter paper in a vacuum filtration funnel, apply vacuum and collect 150.0 ml of the filtrate. Evaporate to dryness and dry the residue at 100-105 °C for 4 h.

Heavy metals (*2.4.8*): maximum 20 ppm.

To the residue obtained in the determination of the sulphated ash add 1 ml of *hydrochloric acid R* and evaporate on a water-bath. Take up the residue in 20 ml of *water R*. 12 ml of the solution complies with test A. Prepare the reference solution using *lead standard solution (1 ppm Pb) R*.

Loss on drying (*2.2.32*): maximum 10.0 per cent, determined on 1.000 g by drying in an oven at 105 °C for 6 h.

Sulphated ash(*2.4.14*): 14.0 per cent to 28.0 per cent (dried substance), determined on 1.0 g, using a mixture of equal volumes of *sulphuric acid R* and *water R*.

Microbial contamination

TAMC: acceptance criterion 10^3 CFU/g (*2.6.12*).

TYMC: acceptance criterion 10^2 CFU/g (*2.6.12*).

Absence of *Escherichia coli* (*2.6.13*).

FUNCTIONALITY-RELATED CHARACTERISTICS

This section provides information on characteristics that are recognised as being relevant control parameters for one or more functions of the substance when used as an excipient (see chapter 5.15). This section is a non-mandatory part of the monograph and it is not necessary to verify the characteristics to demonstrate compliance. Control of these characteristics can however contribute to the quality of a medicinal product by improving the consistency of the manufacturing process and the performance of the medicinal product during use. Where control methods are cited, they are recognised as being suitable for the purpose, but other methods can also be used. Wherever results for a particular characteristic are reported, the control method must be indicated.

The following characteristics may be relevant for croscarmellose sodium used as disintegrant.

Settling volume. Place 75 ml of *water R* in a 100 ml graduated cylinder and add 1.5 g of the substance to be examined in 0.5 g portions, shaking vigorously after each addition. Dilute to 100.0 ml with *water R* and shake again until the substance is homogeneously distributed. Allow to stand for 4 h. The settling volume is between 10.0 ml and 30.0 ml.

Degree of substitution: 0.60 to 0.85 (dried substance).

Place 1.000 g in a 500 ml conical flask, add 300 ml of a 100 g/l solution of *sodium chloride R* and 25.0 ml of *0.1 M sodium hydroxide*, stopper the flask and allow to stand for 5 min, shaking occasionally. Add 0.05 ml of *m-cresol purple solution R* and about 15 ml of *0.1 M hydrochloric acid* from a burette. Insert the stopper and shake. If the solution is violet, add *0.1 M hydrochloric acid* in 1 ml portions until the solution becomes yellow, shaking after each addition. Titrate with *0.1 M sodium hydroxide* until the colour turns to violet.

Calculate the number of milliequivalents (*M*) of base required to neutralise the equivalent of 1 g of dried substance.

Calculate the degree of acid carboxymethyl substitution (*A*) using the following expression:

$$\frac{1150M}{(7102 - 412M - 80C)}$$

C = sulphated ash as a percentage.

Calculate the degree of sodium carboxymethyl substitution (*S*) using the following expression:

$$\frac{(162 + 58A)\,C}{(7102 - 80C)}$$

The degree of substitution is the sum of *A* and *S*.

Particle size distribution (*2.9.31* or *2.9.38*).

Hausner ratio (*2.9.36*).

07/2009:0817

CYPROHEPTADINE HYDROCHLORIDE

Cyproheptadini hydrochloridum

, HCl , $1\frac{1}{2}$ H_2O

$C_{21}H_{22}ClN,1\frac{1}{2}H_2O$ M_r 350.9

[41354-29-4]

DEFINITION

4-(5*H*-Dibenzo[*a,d*][7]annulen-5-ylidene)-1-methylpiperidine hydrochloride sesquihydrate.

Content: 98.5 per cent to 101.0 per cent (anhydrous substance).

CHARACTERS

Appearance: white or slightly yellow, crystalline powder.

Solubility: slightly soluble in water, freely soluble in methanol, sparingly soluble in ethanol (96 per cent).

IDENTIFICATION

A. Infrared absorption spectrophotometry (*2.2.24*).

   Comparison: cyproheptadine hydrochloride CRS.

B. A saturated solution gives reaction (b) of chlorides (*2.3.1*).

TESTS

Acidity. Dissolve 0.10 g in *water R* and dilute to 25 ml with the same solvent. Add 0.1 ml of *methyl red solution R*. Not more than 0.15 ml of *0.01 M sodium hydroxide* is required to change the colour of the indicator.

Related substances. Liquid chromatography (*2.2.29*).

Test solution. Dissolve 40.0 mg of the substance to be examined in mobile phase A and dilute to 20.0 ml with mobile phase A.

Reference solution (a). Dilute 1.0 ml of the test solution to 100.0 ml with mobile phase A. Dilute 1.0 ml of this solution to 10.0 ml with mobile phase A.

Reference solution (b). Dissolve 2.0 mg of dibenzocycloheptene CRS (impurity A), 2.0 mg of dibenzosuberone CRS (impurity B) and 2.0 mg of cyproheptadine impurity C CRS in mobile phase A, add 1.0 ml of the test solution and dilute to 100.0 ml with mobile phase A.

Reference solution (c). Dilute 1.0 ml of reference solution (b) to 10.0 ml with mobile phase A.

Column:

– *size*: *l* = 0.25 m, Ø = 4.6 mm;

– *stationary phase*: *octylsilyl silica gel for chromatography R* (5 μm).

Mobile phase:

– *mobile phase A*: dissolve 6.12 g of *potassium dihydrogen phosphate R* in 900 ml of *water R*, adjust to pH 4.5 with *phosphoric acid R* and dilute to 1000 ml with *water R*; mix 60 volumes of this solution and 40 volumes of *acetonitrile for chromatography R*;

– *mobile phase B*: dissolve 6.12 g of *potassium dihydrogen phosphate R* in 900 ml of *water R*, adjust to pH 4.5 with *phosphoric acid R* and dilute to 1000 ml with *water R*; mix 40 volumes of this solution and 60 volumes of *acetonitrile for chromatography R*;

Time (min)	Mobile phase A (per cent *V/V*)	Mobile phase B (per cent *V/V*)
0 - 10.0	100	0
10.0 - 10.1	100 → 0	0 → 100
10.1 - 35	0	100

Flow rate: 1.0 ml/min.

Detection: spectrophotometer at 230 nm.

Injection: 10 µl.

Relative retention with reference to cyproheptadine (retention time = about 8 min): impurity C = about 0.7; impurity B = about 2.6; impurity A = about 3.9.

System suitability: reference solution (b):

– *resolution*: minimum 7.0 between the peaks due to impurity C and cyproheptadine.

Limits:

– *impurities A, B, C*: for each impurity, not more than 1.5 times the area of the corresponding peak in the chromatogram obtained with reference solution (c) (0.15 per cent);

– *unspecified impurities*: for each impurity, not more than the area of the principal peak in the chromatogram obtained with reference solution (a) (0.10 per cent);

– *total*: not more than 5 times the area of the principal peak in the chromatogram obtained with reference solution (a) (0.5 per cent);

– *disregard limit*: 0.5 times the area of the principal peak in the chromatogram obtained with reference solution (a) (0.05 per cent).

Water (*2.5.12*): 7.0 per cent to 9.0 per cent, determined on 0.200 g.

Sulphated ash (*2.4.14*): maximum 0.1 per cent, determined on 1.0 g.

ASSAY

Dissolve 0.250 g in a mixture of 5.0 ml of *0.01 M hydrochloric acid* and 50 ml of *ethanol (96 per cent) R*. Carry out a potentiometric titration (*2.2.20*), using *0.1 M sodium hydroxide*. Read the volume added between the 2 points of inflexion.

1 ml of *0.1 M sodium hydroxide* is equivalent to 32.39 mg of $C_{21}H_{22}ClN$.

STORAGE

Protected from light.

IMPURITIES

Specified impurities: A, B, C.

A. 5*H*-dibenzo[*a,d*][7]annulene (dibenzocycloheptene),

B. 10,11-dihydro-5*H*-dibenzo[*a,d*][7]annulen-5-one (dibenzosuberone),

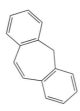

C. 5-(1-methylpiperidin-4-yl)-5*H*-dibenzo[*a,d*][7]annulen-5-ol.

See the information section on general monographs (cover pages)

D

Monographs
D-K

07/2009:1851

DANDELION HERB WITH ROOT

Taraxaci officinalis herba cum radice

DEFINITION

Mixture of whole or fragmented, dried aerial and underground parts of *Taraxacum officinale* F.H. Wiggers.

CHARACTERS

Bitter taste.

IDENTIFICATION

A. The underground parts consist of dark brown or blackish fragments 2-3 cm long, deeply wrinkled longitudinally on the outer surface. The thickened crown shows many scars left by the rosette of leaves. The fracture is short. A transverse section shows a greyish-white or brownish cortex containing concentric layers of brownish laticiferous vessels and a porous, pale yellow, non-radiate wood. Leaf fragments are green, glabrous or densely pilose. They are crumpled and usually show a clearly visible midrib on the inner surface. The lamina, with deeply dentate margins, is crumpled. The solitary flower heads, on hollow stems, consist of an involucre of green, foliaceous bracts surrounding the yellow florets, all of which are ligulate; a few achenes bearing a white, silky, outspread pappus may be present.

B. Reduce to a powder (355) (*2.9.12*). The powder is yellowish-brown. Examine under a microscope using *chloral hydrate solution R*. The powder shows the following diagnostic characters: fragments of cork with flattened, thin-walled cells; reticulate lignified vessels from the roots; fragments of parenchyma containing branched laticiferous vessels; fragments of leaves showing epidermises consisting of interlocking lobed cells, anomocytic stomata (*2.8.3*) and elongated, multicellular covering trichomes with constrictions, which are more or less abundant depending on the variety or sub-variety; fragments of the upper epidermis of the leaf usually accompanied by palisade parenchyma and fragments of the lower epidermis of the leaf accompanied by spongy parenchyma; lignified vessels with spiral or annular thickening; fragments of flower-stem epidermis with stomata and rigid-walled, elongated cells; pollen grains with pitted exines. Examine under a microscope using *glycerol R*. The powder shows angular, irregular inulin fragments, free or included in the parenchyma cells.

C. Thin-layer chromatography (*2.2.27*).

Test solution. To 2.0 g of the powdered herbal drug (355) (*2.9.12*) add 10 ml of *methanol R*. Heat in a water-bath at 60 °C or sonicate for 10 min. Cool and filter.

Reference solution. Dissolve 2 mg of *rutin R* and 2 mg of *chlorogenic acid R* in *methanol R* and dilute to 20 ml with the same solvent.

Plate: *TLC silica gel plate R* (5-40 μm) [or *TLC silica gel plate R* (2-10 μm)].

Mobile phase: *anhydrous formic acid R, water R, ethyl acetate R* (10:10:80 *V/V/V*).

Application: 20 μl [or 5 μl], as bands of 10 mm [or 8 mm].

Development: over a path of 12 cm [or 7 cm].

Drying: in air.

Detection: heat at 100 °C for 5 min; spray with or dip briefly into a 10 g/l solution of *diphenylboric acid aminoethyl ester R* in *methanol R* and dry at 100 °C for 5 min; spray with or dip briefly into a 50 g/l solution of *macrogol 400 R* in *methanol R*; heat at 100 °C for 5 min and examine in ultraviolet light at 365 nm.

Results: see below the sequence of zones present in the chromatograms obtained with the reference solution and the test solution. Furthermore, other faint zones may be present in the chromatogram obtained with the test solution.

Top of the plate	
	A faint red zone
	A faint yellow zone
Chlorogenic acid: a blue zone	2 light blue zones
Rutin: a yellowish-brown zone	
	A light blue zone
Reference solution	**Test solution**

TESTS

Loss on drying (*2.2.32*): maximum 10.0 per cent, determined on 1.000 g of the powdered drug (355) (*2.9.12*) by drying in an oven at 105 °C for 2 h.

Total ash (*2.4.16*): maximum 17.0 per cent.

Ash insoluble in hydrochloric acid (*2.8.1*): maximum 5.0 per cent.

Extractable matter: minimum 30.0 per cent.

To 2.000 g of the powdered herbal drug (250) (*2.9.12*) add 40 g of *water R*. Stir for 1 h and filter. Evaporate 10 g of the filtrate to dryness on a water-bath and dry in an oven at 100-105 °C for 2 h. The residue weighs a minimum of 0.15 g.

Bitterness value (*2.8.15*): minimum 100.

07/2009:0712

DESMOPRESSIN

Desmopressinum

$$\text{Tyr} - \text{Phe} - \text{Gln} - \text{Asn} - \text{Cys} - \text{Pro} - \text{D-Arg} - \text{Gly} - \text{NH}_2$$

$C_{46}H_{64}N_{14}O_{12}S_2$ M_r 1069
[16679-58-6]

DEFINITION

(3-Sulphanylpropanoyl)-L-tyrosyl-L-phenylalanyl-L-glutaminyl-L-asparaginyl-L-cysteinyl-L-prolyl-D-arginylglycinamide cyclic (1→6)-disulfide.

Synthetic cyclic nonapeptide, available as an acetate.

Content: 95.0 per cent to 105.0 per cent (anhydrous and acetic acid-free substance).

CHARACTERS

Appearance: white or almost white, fluffy powder.

Solubility: soluble in water, in ethanol (96 per cent) and in glacial acetic acid.

IDENTIFICATION

A. Examine the chromatograms obtained in the assay.

Results: the retention time and size of the principal peak in the chromatogram obtained with the test solution are approximately the same as those of the principal peak in the chromatogram obtained with the reference solution.

B. Amino acid analysis (*2.2.56*). For hydrolysis use Method 1 and for analysis use Method 1.

Express the content of each amino acid in moles. Calculate the relative proportions of the amino acids, taking 1/6 of the sum of the number of moles of aspartic acid, glutamic acid, proline, glycine, arginine and phenylalanine as equal to 1. The values fall within the following limits: aspartic acid: 0.90 to 1.10; glutamic acid: 0.90 to 1.10; proline: 0.90 to 1.10; glycine: 0.90 to 1.10; arginine: 0.90 to 1.10; phenylalanine: 0.90 to 1.10; tyrosine: 0.70 to 1.05; half-cystine: 0.30 to 1.05. Lysine, isoleucine and leucine are absent; not more than traces of other amino acids are present.

TESTS

Specific optical rotation (*2.2.7*): − 72 to − 82 (anhydrous and acetic acid-free substance).

Dissolve 10.0 mg in a 1 per cent *V/V* solution of *glacial acetic acid R* and dilute to 5.0 ml with the same acid.

Related substances. Liquid chromatography (*2.2.29*): use the normalisation procedure.

Test solution. Dissolve 1.0 mg of the substance to be examined in 2.0 ml of *water R*.

Resolution solution. Dissolve the contents of a vial of *oxytocin/desmopressin validation mixture CRS* in 500 μl of *water R*.

Column:

— *size*: *l* = 0.12 m, Ø = 4.0 mm;

— *stationary phase*: *octadecylsilyl silica gel for chromatography R* (5 μm).

Mobile phase:

— *mobile phase A*: *0.067 M phosphate buffer solution pH 7.0 R*; filter and degas;

— *mobile phase B*: *acetonitrile for chromatography R*, mobile phase A (50:50 *V/V*); filter and degas.

Time (min)	Mobile phase A (per cent *V/V*)	Mobile phase B (per cent *V/V*)
0 - 4	76	24
4 - 18	76 → 58	24 → 42
18 - 35	58 → 48	42 → 52
35 - 40	48 → 76	52 → 24
40 - 50	76	24

Flow rate: 1.5 ml/min.

Detection: spectrophotometer at 220 nm.

Injection: 50 μl.

Retention time: desmopressin = about 16 min; oxytocin = about 17 min.

System suitability: resolution solution:

— *resolution*: minimum 1.5 between the peaks due to desmopressin and oxytoxin.

Limits:

— *unspecified impurities*: for each impurity, maximum 0.5 per cent;

— *total*: maximum 1.5 per cent;

— *disregard limit*: 0.05 per cent.

Acetic acid (*2.5.34*): 3.0 per cent to 8.0 per cent.

Test solution. Dissolve 20.0 mg of the substance to be examined in a mixture of 5 volumes of mobile phase B and 95 volumes of mobile phase A and dilute to 10.0 ml with the same mixture of mobile phases.

Water (*2.5.32*): maximum 6.0 per cent, determined on 20.0 mg.

Bacterial endotoxins (*2.6.14*): less than 500 IU/mg, if intended for use in the manufacture of parenteral preparations without a further appropriate procedure for the removal of bacterial endotoxins.

ASSAY

Liquid chromatography (*2.2.29*) as described in the test for related substances with the following modifications.

Reference solution. Dissolve the contents of a vial of *desmopressin CRS* in *water R* to obtain a concentration of 0.5 mg/ml.

Mobile phase: mobile phase B, mobile phase A (40:60 *V/V*).

Flow rate: 2.0 ml/min.

Retention time: desmopressin = about 5 min.

Calculate the content of desmopressin ($C_{46}H_{64}N_{14}O_{12}S_2$) from the declared content of $C_{46}H_{64}N_{14}O_{12}S_2$ in *desmopressin CRS*.

STORAGE

In an airtight container, protected from light, at a temperature of 2 °C to 8 °C. If the substance is sterile, store in a sterile, airtight, tamper-proof container.

LABELLING

The label states:

— the mass of peptide per container;

— where applicable, that the substance is suitable for use in the manufacture of parenteral preparations.

IMPURITIES

Other detectable impurities (the following substances would, if present at a sufficient level, be detected by one or other of the tests in the monograph. They are limited by the general acceptance criterion for other/unspecified impurities and/or by the general monograph *Substances for pharmaceutical use (2034)*. It is therefore not necessary to identify these impurities for demonstration of compliance. See also *5.10. Control of impurities in substances for pharmaceutical use*): A, B, C, D, E, F, G.

A. X = Gln, Y = Asp, Z = D-Arg: [5-L-aspartic acid]-desmopressin,

B. X = Glu, Y = Asn, Z = D-Arg: [4-L-glutamic acid]-desmopressin,

D. X = Gln, Y = Asn, Z = L-Arg: [8-L-arginine]desmopressin,

C. R = OH, R4 = R5 = H: [9-glycine]desmopressin,

E. R = NH$_2$, R4 = CH$_2$-NH-CO-CH$_3$, R5 = H:
   $N^{5.4}$-[(acetylamino)methyl]desmopressin,

F. R = NH$_2$, R4 = H, R5 = CH$_2$-NH-CO-CH$_3$:
   $N^{4.5}$-[(acetylamino)methyl]desmopressin,

G. R = N(CH$_3$)$_2$, R4 = R5 = H: $N^{1.9}$,$N^{1.9}$-dimethyldesmopressin.

07/2009:0601

DIMENHYDRINATE

Dimenhydrinatum

C$_{24}$H$_{28}$ClN$_5$O$_3$ M_r 470.0
[523-87-5]

DEFINITION

Diphenhydramine [2-(diphenylmethoxy)-N,N-dimethylethanamine] 8-chlorotheophylline (8-chloro-1,3-dimethyl-3,7-dihydro-1H-purine-2,6-dione).

Content:

- *diphenhydramine* (C$_{17}$H$_{21}$NO; M_r 255.4): 53.0 per cent to 55.5 per cent (dried substance);

- *8-chlorotheophylline* (C$_7$H$_7$ClN$_4$O$_2$; M_r 214.6): 44.0 per cent to 46.5 per cent (dried substance).

CHARACTERS

Appearance: white or almost white, crystalline powder or colourless crystals.

Solubility: slightly soluble in water, freely soluble in ethanol (96 per cent).

IDENTIFICATION

First identification: C.

Second identification: A, B, D.

A. Melting point (*2.2.14*): 102 °C to 106 °C.

B. Dissolve 0.1 g in a mixture of 3 ml of *water R* and 3 ml of *ethanol (96 per cent) R*, add 6 ml of *water R* and 1 ml of *dilute hydrochloric acid R* and cool in iced water for 30 min, scratching the wall of the tube with a glass rod if necessary to initiate crystallisation. Dissolve about 10 mg of the precipitate obtained in 1 ml of *hydrochloric acid R*, add 0.1 g of *potassium chlorate R* and evaporate to dryness in a porcelain dish. A reddish residue is obtained that becomes violet-red when exposed to ammonia vapour.

C. Infrared absorption spectrophotometry (*2.2.24*).
   Comparison: dimenhydrinate CRS.

D. Dissolve 0.2 g in 10 ml of *ethanol (96 per cent) R*. Add 10 ml of *picric acid solution R* and initiate crystallisation by scratching the wall of the tube with a glass rod. The precipitate, washed with *water R* and dried at 100-105 °C, melts (*2.2.14*) at 130 °C to 134 °C.

TESTS

Appearance of solution. The solution is clear (*2.2.1*) and colourless (*2.2.2, Method II*).

Dissolve 1.0 g in *ethanol (96 per cent) R* and dilute to 20 ml with the same solvent.

pH (*2.2.3*): 7.1 to 7.6 for the filtrate.

To 0.4 g add 20 ml of *carbon dioxide-free water R*, shake for 2 min and filter.

Related substances. Liquid chromatography (*2.2.29*).

Solvent mixture: acetonitrile R, water R (18:82 V/V).

Test solution. Dissolve 0.100 g of the substance to be examined in the solvent mixture and dilute to 100.0 ml with the solvent mixture.

Reference solution (a). Dissolve 57 mg of *diphenhydramine hydrochloride CRS* in the solvent mixture and dilute to 50.0 ml with the solvent mixture.

Reference solution (b). Dilute 1.0 ml of reference solution (a) to 100.0 ml with the solvent mixture. Dilute 2.0 ml of this solution to 10.0 ml with the solvent mixture.

Reference solution (c). Dissolve 5.0 mg of *diphenhydramine impurity A CRS* (impurity F) in 5.0 ml of reference solution (a) and dilute to 50.0 ml with the solvent mixture.

Reference solution (d). Dissolve the contents of a vial of *dimenhydrinate for peak identification CRS* (containing impurities A and E) in 1.0 ml of the solvent mixture.

Column:

- *size*: l = 0.25 m, Ø = 4.6 mm;

- *stationary phase*: end-capped octadecylsilyl silica gel for chromatography R (5 µm);

- *temperature*: 30 °C.

Mobile phase:

- *mobile phase A*: dissolve 10.0 g of *triethylamine R2* in 950 ml of *water R*, adjust to pH 2.5 with *phosphoric acid R* and dilute to 1000 ml with *water R*;

- *mobile phase B*: acetonitrile R1;

Time (min)	Mobile phase A (per cent V/V)	Mobile phase B (per cent V/V)	Flow rate (ml/min)
0 - 2	82	18	1.2
2 - 15	82 → 50	18 → 50	1.2
15 - 20	50 → 20	50 → 80	1.2 → 2.0
20 - 30	20	80	2.0

Detection: spectrophotometer at 225 nm.

Injection: 10 µl.

Identification of impurities: use the chromatogram supplied with *dimenhydrinate for peak identification CRS* and the chromatogram obtained with reference solution (d) to identify the peaks due to impurities A and E; use the chromatogram obtained with reference solution (c) to identify impurity F.

Relative retention with reference to diphenhydramine (retention time = about 13 min): impurity A = about 0.3; impurity E = about 0.7; impurity F = about 0.95.

System suitability: reference solution (c):

- *resolution*: minimum 1.5 between the peaks due to impurity F and diphenhydramine.

Limits:

- *impurities A, F*: for each impurity, not more than the area of the principal peak in the chromatogram obtained with reference solution (b) (0.2 per cent);

— *impurity E*: not more than 0.75 times the area of the principal peak in the chromatogram obtained with reference solution (b) (0.15 per cent);

— *unspecified impurities*: for each impurity, not more than 0.5 times the area of the principal peak in the chromatogram obtained with reference solution (b) (0.10 per cent);

— *total*: not more than 2.5 times the area of the principal peak in the chromatogram obtained with reference solution (b) (0.5 per cent);

— *disregard limit*: 0.25 times the area of the principal peak in the chromatogram obtained with reference solution (b) (0.05 per cent).

Loss on drying (*2.2.32*): maximum 0.5 per cent, determined on 1.000 g by drying *in vacuo*.

Sulphated ash (*2.4.14*): maximum 0.2 per cent, determined on 1.0 g.

ASSAY

Diphenhydramine. Dissolve 0.200 g in 60 ml of *anhydrous acetic acid R*. Titrate with *0.1 M perchloric acid*, determining the end-point potentiometrically (*2.2.20*).

1 ml of *0.1 M perchloric acid* is equivalent to 25.54 mg of $C_{17}H_{21}NO$.

8-Chlorotheophylline. To 0.800 g add 50 ml of *water R*, 3 ml of *dilute ammonia R1* and 0.6 g of *ammonium nitrate R* and heat on a water-bath for 5 min. Add 25.0 ml of *0.1 M silver nitrate* and continue heating on a water-bath for 15 min with frequent swirling. Cool, add 25 ml of *dilute nitric acid R* and dilute to 250.0 ml with *water R*. Filter and discard the first 25 ml of the filtrate. Using 5 ml of *ferric ammonium sulphate solution R2* as indicator, titrate 100.0 ml of the filtrate with *0.1 M ammonium thiocyanate* until a yellowish-brown colour is obtained.

1 ml of *0.1 M silver nitrate* is equivalent to 21.46 mg of $C_7H_7ClN_4O_2$.

IMPURITIES

Specified impurities: A, E, F.

Other detectable impurities (the following substances would, if present at a sufficient level, be detected by one or other of the tests in the monograph. They are limited by the general acceptance criterion for other/unspecified impurities and/or by the general monograph *Substances for pharmaceutical use (2034)*. It is therefore not necessary to identify these impurities for demonstration of compliance. See also *5.10*. *Control of impurities in substances for pharmaceutical use): C, D, G, H, I, J, K.*

A. theophylline,

C. caffeine,

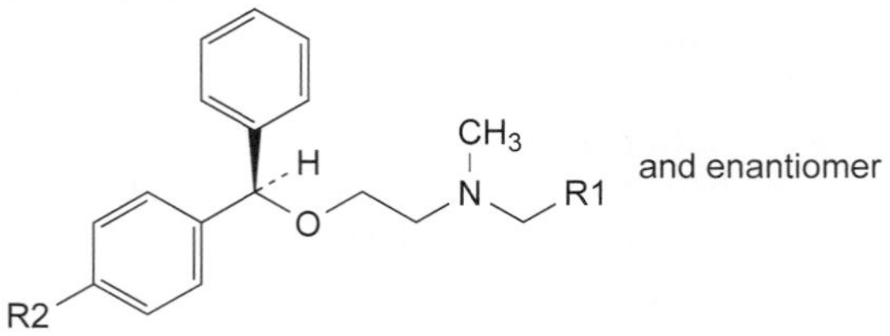

D. R1 = CH₂-N(CH₃)₂, R2 = H: *N*-[2-(diphenylmethoxy)ethyl]-*N,N',N'*-trimethylethane-1,2-diamine,

G. R1 = H, R2 = CH₃: *N,N*-dimethyl-2-[(*RS*)-(4-methylphenyl)(phenyl)methoxy]ethanamine (4-methyldiphenhydramine),

H. R1 = H, R2 = Br: 2-[(*RS*)-(4-bromophenyl)-(phenyl)methoxy]-*N,N*-dimethylethanamine (4-bromodiphenhydramine),

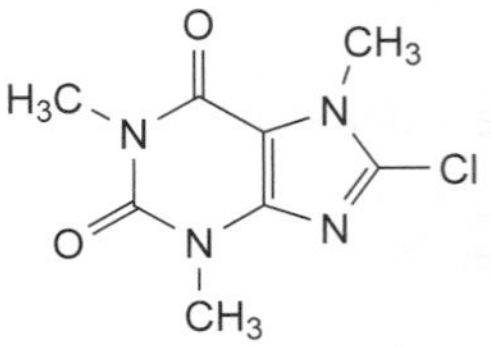

E. 8-chloro-1,3,7-trimethyl-3,7-dihydro-1*H*-purine-2,6-dione (8-chlorocaffeine),

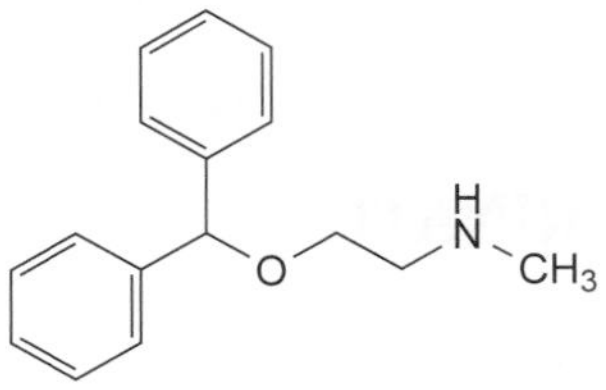

F. 2-(diphenylmethoxy)-*N*-methylethanamine (diphenhydramine impurity A),

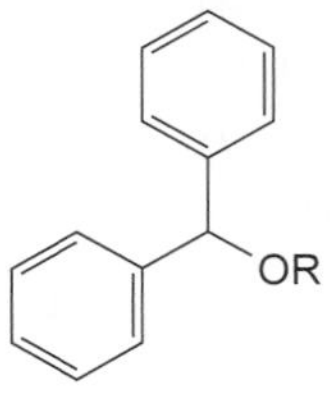

I. R = H: diphenylmethanol (benzhydrol),

K. R = CH(C₆H₅)₂: [oxybis(methanetriyl)]tetrabenzene,

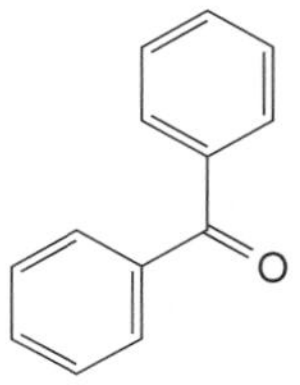

J. diphenylmethanone(benzophenone).

07/2009:2404

DROSPIRENONE

Drospirenonum

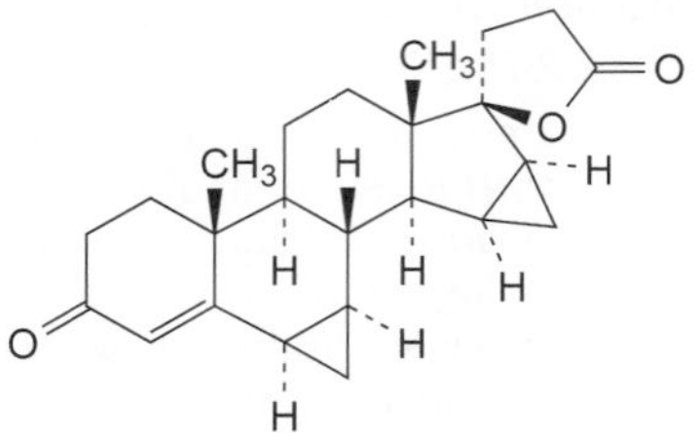

$C_{24}H_{30}O_3$
[67392-87-4]

M_r 366.5

DEFINITION

3-Oxo-6α,7α,15α,16α-tetrahydro-3'*H*,3''*H*-dicyclopropa-[6,7:15,16]-17α-pregn-4-en-21,17-carbolactone.

Content: 98.0 per cent to 102.0 per cent (dried substance).

CHARACTERS

Appearance: white or almost white powder.

Solubility: practically insoluble in water, freely soluble in methylene chloride, soluble in methanol, sparingly soluble in ethanol (96 per cent).

IDENTIFICATION

A. Specific optical rotation (see Tests).

B. Infrared absorption spectrophotometry (*2.2.24*).

   Comparison: *drospirenone CRS*.

TESTS

Specific optical rotation (*2.2.7*): − 187 to − 193 (dried substance).

Dissolve 0.100 g in *methanol R* and dilute to 10.0 ml with the same solvent.

Related substances. Liquid chromatography (*2.2.29*).

Solvent mixture: acetonitrile R, water R (50:50 *V/V*).

Test solution. Dissolve 30.0 mg of the substance to be examined in the solvent mixture and dilute to 50.0 ml with the solvent mixture.

Reference solution (a). Dilute 1.0 ml of the test solution to 10.0 ml with the solvent mixture. Use 1.0 ml of this solution to dissolve the contents of a vial of *drospirenone impurity E CRS*.

Reference solution (b). Dilute 1.0 ml of the test solution to 100.0 ml with the solvent mixture. Dilute 1.0 ml of this solution to 10.0 ml with the solvent mixture.

Reference solution (c). Dissolve 30.0 mg of *drospirenone CRS* in the solvent mixture and dilute to 50.0 ml with the solvent mixture.

Column:

– *size*: l = 0.25 m, Ø = 4.6 mm;
– *stationary phase*: spherical *end-capped octadecylsilyl silica gel for chromatography R* (3 µm);
– *temperature*: 35 °C.

Mobile phase:

– *mobile phase A*: water R;
– *mobile phase B*: acetonitrile R;

Time (min)	Mobile phase A (per cent *V/V*)	Mobile phase B (per cent *V/V*)
0 - 2	63	37
2 - 16	63 → 52	37 → 48
16 - 23	52	48
23 - 31	52 → 20	48 → 80
31 - 39	20	80

Flow rate: 1.0 ml/min.

Detection: spectrophotometer at 245 nm.

Injection: 10 µl of the test solution and reference solutions (a) and (b).

Relative retention with reference to drospirenone (retention time = about 22 min): impurity E = about 1.1.

System suitability: reference solution (a):

– *resolution*: minimum 5.0 between the peaks due to drospirenone and impurity E.

Limits:

– *unspecified impurities*: for each impurity, not more than the area of the principal peak in the chromatogram obtained with reference solution (b) (0.10 per cent);
– *total*: not more than 3 times the area of the principal peak in the chromatogram obtained with reference solution (b) (0.3 per cent);

– *disregard limit*: 0.5 times the area of the principal peak in the chromatogram obtained with reference solution (b) (0.05 per cent).

Loss on drying (*2.2.32*): maximum 0.5 per cent, determined on 1.000 g by drying in an oven at 105 °C for 3 h.

ASSAY

Liquid chromatography (*2.2.29*) as described in the test for related substances with the following modification.

Injection: 10 µl of the test solution and reference solution (c).

Calculate the percentage content of $C_{24}H_{30}O_3$ from the declared content of *drospirenone CRS*.

IMPURITIES

Other detectable impurities (the following substances would, if present at a sufficient level, be detected by one or other of the tests in the monograph. They are limited by the general acceptance criterion for other/unspecified impurities and/or by the general monograph *Substances for pharmaceutical use (2034)*. It is therefore not necessary to identify these impurities for demonstration of compliance. See also *5.10. Control of impurities in substances for pharmaceutical use*): A, B, C, D, E, F, G, H, I, K.

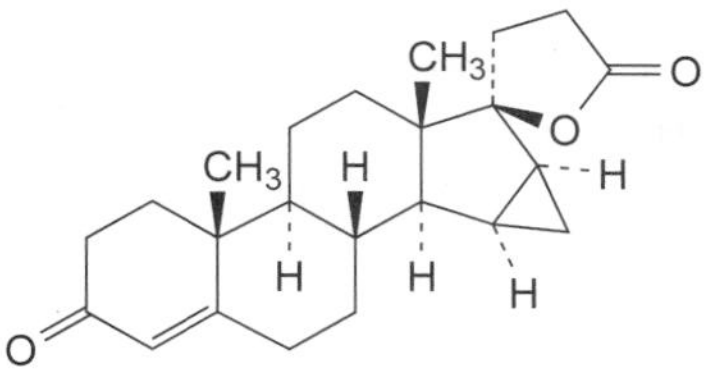

A. 3-oxo-15α,16α-dihydro-3'*H*-cyclopropa[15,16]-17α-pregn-4-ene-21,17-carbolactone (6,7-desmethylenedrospirenone),

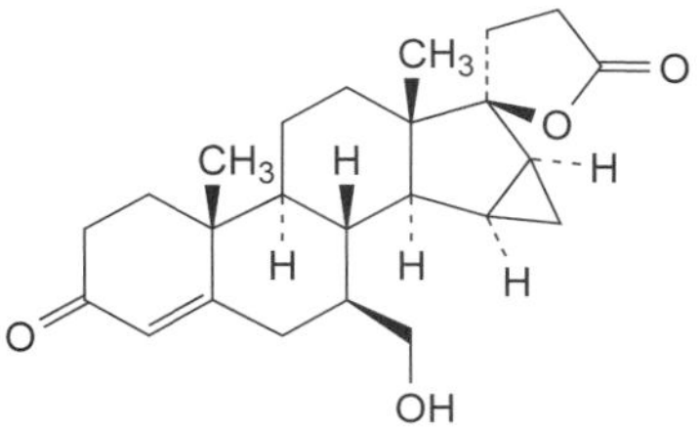

B. 7β-(hydroxymethyl)-3-oxo-15α,16α-dihydro-3'*H*-cyclopropa[15,16]-17α-pregn-4-ene-21,17-carbolactone (7β-hydroxymethyl derivative),

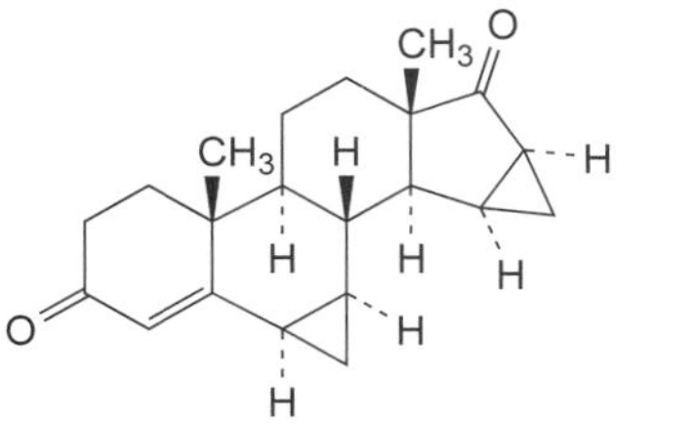

C. 6α,7α,15α,16α-tetrahydro-3'*H*,3''*H*-dicyclopropa-[6,7:15,16]androst-4-ene-3,17-dione (17-keto derivative),

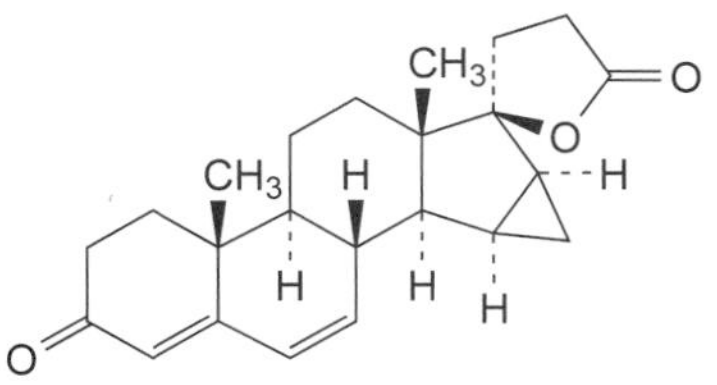

D. 3-oxo-15α,16α-dihydro-3'*H*-cyclopropa[15,16]-17α-pregna-4,6-diene-21,17-carbolactone (Δ6-drospirenone),

E. 3-oxo-6α,7α,15α,16α-tetrahydro-3'H,3"H -
dicyclopropa[6,7:15,16]pregn-4-ene-21,17-carbolactone
(17-epidrospirenone),

F. 15β-methyl-3-oxo-6α,7α-dihydro-3'H-cyclopropa[6,7]-17α-
pregn-4-ene-21,17-carbolactone (3"-16-secodrospirenone),

G. 7β-(chloromethyl)-3-oxo-15α,16α-dihydro-3'H-
cyclopropa[15,16]-17α-pregn-4-ene-21,17-carbolactone
(3'-chloro-3',6-secodrospirenone),

H. 7β-(chloromethyl)-3-oxo-15α,16α-dihydro-3'H-
cyclopropa[15,16]pregn-4-ene-21,17-carbolactone
(3'-chloro-3',6-seco-17-epidrospirenone),

I. 7β-(hydroxymethyl)-15α,16α-dihydro-3'H-cyclopropa[15,
16]-17α-pregna-3,5-diene-21,17-carbolactone
(7β-hydroxymethyldiene derivative),

K. 3-oxo-6β,7β,15α,16α-tetrahydro-3'H,3"H-dicyclopropa-
[6,7:15,16]-17α-pregn-4-ene-21,17-carbolactone
(6α,7α-drospirenone).

E

Monographs D-K

07/2009:0457

ETACRYNIC ACID

Acidum etacrynicum

C$_{13}$H$_{12}$Cl$_2$O$_4$ M$_r$ 303.1
[58-54-8]

DEFINITION

[2,3-Dichloro-4-(2-methylenebutanoyl)phenoxy]acetic acid

Content: 98.0 per cent to 102.0 per cent (dried substance).

CHARACTERS

Appearance: white or almost white, crystalline powder.

Solubility: very slightly soluble in water, freely soluble in ethanol (96 per cent). It dissolves in ammonia and in dilute solutions of alkali hydroxides and carbonates.

IDENTIFICATION

First identification: C.

Second identification: A, B, D, E.

A. Melting point (2.2.14): 121 °C to 124 °C.

B. Ultraviolet and visible absorption spectrophotometry (2.2.25).

   Solvent mixture: 103 g/l solution of hydrochloric acid R, methanol R (1:99 V/V).

   Test solution: Dissolve 50.0 mg in the solvent mixture and dilute to 100.0 ml with the solvent mixture. Dilute 10.0 ml of this solution to 100.0 ml with the solvent mixture.

   Spectral range: 230-350 nm.

   Absorption maximum: at 270 nm.

   Shoulder: at about 285 nm.

   Specific absorbance at the absorption maximum: 110 to 120.

C. Infrared absorption spectrophotometry (2.2.24).

   Comparison: etacrynic acid CRS.

D. Dissolve about 30 mg in 2 ml of aldehyde-free alcohol R. Dissolve 70 mg of hydroxylamine hydrochloride R in 0.1 ml of water R, add 7 ml of alcoholic potassium hydroxide solution R and dilute to 10 ml with aldehyde-free alcohol R. Allow to stand and add 1 ml of the supernatant liquid to the solution of the substance to be examined. Heat the mixture on a water-bath for 3 min. After cooling, add 3 ml of water R and 0.15 ml of hydrochloric acid R. Examined in ultraviolet light at 254 nm, the mixture shows an intense blue fluorescence.

E. Dissolve about 25 mg in 2 ml of a 42 g/l solution of sodium hydroxide R and heat in a water-bath for 5 min. Cool and add 0.25 ml of a mixture of equal volumes of sulphuric acid R and water R. Add 0.5 ml of a 100 g/l solution of chromotropic acid, sodium salt R and, carefully, 2 ml of sulphuric acid R. An intense violet colour is produced.

TESTS

Related substances. Liquid chromatography (2.2.29).

Solvent mixture: acetonitrile R, water R (40:60 V/V).

Test solution. Dissolve 25 mg of the substance to be examined in the solvent mixture and dilute to 25.0 ml with the solvent mixture.

Reference solution (a). Dilute 1.0 ml of the test solution to 100.0 ml with the solvent mixture. Dilute 1.0 ml of this solution to 10.0 ml with the solvent mixture.

Reference solution (b). Dissolve 5 mg of etacrynic acid for system suitability CRS (containing impurities A, B and C) in 5.0 ml of the solvent mixture.

Column:
— size: l = 0.25 m, Ø = 4.0 mm;
— stationary phase: end-capped octadecylsilyl silica gel for chromatography R (5 µm);
— temperature: 25 °C.

Mobile phase:
— mobile phase A: 1 per cent V/V solution of triethylamine R adjusted to pH 6.8 with phosphoric acid R;
— mobile phase B: acetonitrile R;

Time (min)	Mobile phase A (per cent V/V)	Mobile phase B (per cent V/V)
0-2.5	70	30
2.5-3	70→65	30→35
3-6	65	35
6-7	65→45	35→55
7-22	45	55

Flow rate: 0.8 ml/min.

Detection: spectrophotometer at 280 nm.

Injection: 10 µl.

Identification of impurities: use the chromatogram supplied with etacrynic acid for system suitability CRS and the chromatogram obtained with reference solution (b) to identify the peaks due to impurities A, B and C.

Relative retention with reference to etacrynic acid (retention time = about 9 min): impurity A = about 0.8; impurity B = about 1.3; impurity C = about 1.7.

System suitability: reference solution (b):
— resolution: minimum 4.0 between the peaks due to impurity A and etacrynic acid.

Limits:
— correction factors: for the calculation of contents, multiply the peak areas of the following impurities by the corresponding correction factor: impurity A = 0.6; impurity B = 0.6; impurity C = 1.3;
— impurity C: not more than 3 times the area of the principal peak in the chromatogram obtained with reference solution (a) (0.3 per cent);
— impurities A, B: for each impurity, not more than 1.5 times the area of the principal peak in the chromatogram obtained with reference solution (a) (0.15 per cent);
— unspecified impurities: for each impurity, not more than the area of the principal peak in the chromatogram obtained with reference solution (a) (0.10 per cent);
— total: not more than 8 times the area of the principal peak in the chromatogram obtained with reference solution (a) (0.8 per cent);
— disregard limit: 0.5 times the area of the principal peak in the chromatogram obtained with reference solution (a) (0.05 per cent).

Heavy metals (*2.4.8*): maximum 20 ppm.

1.0 g complies with test F. Prepare the reference solution using 2 ml of *lead standard solution (10 ppm Pb) R*.

Loss on drying (*2.2.32*): maximum 0.5 per cent, determined on 2.000 g by drying at 60 °C over *diphosphorus pentoxide R* at a pressure of 0.1-0.5 kPa.

Sulphated ash (*2.4.14*): maximum 0.1 per cent, determined on 1.0 g.

ASSAY

Dissolve 0.250 g in 100 ml of *methanol R* and add 5 ml of *water R*. Titrate with *0.1 M sodium hydroxide*, determining the end-point potentiometrically (*2.2.20*).

1 ml of *0.1 M sodium hydroxide* is equivalent to 30.31 mg of $C_{13}H_{12}Cl_2O_4$.

IMPURITIES

Specified impurities: A, B, C.

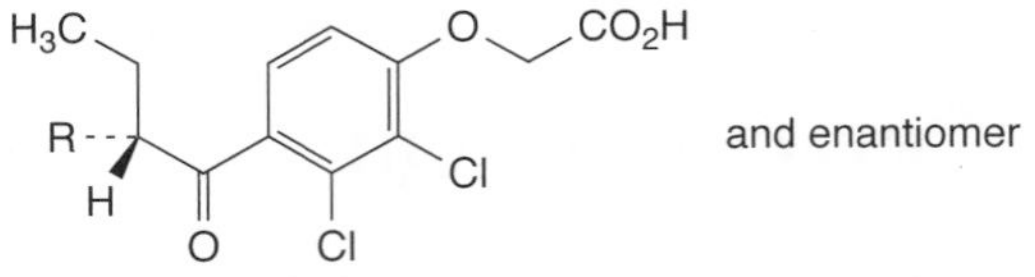

and enantiomer

A. R = H: (4-butanoyl-2,3-dichlorophenoxy)acetic acid,

B. R = CH$_2$Cl: [2,3-dichloro-4-[2-(chloromethyl)butanoyl]-phenoxy]acetic acid,

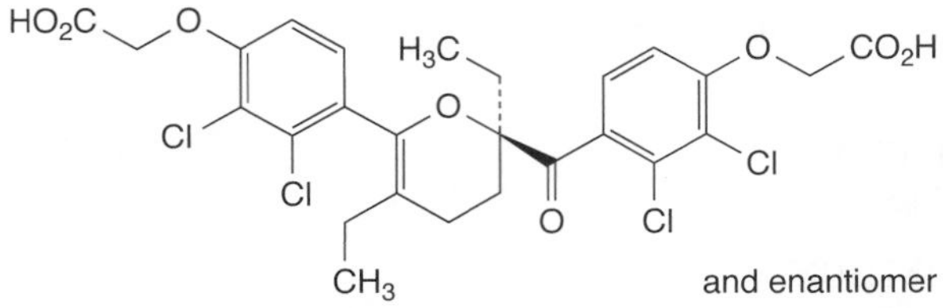

and enantiomer

C. [4-[2-[4-(carboxymethoxy)-2,3-dichlorobenzoyl]-2,5-diethyl-3,4-dihydro-2*H*-pyran-6-yl]-2,3-dichlorophenoxy]acetic acid.

F

Monographs
D-K

01/2008:1519
corrected 6.5

FLURBIPROFEN

Flurbiprofenum

and enantiomer

$C_{15}H_{13}FO_2$ M_r 244.3
[5104-49-4]

DEFINITION

(2*RS*)-2-(2-Fluorobiphenyl-4-yl)propanoic acid.

Content: 99.0 per cent to 101.0 per cent (dried substance).

CHARACTERS

Appearance: white or almost white, crystalline powder.

Solubility: practically insoluble in water, freely soluble in ethanol (96 per cent) and in methylene chloride. It dissolves in aqueous solutions of alkali hydroxides and carbonates.

IDENTIFICATION

First identification: C, D.

Second identification: A, B, D.

A. Melting point (*2.2.14*): 114 °C to 117 °C.

B. Ultraviolet and visible absorption spectrophotometry (*2.2.25*).

   Test solution. Dissolve 0.10 g in *0.1 M sodium hydroxide* and dilute to 100.0 ml with the same alkaline solution. Dilute 1.0 ml of this solution to 100.0 ml with *0.1 M sodium hydroxide*.

   Spectral range: 230-350 nm.

   Absorption maximum: at 247 nm.

   Specific absorbance at the absorption maximum: 780 to 820.

C. Infrared absorption spectrophotometry (*2.2.24*).

   Comparison: flurbiprofen CRS.

D. Mix about 5 mg with 45 mg of *heavy magnesium oxide R* and ignite in a crucible until an almost white residue is obtained (usually less than 5 min). Allow to cool, add 1 ml of *water R*, 0.05 ml of *phenolphthalein solution R1* and about 1 ml of *dilute hydrochloric acid R* to render the solution colourless. Filter. To a freshly prepared mixture of 0.1 ml of *alizarin S solution R* and 0.1 ml of *zirconyl nitrate solution R* add 1.0 ml of the filtrate. Mix, allow to stand for 5 min and compare the colour of the solution with that of a blank prepared in the same manner. The test solution is yellow and the blank is red.

TESTS

Appearance of solution. The solution is clear (*2.2.1*) and colourless (*2.2.2, Method I*).

Dissolve 1.0 g in *methanol R* and dilute to 10 ml with the same solvent.

Optical rotation (*2.2.7*): − 0.1° to + 0.1°.

Dissolve 0.50 g in *methanol R* and dilute to 20.0 ml with the same solvent.

Related substances. Liquid chromatography (*2.2.29*).

Solvent mixture: acetonitrile R, water R (45:55 V/V).

Test solution. Dissolve 0.20 g of the substance to be examined in the solvent mixture and dilute to 100.0 ml with the solvent mixture.

Reference solution (a). Dilute 1.0 ml of the test solution to 50.0 ml with the solvent mixture. Dilute 1.0 ml of this solution to 10.0 ml with the solvent mixture.

Reference solution (b). Dissolve 10.0 mg of *flurbiprofen impurity A CRS* in the solvent mixture and dilute to 100.0 ml with the solvent mixture. Dilute 10.0 ml of this solution to 100.0 ml with the solvent mixture.

Reference solution (c). Dissolve 10 mg of the substance to be examined in the solvent mixture and dilute to 100.0 ml with the solvent mixture. Dilute 1.0 ml of this solution to 10.0 ml with reference solution (b).

Column:

— *size*: *l* = 0.15 m, Ø = 3.9 mm;

— *stationary phase*: *octadecylsilyl silica gel for chromatography R* (5 µm).

Mobile phase: *glacial acetic acid R, acetonitrile R, water R* (5:35:60 V/V/V).

Flow rate: 1 ml/min.

Detection: spectrophotometer at 254 nm.

Injection: 10 µl.

Run time: twice the retention time of flurbiprofen.

System suitability: reference solution (c):

— *resolution*: minimum 1.5 between the peaks due to impurity A and flurbiprofen.

Limits:

— *impurity A*: not more than the area of the corresponding peak in the chromatogram obtained with reference solution (b) (0.5 per cent);

— *impurities B, C, D, E*: for each impurity, not more than the area of the principal peak in the chromatogram obtained with reference solution (a) (0.2 per cent);

— *sum of impurities other than A*: not more than 5 times the area of the principal peak in the chromatogram obtained with reference solution (a) (1.0 per cent);

— *disregard limit*: 0.1 times the area of the principal peak in the chromatogram obtained with reference solution (a) (0.02 per cent).

Heavy metals (*2.4.8*): maximum 10 ppm.

Dissolve 2.0 g in a mixture of 10 volumes of *water R* and 90 volumes of *methanol R* and dilute to 20 ml with the same mixture of solvents. 12 ml of the solution complies with test B. Prepare the reference solution using lead standard solution (1 ppm Pb) obtained by diluting *lead standard solution (100 ppm Pb) R* with a mixture of 10 volumes of *water R* and 90 volumes of *methanol R*.

Loss on drying (*2.2.32*): maximum 0.5 per cent, determined on 1.000 g by drying at 60 °C at a pressure not exceeding 0.7 kPa for 3 h.

Sulphated ash (*2.4.14*): maximum 0.1 per cent, determined on 1.0 g in a platinum crucible.

ASSAY

Dissolve 0.200 g in 50 ml of *ethanol (96 per cent) R*. Titrate with *0.1 M sodium hydroxide*, determining the end-point potentiometrically (*2.2.20*).

1 ml of *0.1 M sodium hydroxide* is equivalent to 24.43 mg of $C_{15}H_{13}FO_2$.

IMPURITIES

Specified impurities: A, B, C, D, E.

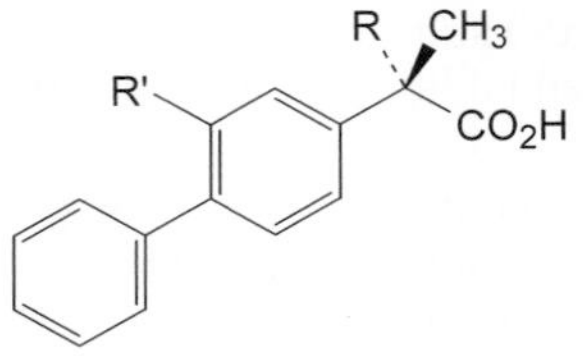

and enantiomer

A. R = R′ = H: (2RS)-2-(biphenyl-4-yl)propanoic acid,

B. R = CH(CH₃)-CO₂H, R′ = F: 2-(2-fluorobiphenyl-4-yl)-2,3-dimethylbutanedioic acid,

C. R = OH, R′ = F: (2RS)-2-(2-fluorobiphenyl-4-yl)-2-hydroxypropanoic acid,

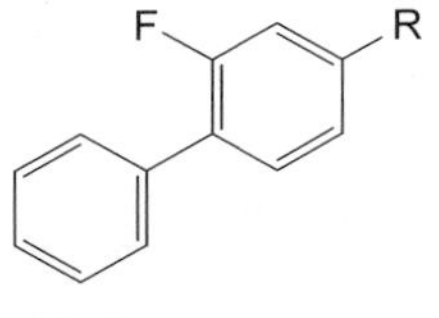

D. R = CO-CH₃: 1-(2-fluorobiphenyl-4-yl)ethanone,

E. R = CO₂H: 2-fluorobiphenyl-4-carboxylic acid.

01/2008:1520
corrected 6.5

FOSCARNET SODIUM HEXAHYDRATE

Foscarnetum natricum hexahydricum

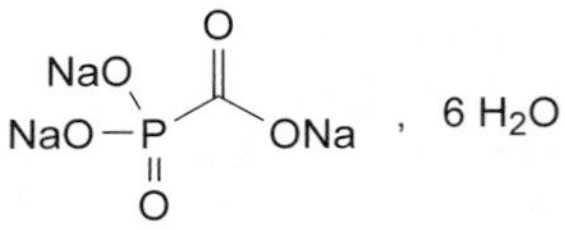

$CNa_3O_5P,6H_2O$ M_r 300.0

[34156-56-4]

DEFINITION

Trisodium phosphonatoformate hexahydrate.

Content: 98.5 per cent to 101.0 per cent (dried substance).

CHARACTERS

Appearance: white or almost white, crystalline powder.

Solubility: soluble in water, practically insoluble in ethanol (96 per cent).

IDENTIFICATION

A. Infrared absorption spectrophotometry (*2.2.24*).

    Comparison: foscarnet sodium hexahydrate CRS.

B. It gives reaction (a) of sodium (*2.3.1*).

TESTS

Solution S. Dissolve 0.5 g in *carbon dioxide-free water R* and dilute to 25 ml with the same solvent.

Appearance of solution. Solution S is not more opalescent than reference suspension I (*2.2.1*) and is colourless (*2.2.2*, *Method II*).

pH (*2.2.3*): 9.0 to 11.0 for solution S.

Impurity D. Gas chromatography (*2.2.28*).

Test solution. Dissolve 0.25 g of the substance to be examined in 9.0 ml of *0.1 M acetic acid* using a magnetic stirrer. Add 1.0 ml of *anhydrous ethanol R* and mix.

Reference solution. Dissolve 25 mg of *triethyl phosphonoformate R* in *anhydrous ethanol R* and dilute to 100 ml with the same solvent. Dilute 1 ml of this solution to 10 ml with *anhydrous ethanol R*.

Column:

— *material*: fused silica;

— *size*: l = 25 m, Ø = 0.31 mm;

— *stationary phase*: poly(dimethyl)(diphenyl)(divinyl)-siloxane R (film thickness 0.5 µm).

Carrier gas: helium for chromatography R.

Split ratio: 1:20.

Temperature:

	Time (min)	Temperature (°C)
Column	0 - 8	100 → 180
Injection port		200
Detector		250

Detection: flame ionisation.

Injection: 3 µl.

Limit:

— *impurity D*: not more than the area of the principal peak in the chromatogram obtained with the reference solution (0.1 per cent).

Related substances. Liquid chromatography (*2.2.29*).

Test solution. Dissolve 25 mg of the substance to be examined in the mobile phase and dilute to 10.0 ml with the mobile phase.

Reference solution (a). Dilute 1.0 ml of the test solution to 50.0 ml with the mobile phase. Dilute 1.0 ml of this solution to 10.0 ml with the mobile phase.

Reference solution (b). Dissolve 5.0 mg of *foscarnet impurity B CRS* in the mobile phase, add 2.0 ml of the test solution and dilute to 50.0 ml with the mobile phase.

Column:

— *size*: l = 0.10 m, Ø = 4.6 mm;

— *stationary phase*: octadecylsilyl silica gel for chromatography R (3 µm).

Mobile phase: dissolve 3.22 g of *sodium sulphate decahydrate R* in *water R*, add 3 ml of *glacial acetic acid R* and 6 ml of a 44.61 g/l solution of *sodium pyrophosphate R* and dilute to 1000 ml with *water R* (solution A); dissolve 3.22 g of *sodium sulphate decahydrate R* in *water R*, add 6.8 g of *sodium acetate R* and 6 ml of a 44.61 g/l solution of *sodium pyrophosphate R* and dilute to 1000 ml with *water R* (solution B). Mix about 700 ml of solution A and about 300 ml of solution B to obtain a solution of pH 4.4. To 1000 ml of this solution, add 0.25 g of *tetrahexylammonium hydrogen sulphate R* and 100 ml of *methanol R*.

Flow rate: 1.0 ml/min.

Detection: spectrophotometer at 230 nm.

Injection: 20 µl.

Run time: 2.5 times the retention time of foscarnet.

System suitability: reference solution (b):

— *resolution*: minimum 7 between the peaks due to foscarnet and impurity B.

Limits:

— *impurities A, B, C*: for each impurity, not more than the area of the principal peak in the chromatogram obtained with reference solution (a) (0.2 per cent);

- *total*: not more than twice the area of the principal peak in the chromatogram obtained with reference solution (a) (0.4 per cent);
- *disregard limit*: 0.2 times the area of the principal peak in the chromatogram obtained with reference solution (a) (0.04 per cent); disregard any peak with a relative retention time less than 0.6.

Phosphate and phosphite. Liquid chromatography (*2.2.29*).

Test solution. Dissolve 60.0 mg of the substance to be examined in *water R* and dilute to 25.0 ml with the same solvent.

Reference solution (a). Dissolve 28 mg of *sodium dihydrogen phosphate monohydrate R* in *water R* and dilute to 100 ml with the same solvent.

Reference solution (b). Dissolve 43 mg of *sodium phosphite pentahydrate R* in *water R* and dilute to 100 ml with the same solvent.

Reference solution (c). Dilute 1.0 ml of reference solution (a) and 1.0 ml of reference solution (b) to 25 ml with *water R*.

Reference solution (d). Dilute 3 ml of reference solution (a) and 3 ml of reference solution (b) to 25 ml with *water R*.

Column:
- *size*: l = 0.05 m, Ø = 4.6 mm;
- *stationary phase*: *anion exchange resin R*.

Mobile phase: dissolve 0.102 g of *potassium hydrogen phthalate R* in *water R*, add 2.5 ml of *1 M nitric acid* and dilute to 1000 ml with *water R*.

Flow rate: 1.4 ml/min.

Detection: spectrophotometer at 290 nm (indirect detection).

Injection: 20 µl of the test solution and reference solutions (c) and (d).

System suitability: reference solution (d):
- *resolution*: minimum 2.0 between the peaks due to phosphate (1st peak) and phosphite;
- *signal-to-noise ratio*: minimum 10 for the principal peak.

Limits:
- *phosphate*: not more than the area of the corresponding peak in the chromatogram obtained with reference solution (c) (0.3 per cent);
- *phosphite*: not more than the area of the corresponding peak in the chromatogram obtained with reference solution (c) (0.3 per cent).

Heavy metals: maximum 10 ppm.

Dissolve 1.25 g in 12.5 ml of *1 M hydrochloric acid*. Warm on a water-bath for 3 min and cool to room temperature. Transfer to a beaker, adjust to about pH 3.5 with *dilute ammonia R1* and dilute to 25 ml with *water R* (solution A). To 12 ml of solution A, add 2.0 ml of *buffer solution pH 3.5 R*. Rapidly pour the mixture into a test tube containing 1 drop of *sodium sulphide solution R*. The solution is not more intensely coloured than a reference solution prepared simultaneously and in the same manner by pouring a mixture of 5.0 ml of *lead standard solution (1 ppm Pb) R*, 5.0 ml of *water R*, 2.0 ml of solution A and 2.0 ml of *buffer solution pH 3.5 R* into a test tube containing 1 drop of *sodium sulphide solution R*.

Loss on drying (*2.2.32*): 35.0 per cent to 37.0 per cent, determined on 1.000 g by drying in an oven at 150 °C.

Bacterial endotoxins (*2.6.14*): less than 83.3 IU/g, if intended for use in the manufacture of parenteral preparations without a further appropriate procedure for the removal of bacterial endotoxins.

ASSAY

Dissolve 0.200 g in 50 ml of *water R*. Titrate with *0.05 M sulphuric acid*, determining the end-point potentiometrically (*2.2.20*) at the 1st point of inflexion.

1 ml of *0.05 M sulphuric acid* is equivalent to 19.20 mg of CNa_3O_5P.

STORAGE

Protected from light.

IMPURITIES

Specified impurities: A, B, C, D.

A. R1 = OC_2H_5, R2 = R3 = ONa: disodium (ethoxycarbonyl)phosphonate,

B. R1 = R2 = ONa, R3 = OC_2H_5: disodium (ethoxyoxydophosphanyl)formate,

C. R1 = R2 = OC_2H_5, R3 = ONa: ethyl sodium (ethoxycarbonyl)phosphonate,

D. R1 = R2 = R3 = OC_2H_5: methyl (diethoxyphosphoryl)-formate.

07/2009:1214

FRANGULA BARK DRY EXTRACT, STANDARDISED

Frangulae corticis extractum siccum normatum

DEFINITION

Standardised dry extract obtained from *Frangula bark (0025)*.

Content: 15.0 per cent to 30.0 per cent of glucofrangulins, expressed as glucofrangulin A ($C_{27}H_{30}O_{14}$; M_r 578.5) (dried extract); the measured content does not deviate from that stated on the label by more than ± 10 per cent.

PRODUCTION

The extract is produced from the herbal drug by a suitable procedure using ethanol (50-90 per cent *V/V*).

CHARACTERS

Appearance: yellowish-brown, fine powder.

IDENTIFICATION

A. Thin-layer chromatography (*2.2.27*).

    Test solution. To 0.05 g of the extract to be examined add 5 ml of *ethanol (70 per cent V/V) R* and heat to boiling. Cool and centrifuge. Decant the supernatant solution immediately and use within 30 min.

    Reference solution. Dissolve 20 mg of *barbaloin R* in *ethanol (70 per cent V/V) R* and dilute to 10 ml with the same solvent.

    Plate: *TLC silica gel plate R*.

    Mobile phase: *water R, methanol R, ethyl acetate R* (13:17:100 *V/V/V*).

    Application: 10 µl as bands.

    Development: over a path of 10 cm.

Drying: in air for 5 min.

Detection: spray with a 50 g/l solution of *potassium hydroxide R* in *ethanol (50 per cent V/V) R* and heat at 100-105 °C for 15 min; examine immediately after heating.

Results: the chromatogram obtained with the reference solution shows in the middle third a reddish-brown zone due to barbaloin. The chromatogram obtained with the test solution shows 2 orange-brown zones (glucofrangulins) in the lower third and 2-4 red zones (frangulins, not always clearly separated, and above them frangula-emodin) in the upper third.

B. To about 25 mg add 25 ml of *dilute hydrochloric acid R* and heat the mixture on a water-bath for 15 min. Allow to cool, shake with 20 ml of *ether R* and discard the aqueous layer. Shake the ether layer with 10 ml of *dilute ammonia R1*. The aqueous layer becomes reddish-violet.

TESTS

Loss on drying (*2.8.17*): maximum 5.0 per cent.

Microbial contamination

TAMC: acceptance criterion 10^4 CFU/g (*2.6.12*).

TYMC: acceptance criterion 10^2 CFU/g (*2.6.12*).

Absence of *Escherichia coli* (*2.6.13*).

Absence of *Salmonella* (*2.6.13*).

ASSAY

Carry out the assay protected from bright light.

Into a tared round-bottomed flask with a ground-glass neck, weigh 0.100 g. Add 25.0 ml of a 70 per cent *V/V* solution of *methanol R*, mix and weigh again. Heat the flask in a water-bath under a reflux condenser at 70 °C for 15 min. Allow to cool, weigh and adjust to the original mass with a 70 per cent *V/V* solution of *methanol R*. Filter and transfer 5.0 ml of the filtrate to a separating funnel. Add 50 ml of *water R* and 0.1 ml of *hydrochloric acid R*. Shake with 5 quantities, each of 20 ml, of *light petroleum R1*. Allow the layers to separate and transfer the aqueous layer to a 100 ml volumetric flask. Combine the light petroleum layers and wash with 2 quantities, each of 15 ml, of *water R*. Use this water for washing the separating funnel and add it to the aqueous solution in the volumetric flask. Add 5 ml of a 50 g/l solution of *sodium carbonate R* and dilute to 100.0 ml with *water R*. Discard the light petroleum layer. Transfer 40.0 ml of the aqueous solution to a 200 ml round-bottomed flask with a ground-glass neck. Add 20 ml of a 200 g/l solution of *ferric chloride R* and heat under a reflux condenser for 20 min in a water-bath with the water level above that of the liquid in the flask. Add 2 ml of *hydrochloric acid R* and continue heating for 20 min, shaking frequently, until the precipitate is dissolved. Allow to cool, transfer the mixture to a separating funnel and shake with 3 quantities, each of 25 ml, of *ether R*, previously used to rinse the flask. Combine the ether extracts and wash with 2 quantities, each of 15 ml, of *water R*. Transfer the ether layer to a volumetric flask and dilute to 100.0 ml with *ether R*. Evaporate 20.0 ml carefully to dryness and dissolve the residue in 10.0 ml of a 5 g/l solution of *magnesium acetate R* in *methanol R*. Measure the absorbance (*2.2.25*) at 515 nm using *methanol R* as the compensation liquid.

Calculate the percentage content of glucofrangulins, expressed as glucofrangulin A, using the following expression:

$$\frac{A \times 3.06}{m}$$

i.e. taking the specific absorbance of glucofrangulin A to be 204, calculated on the basis of the specific absorbance of barbaloin.

A = absorbance at 515 nm;

m = mass of the preparation to be examined, in grams.

LABELLING

The label states the content of glucofrangulins.

G

See the information section on general monographs (cover pages)

07/2009:1726

GESTODENE

Gestodenum

$C_{21}H_{26}O_2$ M_r 310.4
[60282-87-3]

DEFINITION

13-Ethyl-17-hydroxy-18,19-dinor-17α-pregna-4,15-dien-20-yn-3-one.

Content: 97.5 per cent to 102.0 per cent (dried substance).

CHARACTERS

Appearance: white or yellowish, crystalline powder.

Solubility: practically insoluble in water, freely soluble in methylene chloride, soluble in methanol, sparingly soluble in ethanol (96 per cent).

It shows polymorphism (5.9).

IDENTIFICATION

A. Specific optical rotation (see Tests).

B. Infrared absorption spectrophotometry (2.2.24).

   Comparison: gestodene CRS.

   If the spectra obtained in the solid state show differences, dissolve the substance to be examined and the reference substance separately in acetone R, evaporate to dryness and record new spectra using the residues.

TESTS

Specific optical rotation (2.2.7): − 188 to − 198 (dried substance).

Dissolve 0.100 g in methanol R and dilute to 10.0 ml with the same solvent.

Related substances. Liquid chromatography (2.2.29).

Solvent mixture: acetonitrile R1, water R (50:50 V/V).

Test solution (a). Dissolve 30.0 mg of the substance to be examined in 5 ml of acetonitrile R1 and dilute to 10.0 ml with water R.

Test solution (b). Dilute 1.0 ml of test solution (a) to 10.0 ml with the solvent mixture.

Reference solution (a). Dissolve 3 mg of gestodene for system suitability CRS (containing impurities A, B, C and L) in 0.5 ml of acetonitrile R1 and dilute to 1.0 ml with water R.

Reference solution (b). Dilute 1.0 ml of test solution (a) to 100.0 ml with the solvent mixture. Dilute 1.0 ml of this solution to 10.0 ml with the solvent mixture.

Reference solution (c). Dissolve 30.0 mg of gestodene CRS in 5 ml of acetonitrile R1 and dilute to 10.0 ml with water R. Dilute 1.0 ml of this solution to 10.0 ml with the solvent mixture.

Reference solution (d). Dissolve the contents of a vial of gestodene impurity I CRS in 1.0 ml of the solvent mixture.

Column:
— size: l = 0.15 m, Ø = 4.6 mm;

— stationary phase: spherical end-capped octylsilyl silica gel for chromatography R (3.5 µm).

Mobile phase:
— mobile phase A: water R;
— mobile phase B: acetonitrile R1;

Time (min)	Mobile phase A (per cent V/V)	Mobile phase B (per cent V/V)
0 - 2	62	38
2 - 20	62 → 58	38 → 42
20 - 24	58 → 30	42 → 70
24 - 32	30	70

Flow rate: 1.0 ml/min.

Detection: spectrophotometer at 205 nm and at 254 nm.

Injection: 10 µl of test solution (a) and reference solutions (a), (b) and (d).

Identification of impurities: use the chromatogram supplied with gestodene for system suitability CRS and the chromatogram obtained with reference solution (a) to identify the peaks due to impurities A, B, C and L; use the chromatogram obtained with reference solution (d) to identify the peak due to impurity I.

Relative retention with reference to gestodene (retention time = about 12.5 min): impurity A = about 0.9; impurity C = about 1.1; impurity I = about 1.2; impurity L = about 1.46; impurity B = about 1.53.

System suitability: reference solution (a):

— resolution: minimum 2.0 between the peaks due to impurity A and gestodene.

Limits:

— correction factors: for the calculation of content, multiply the peak areas of the following impurities by the corresponding correction factor: impurity A = 2.2; impurity I = 1.3;

— impurity A at 254 nm: not more than 3 times the area of the principal peak in the chromatogram obtained with reference solution (b) (0.3 per cent);

— impurity B at 205 nm: not more than twice the area of the principal peak in the chromatogram obtained with reference solution (b) (0.2 per cent);

— impurity C at 254 nm: not more than twice the area of the principal peak in the chromatogram obtained with reference solution (b) (0.2 per cent);

— impurities I, L at 205 nm: for each impurity, not more than 1.5 times the area of the principal peak in the chromatogram obtained with reference solution (b) (0.15 per cent);

— unspecified impurities at 254 nm: for each impurity, not more than the area of the principal peak in the chromatogram obtained with reference solution (b) (0.10 per cent);

— total at 254 nm: not more than 5 times the area of the principal peak in the chromatogram obtained with reference solution (b) (0.5 per cent);

— disregard limit at 254 nm: 0.5 times the area of the principal peak in the chromatogram obtained with reference solution (b) (0.05 per cent).

Loss on drying (2.2.32): maximum 0.5 per cent, determined on 1.000 g by drying in an oven at 105 °C for 3 h.

ASSAY

Liquid chromatography (2.2.29) as described in the test for related substances with the following modification.

Injection: test solution (b) and reference solution (c).

Calculate the percentage content of $C_{21}H_{26}O_2$ from the declared content of *gestodene CRS*.

IMPURITIES

Specified impurities: A, B, C, I, L.

Other detectable impurities (the following substances would, if present at a sufficient level, be detected by one or other of the tests in the monograph. They are limited by the general acceptance criterion for other/unspecified impurities and/or by the general monograph *Substances for pharmaceutical use (2034)*. It is therefore not necessary to identify these impurities for demonstration of compliance. See also *5.10. Control of impurities in substances for pharmaceutical use*):

— at 205 nm: G, J, K;

— at 254 nm: D, E, F, H.

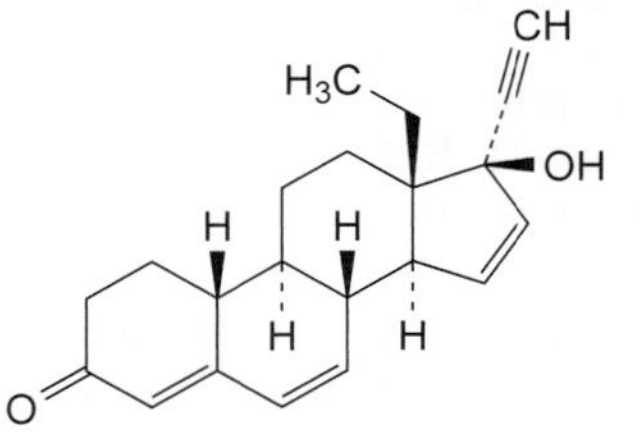

A. 13-ethyl-17-hydroxy-18,19-dinor-17α-pregna-4,6,15-trien-20-yn-3-one (Δ6-gestodene),

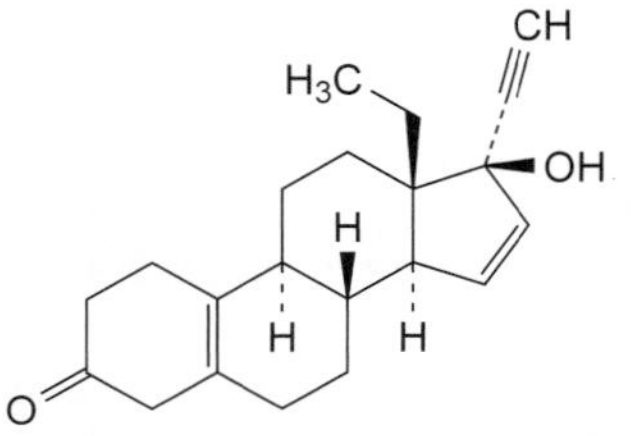

B. 13-ethyl-17-hydroxy-18,19-dinor-17α-pregna-5(10),15-dien-20-yn-3-one (Δ5(10)-gestodene),

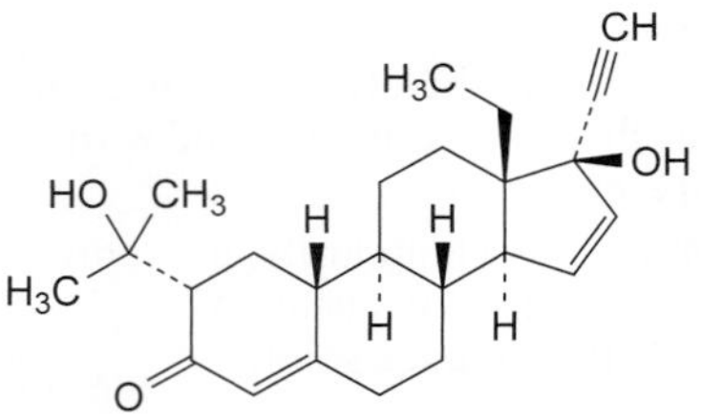

C. 13-ethyl-17-hydroxy-2α-(1-hydroxy-1-methylethyl)-18,19-dinor-17α-pregna-4,15-dien-20-yn-3-one (2-isopropanol-gestodene),

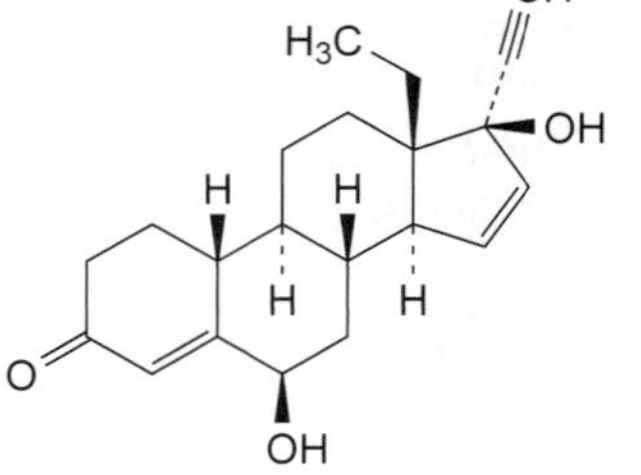

D. 13-ethyl-6β,17-dihydroxy-18,19-dinor-17α-pregna-4,15-dien-20-yn-3-one (6β-hydroxy-gestodene),

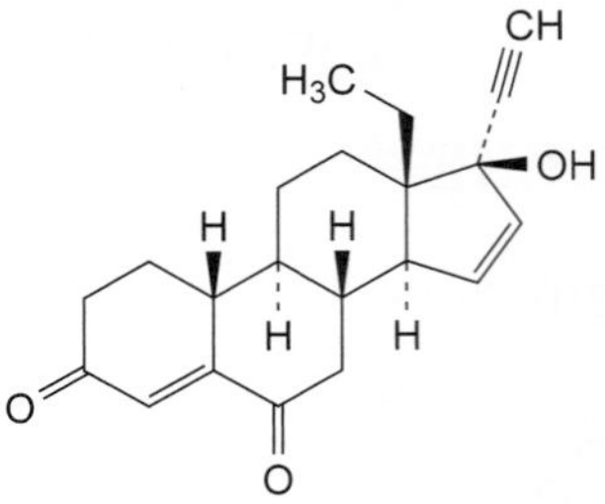

E. 13-ethyl-17-hydroxy-18,19-dinor-17α-pregna-4,15-dien-20-yne-3,6-dione (6-keto-gestodene),

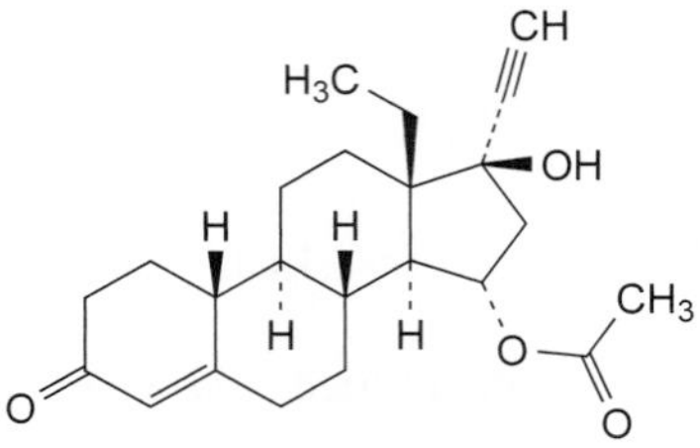

F. 13-ethyl-17-hydroxy-3-oxo-18,19-dinor-17α-pregn-4-en-20-yn-15α-yl acetate (15α-acetoxy-gestodene),

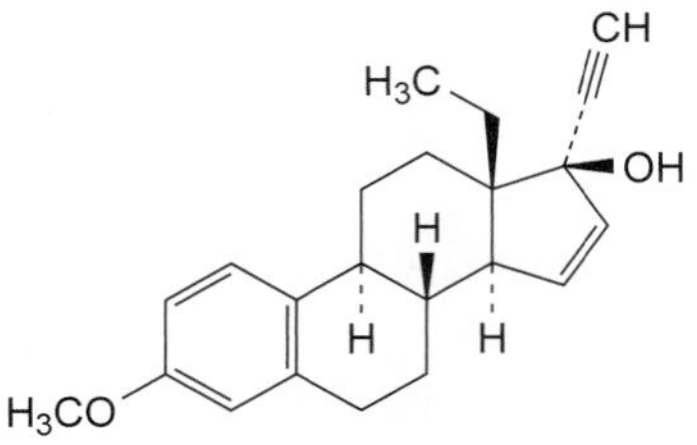

G. 13-ethyl-3-methoxy-18,19-dinor-17α-pregna-1,3,5(10),15-tetraen-20-yn-17-ol (A-aromatic-gestodene),

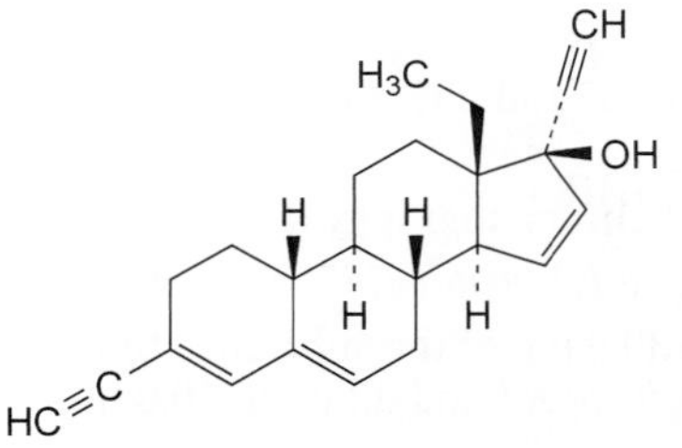

H. 13-ethyl-3-ethynyl-18,19-dinor-17α-pregna-3,5,15-trien-20-yn-17-ol (diethynyl-gestodene),

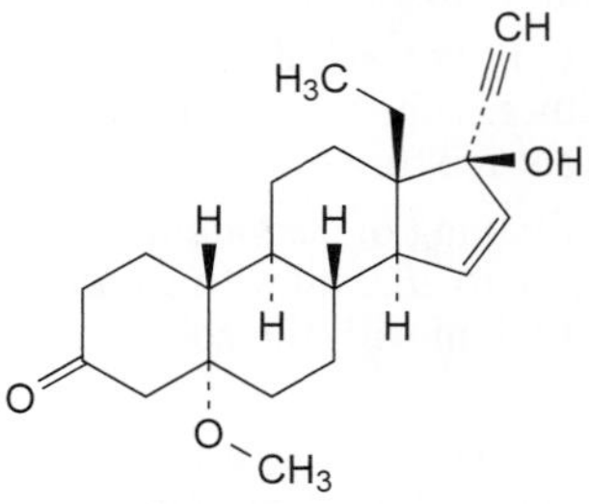

I. 13-ethyl-17-hydroxy-5-methoxy-18,19-dinor-5α,17α-pregn-15-en-20-yn-3-one (5-methoxy-gestodene),

J. 13-ethylspiro(18,19-dinor-17α-pregna-5,15-dien-20-yne-3,2'-[1,3]dioxolan)-17-ol and 13-ethylspiro(18,19-dinor-17α-pregna-5(10),15-dien-20-yne-3,2'-[1,3]dioxolan)-17-ol (gestodene ketal),

K. 13-ethyl-3,17-dihydroxy-18,19-dinor-17α-pregna-1,3,5(10),15-tetraen-20-yn-6-one (aromatic 6-keto-gestodene),

L. 13-ethyl-17-hydroxy-18,19-dinor-17α-pregna-5,15-dien-20-yn-3-one (Δ5(6)-gestodene).

07/2009:1828

GINKGO LEAF

Ginkgonis folium

DEFINITION

Whole or fragmented, dried leaf of *Ginkgo biloba* L.

Content: not less than 0.5 per cent of flavonoids, expressed as flavone glycosides (M_r 757) (dried drug).

IDENTIFICATION

A. The leaf is greyish or yellowish-green or yellowish-brown. The upper surface is slightly darker than the lower surface. The petioles are about 4-9 cm long. The lamina is about 4-10 cm wide, fan-shaped, usually bilobate or sometimes undivided. Both surfaces are smooth, and the venation dichotomous, the veins appearing to radiate from the base; they are equally prominent on both surfaces. The distal margin is incised, irregularly and to different degrees, and irregularly lobate or emarginate. The lateral margins are entire and taper towards the base.

B. Reduce to a powder (355) (*2.9.12*). The powder is greyish or yellowish-green or yellowish-brown. Examine under a microscope using *chloral hydrate solution R*. The powder shows the following diagnostic characters:

irregularly-shaped fragments of the lamina in surface view, the upper epidermis consisting of elongated cells with irregularly sinuous walls, the lower epidermal cells smaller, with a finely striated cuticle and each cell shortly papillose; stomata about 60 µm, wide, deeply sunken with 6-8 subsidiary cells, are more numerous in the lower epidermis; abundant large cluster crystals of calcium oxalate of various sizes in the mesophyll; fragments of vascular tissue from the petiole and veins.

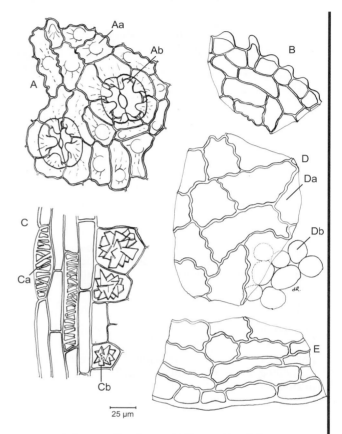

25 µm

A. Lower epidermis in surface view with papillose cells (Aa) and stomata (Ab)

B. Lower epidermis in side view

C. Vascular tissue with xylem (Ca) and cluster crystals of calcium oxalate (Cb)

D. Upper epidermis in surface view (Da) with palisade parenchyma (Db)

E. Margin of lamina, upper surface, in side view

Figure 1828.-1. — *Illustration of powdered herbal drug of ginkgo leaf (see Identification B)*

C. Thin-layer chromatography (*2.2.27*).

Test solution. To 2.0 g of the powdered drug (710) (*2.9.12*) add 10 ml of *methanol R*. Heat in a water-bath at 65 °C for 10 min. Shake frequently. Allow to cool to room temperature and filter.

Reference solution. Dissolve 1.0 mg of *chlorogenic acid R* and 3.0 mg of *rutin R* in 20 ml of *methanol R*.

Plate: TLC silica gel plate R.

Mobile phase: anhydrous formic acid R, glacial acetic acid R, water R, ethyl acetate R (7.5:7.5:17.5:67.5 V/V/V/V).

Application: 20 µl as bands.

Development: over a path of 17 cm.

Drying: at 100-105 °C.

Monographs D-K

Detection: spray the warm plate with a 10 g/l solution of *diphenylboric acid aminoethyl ester R* in *methanol R*. Subsequently spray with the same volume of a 50 g/l solution of *macrogol 400 R* in *methanol R*. Allow to dry in air for about 30 min. Examine in ultraviolet light at 365 nm.

Results: see below the sequence of the zones present in the chromatograms obtained with the reference solution and the test solution. Furthermore, other weaker fluorescent zones may be present in the chromatogram obtained with the test solution.

Top of the plate	
	A yellowish-brown fluorescent zone
	A green fluorescent zone
	2 yellowish-brown fluorescent zones
	An intense light blue fluorescent zone sometimes overlapped by a greenish-brown fluorescent zone
Chlorogenic acid: a light blue fluorescent zone	A green fluorescent zone
Rutin: a yellowish-brown fluorescent zone	2 yellowish-brown fluorescent zones
	A green fluorescent zone
	A yellowish-brown fluorescent zone
Reference solution	**Test solution**

TESTS

Foreign matter (*2.8.2*): maximum 5 per cent of stems and 2 per cent of other foreign matter.

Loss on drying (*2.2.32*): maximum 11.0 per cent, determined on 1.000 g of the powdered drug (355) (*2.9.12*) by drying in an oven at 105 °C for 2 h.

Total ash (*2.4.16*): maximum 11.0 per cent.

ASSAY

Flavonoids. Liquid chromatography (*2.2.29*).

Test solution. Heat 2.500 g of the powdered drug (710) (*2.9.12*) in 50 ml of a 60 per cent *V/V* solution of *acetone R* under a reflux condenser for 30 min. Filter and collect the filtrate. Extract the drug residue a 2nd time in the same manner, using 40 ml of a 60 per cent *V/V* solution of *acetone R* and filter. Collect the filtrates and dilute to 100.0 ml with a 60 per cent *V/V* solution of *acetone R*. Evaporate 50.0 ml of the solution to eliminate the acetone and transfer to a 50.0 ml vial, rinsing with 30 ml of *methanol R*. Add 4.4 ml of *hydrochloric acid R1*, dilute to 50.0 ml with *water R* and centrifuge. Place 10 ml of the supernatant liquid in a 10 ml brown-glass vial. Close with a rubber seal and an aluminium cap and heat on a water-bath for 25 min. Allow to cool to room temperature.

Reference solution. Dissolve 10.0 mg of *quercetin dihydrate R* in 20 ml of *methanol R*. Add 15.0 ml of *dilute hydrochloric acid R* and 5 ml of *water R* and dilute to 50.0 ml with *methanol R*.

Column:
- *size*: l = 0.125 m, Ø = 4 mm;
- *stationary phase*: *octadecylsilyl silica gel for chromatography R* (5 µm);
- *temperature*: 25 °C.

Mobile phase:
- *mobile phase A*: 0.3 g/l solution of *phosphoric acid R* adjusted to pH 2.0,
- *mobile phase B*: methanol R,

Time (min)	Mobile phase A (per cent *V/V*)	Mobile phase B (per cent *V/V*)
0 - 1	60	40
1 - 20	60 → 45	40 → 55
20 - 21	45 → 0	55 → 100
21 - 25	0	100

Flow rate: 1.0 ml/min.

Detection: spectrophotometer at 370 nm.

Injection: 10 µl.

Relative retention with reference to quercetin (retention time = about 12.5 min): kaempferol = about 1.4; isorhamnetin = about 1.5.

System suitability:
- *resolution*: minimum 1.5 between the peaks due to kaempferol and to isorhamnetin.

Do not take into account peaks eluting before the quercetin peak or after the isorhamnetin peak in the chromatogram obtained with the test solution.

Calculate the percentage content of flavonoids, expressed as flavone glycosides, using the following expression:

$$2 \times \frac{F_1 \times m_1 \times 2.514 \times p}{F_2 \times m_2}$$

F_1 = sum of the areas of all the considered peaks in the chromatogram obtained with the test solution;

F_2 = area of the peak corresponding to quercetin in the chromatogram obtained with the reference solution;

m_1 = mass of quercetin used to prepare the reference solution, in grams;

m_2 = mass of the drug to be examined used to prepare the test solution, in grams;

p = percentage content of anhydrous quercetin in *quercetin dihydrate R*.

07/2009:1978

GUAIACOL

Guaiacolum

$C_7H_8O_2$ M_r 124.1
[90-05-1]

DEFINITION

2-Methoxyphenol.

Content: 97.0 per cent to 102.0 per cent (anhydrous substance).

CHARACTERS

Appearance: crystalline mass or colourless or yellowish liquid, hygroscopic.

Solubility: sparingly soluble in water, very soluble in methylene chloride, freely soluble in ethanol (96 per cent).

mp: about 28 °C.

IDENTIFICATION

First identification: A.

Second identification: B.

A. Infrared absorption spectrophotometry (2.2.24).

   Comparison: guaiacol CRS.

B. Thin-layer chromatography (2.2.27).

   Test solution. Dissolve 0.5 g of the substance to be examined in *methanol R* and dilute to 25 ml with the same solvent.

   Reference solution. Dissolve 0.5 g of *guaiacol CRS* in *methanol R* and dilute to 25 ml with the same solvent.

   Plate: TLC silica gel plate R.

   Mobile phase: anhydrous acetic acid R, methanol R, toluene R (6:14:80 V/V/V).

   Application: 5 µl.

   Development: over 2/3 of the plate.

   Drying: in air.

   Detection: spray with *ferric chloride solution R1.*

   Results: the principal spot in the chromatogram obtained with the test solution is similar in position, colour and size to the principal spot in the chromatogram obtained with the reference solution.

TESTS

Solution S. Dissolve 1.00 g in *ethanol (96 per cent) R* and dilute to 10.0 ml with the same solvent.

Appearance of solution. Solution S is clear (2.2.1) and not more intensely coloured than reference solution BY_6 (2.2.2, Method I).

Acidity or alkalinity. To 5.0 ml of solution S, add 10 ml of *carbon dioxide-free water R* and 0.1 ml of *methyl red mixed solution R.* Not more than 0.05 ml of *0.1 M hydrochloric acid* or *0.1 M sodium hydroxide* is required to change the colour of the indicator.

Impurity A. Liquid chromatography (2.2.29).

Solvent mixture: phosphoric acid R, water R, methanol R (1:499:500 V/V/V).

Test solution (a). Dissolve 1.0 g of the substance to be examined in the solvent mixture and dilute to 25.0 ml with the solvent mixture.

Test solution (b). Dissolve 20.0 mg of the substance to be examined in the solvent mixture and dilute to 100.0 ml with the solvent mixture.

Reference solution (a). Dilute 1.0 ml of test solution (a) to 100.0 ml with the solvent mixture. Dilute 1.0 ml of this solution to 20.0 ml with the solvent mixture.

Reference solution (b). Dissolve 0.20 g of *pyrocatechol R* (impurity A) and 0.20 g of *phenol R* (impurity B) in the solvent mixture and dilute to 100 ml with the solvent mixture. Dilute 1 ml of this solution to 10 ml with the solvent mixture.

Reference solution (c). Dissolve 20.0 mg of *guaiacol CRS* in the solvent mixture and dilute to 100.0 ml with the solvent mixture.

Column:

— *size: l = 0.15 m, Ø = 4.6 mm;*

— *stationary phase: octadecylsilyl silica gel for chromatography R (5 µm).*

Mobile phase:

— *mobile phase A: phosphoric acid R, methanol R, water R (1:150:849 V/V/V);*

— *mobile phase B: methanol R;*

Time (min)	Mobile phase A (per cent V/V)	Mobile phase B (per cent V/V)
0 - 28	100	0
28 - 30	100 → 35	0 → 65
30 - 40	35	65

Flow rate: 1 ml/min.

Detection: spectrophotometer at 270 nm.

Injection: 20 µl of test solution (a) and reference solutions (a) and (b).

Retention time: guaiacol = about 20 min.

System suitability: reference solution (b):

— *resolution:* minimum 5.0 between the peaks due to impurities A (1st peak) and B (2nd peak).

Limit:

— *impurity A:* not more than the area of the principal peak in the chromatogram obtained with reference solution (a) (0.05 per cent).

Related substances. Gas chromatography (2.2.28): use the normalisation procedure.

Test solution. Dissolve 1.00 g of the substance to be examined in *acetonitrile R* and dilute to 10.0 ml with the same solvent.

Reference solution (a). Dissolve 0.20 g of *phenol R* (impurity B) and 0.40 g of *methyl benzoate R* (impurity E) in *acetonitrile R* and dilute to 50 ml with the same solvent. Dilute 1 ml of this solution to 20 ml with *acetonitrile R.*

Reference solution (b). Dilute 0.5 ml of the test solution to 100.0 ml with *acetonitrile R.* Dilute 1.0 ml of this solution to 10.0 ml with *acetonitrile R.*

Reference solution (c). Dissolve 10 mg of *veratrole R* (impurity C) in *acetonitrile R* and dilute to 10 ml with the same solvent.

Column:

— *material:* fused silica;

— *size: l = 25 m, Ø = 0.53 mm;*

— *stationary phase: poly(cyanopropyl)(7)(phenyl)-(7)(methyl)(86)siloxane R (film thickness 2 µm).*

Carrier gas: helium for chromatography R.

Flow rate: 5 ml/min.

Split ratio: 1:5.

Temperature:

	Time (min)	Temperature (°C)
Column	0 - 15	90
	15 - 45	90 → 180
Injection port		200
Detector		220

Detection: flame ionisation.

Injection: 1 µl.

Relative retention with reference to guaiacol (retention time = about 25 min): impurity E = about 0.88; impurity B = about 0.92; impurity C = about 1.1.

System suitability: reference solution (a):

— *resolution:* minimum 2.0 between the peaks due to impurities E (1st peak) and B (2nd peak).

Limits:

— *impurity C:* maximum 0.4 per cent;

— *impurity E*: maximum 0.2 per cent;

— *impurity B*: maximum 0.15 per cent;

— *unspecified impurities*: for each impurity, maximum 0.10 per cent;

— *total*: maximum 1.0 per cent;

— *disregard limit*: the area of the principal peak in the chromatogram obtained with reference solution (b) (0.05 per cent).

Water (*2.5.12*): maximum 0.5 per cent, determined on 2.000 g.

ASSAY

Liquid chromatography (*2.2.29*) as described in the test for impurity A with the following modification.

Injection: test solution (b) and reference solution (c).

Calculate the percentage content of $C_7H_8O_2$ from the declared content of *guaiacol CRS*.

STORAGE

In an airtight container, protected from light.

IMPURITIES

Specified impurities: A, B, C, E.

Other detectable impurities (the following substances would, if present at a sufficient level, be detected by one or other of the tests in the monograph. They are limited by the general acceptance criterion for other/unspecified impurities and/or by the general monograph *Substances for pharmaceutical use (2034)*. It is therefore not necessary to identify these impurities for demonstration of compliance. See also *5.10. Control of impurities in substances for pharmaceutical use*): *D, F, G, H.*

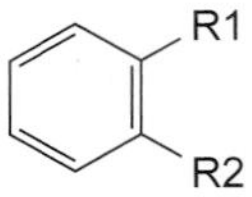

A. R1 = R2 = OH: benzene-1,2-diol (pyrocatechol),

B. R1 = OH, R2 = H: phenol,

C. R1 = R2 = OCH$_3$: 1,2-dimethoxybenzene (veratrole),

E. R1 = CO-O-CH$_3$, R2 = H: methyl benzoate,

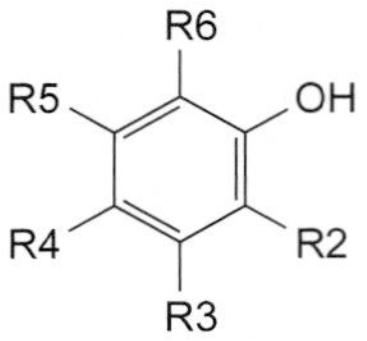

D. R2 = R5 = OCH$_3$, R3 = R4 = R6 = H: 2,5-dimethoxyphenol,

F. R2 = OCH$_3$, R3 = R4 = R5 = H, R6 = CH$_3$: 2-methoxy-6-methylphenol (6-methylguaiacol),

G. R2 = R3 = R5 = R6 = H, R4 = OCH$_3$: 4-methoxyphenol,

H. R2 = R4 = R5 = R6 = H, R3 = OCH$_3$: 3-methoxyphenol.

H

07/2009:0335

HYDROCORTISONE

Hydrocortisonum

$C_{21}H_{30}O_5$ M_r 362.5

[50-23-7]

DEFINITION

11β,17,21-Trihydroxypregn-4-ene-3,20-dione.

Content: 97.0 per cent to 103.0 per cent (dried substance).

CHARACTERS

Appearance: white or almost white, crystalline powder.

Solubility: practically insoluble in water, sparingly soluble in acetone and in ethanol (96 per cent), slightly soluble in methylene chloride.

It shows polymorphism (*5.9*).

IDENTIFICATION

First identification: A, B.

Second identification: C, D.

A. Infrared absorption spectrophotometry (*2.2.24*).

   Comparison: hydrocortisone CRS.

   If the spectra obtained in the solid state show differences, dissolve the substance to be examined and the reference substance separately in the minimum volume of *acetone R*, evaporate to dryness on a water-bath and record new spectra using the residues.

B. Liquid chromatography (*2.2.29*) as described in the test for related substances with the following modification.

   Injection: test solution and reference solution (c).

   Results: the principal peak in the chromatogram obtained with the test solution is similar in retention time and size to the principal peak in the chromatogram obtained with reference solution (c).

C. Thin-layer chromatography (*2.2.27*).

   Solution A. Dissolve 25 mg of the substance to be examined in *methanol R* and dilute to 5 ml with the same solvent.

   Solution B. Dissolve 25 mg of *hydrocortisone CRS* in *methanol R* and dilute to 5 ml with the same solvent.

   Test solution (a). Dilute 2 ml of solution A to 10 ml with *methylene chloride R*.

   Test solution (b). Transfer 0.4 ml of solution A to a glass tube 100 mm long and 20 mm in diameter and fitted with a ground-glass stopper or a polytetrafluoroethylene cap. Evaporate the solvent with gentle heating under a stream of *nitrogen R*. Add 2 ml of a 15 per cent *V/V* solution of *glacial acetic acid R* and 50 mg of *sodium bismuthate R*. Stopper the tube and shake the suspension in a mechanical shaker, protected from light, for 1 h. Add

2 ml of a 15 per cent *V/V* solution of *glacial acetic acid R* and filter into a 50 ml separating funnel, washing the filter with 2 quantities, each of 5 ml, of *water R*. Shake the clear filtrate with 10 ml of *methylene chloride R*. Wash the organic layer with 5 ml of *1 M sodium hydroxide* and then with 2 quantities, each of 5 ml, of *water R*. Dry over *anhydrous sodium sulphate R*.

Reference solution (a). Dilute 2 ml of solution B to 10 ml with *methylene chloride R*.

Reference solution (b). Transfer 0.4 ml of solution B to a glass tube 100 mm long and 20 mm in diameter and fitted with a ground-glass stopper or a polytetrafluoroethylene cap. Evaporate the solvent with gentle heating under a stream of *nitrogen R*. Add 2 ml of a 15 per cent *V/V* solution of *glacial acetic acid R* and 50 mg of *sodium bismuthate R*. Stopper the tube and shake the suspension in a mechanical shaker, protected from light, for 1 h. Add 2 ml of a 15 per cent *V/V* solution of *glacial acetic acid R* and filter into a 50 ml separating funnel, washing the filter with 2 quantities, each of 5 ml, of *water R*. Shake the clear filtrate with 10 ml of *methylene chloride R*. Wash the organic layer with 5 ml of *1 M sodium hydroxide* and then with 2 quantities, each of 5 ml, of *water R*. Dry over *anhydrous sodium sulphate R*.

Plate: TLC silica gel F$_{254}$ plate R.

Mobile phase A: add a mixture of 1.2 volumes of *water R* and 8 volumes of *methanol R* to a mixture of 15 volumes of *ether R* and 77 volumes of *methylene chloride R*.

Mobile phase B: *butanol R* saturated with *water R*, *toluene R*, *ether R* (5:15:80 *V/V/V*).

Application: 5 µl of test solution (a) and reference solution (a), 25 µl of test solution (b) and reference solution (b), applying the latter 2 in small quantities to obtain small spots.

Development: over a path of 15 cm with mobile phase A, and then over a path of 15 cm with mobile phase B.

Drying: in air.

Detection A: examine in ultraviolet light at 254 nm.

Results A: the principal spot in each of the chromatograms obtained with test solutions (a) and (b) is similar in position and size to the principal spot in the chromatogram obtained with the corresponding reference solution.

Detection B: spray with *alcoholic solution of sulphuric acid R* and heat at 120 °C for 10 min or until the spots appear; allow to cool, and examine in daylight and in ultraviolet light at 365 nm.

Results B: the principal spot in each of the chromatograms obtained with test solutions (a) and (b) is similar in position, colour in daylight, fluorescence in ultraviolet light at 365 nm and size to the principal spot in the chromatogram obtained with the corresponding reference solution. The principal spots in the chromatograms obtained with test solution (b) and reference solution (b) have an R_F value distinctly higher than that of the principal spots in the chromatograms obtained with test solution (a) and reference solution (a).

D. Add about 2 mg to 2 ml of *sulphuric acid R* and shake to dissolve. Within 5 min, an intense brownish-red colour develops with a green fluorescence that is particularly intense when examined in ultraviolet light at 365 nm. Add the solution to 10 ml of *water R* and mix. The colour fades and a clear solution remains. The fluorescence in ultraviolet light does not disappear.

TESTS

Specific optical rotation (*2.2.7*): + 162 to + 168 (dried substance).

Dissolve 0.200 g in *methanol R*, dilute to 25.0 ml with the same solvent and sonicate for 10 min.

Related substances. Liquid chromatography (*2.2.29*).

Solvent mixture: acetonitrile R, water R (40:60 V/V).

Test solution. Dissolve 20 mg of the substance to be examined in the solvent mixture, dilute to 10.0 ml with the solvent mixture and sonicate for 10 min.

Reference solution (a). Dissolve 4 mg of *prednisolone CRS* (impurity A), 2 mg of *cortisone R* (impurity B), 8 mg of *hydrocortisone acetate CRS* (impurity C) and 6 mg of *Reichstein's substance S R* (impurity F) in 40 ml of *acetonitrile R* and dilute to 100.0 ml with *water R*. Dilute 0.5 ml of this solution to 5.0 ml with the test solution.

Reference solution (b). Dilute 1.0 ml of the test solution to 100.0 ml with the solvent mixture. Dilute 1.0 ml of this solution to 10.0 ml with the solvent mixture.

Reference solution (c). Dissolve 2 mg of *hydrocortisone CRS* in 1.0 ml of the solvent mixture and sonicate for 10 min.

Reference solution (d). Dissolve 2 mg of *hydrocortisone for peak identification CRS* (containing impurities D, E, G, H, I and N) in 1.0 ml of the solvent mixture and sonicate for 10 min.

Column:
- *size*: l = 0.25 m, Ø = 4.6 mm;
- *stationary phase*: base-deactivated end-capped octadecylsilyl silica gel for chromatography R (5 µm).

Mobile phase:
- *mobile phase A*: water R;
- *mobile phase B*: acetonitrile R;

Time (min)	Mobile phase A (per cent V/V)	Mobile phase B (per cent V/V)
0 - 18	74	26
18 - 32	74 → 55	26 → 45
32 - 48	55 → 30	45 → 70

Flow rate: 0.8 ml/min.

Detection: spectrophotometer at 254 nm.

Injection: 10 µl of the test solution and reference solutions (a), (b) and (d).

Identification of impurities: use the chromatogram supplied with *hydrocortisone for peak identification CRS* and the chromatogram obtained with reference solution (d) to identify the peaks due to impurities D, E, G, H, I and N; use the chromatogram obtained with reference solution (a) to identify the peaks due to impurities A, B, C and F.

Relative retention with reference to hydrocortisone (retention time = about 24 min): impurity D = about 0.2; impurity H = about 0.3; impurity I = about 0.5; impurity G = about 0.8; impurity E = about 0.86; impurity A = about 0.96; impurity B = about 1.1; impurity F = about 1.4; impurity C = about 1.5; impurity N = about 1.7.

System suitability: reference solution (a):
- *peak-to-valley ratio*: minimum 3.0, where H_p = height above the baseline of the peak due to impurity A and H_v = height above the baseline of the lowest point of the curve separating this peak from the peak due to hydrocortisone.

Limits:
- *correction factors*: for the calculation of content, multiply the peak areas of the following impurities by the corresponding correction factor: impurity D = 1.8; impurity E = 2.7;
- *impurities C, D, E, I*: for each impurity, not more than 5 times the area of the principal peak in the chromatogram obtained with reference solution (b) (0.5 per cent);
- *impurity F*: not more than 3 times the area of the principal peak in the chromatogram obtained with reference solution (b) (0.3 per cent);
- *impurities A, B, G*: for each impurity, not more than twice the area of the principal peak in the chromatogram obtained with reference solution (b) (0.2 per cent);
- *impurities H, N*: for each impurity, not more than 1.5 times the area of the principal peak in the chromatogram obtained with reference solution (b) (0.15 per cent);
- *unspecified impurities*: for each impurity, not more than the area of the principal peak in the chromatogram obtained with reference solution (b) (0.10 per cent);
- *total*: not more than 20 times the area of the principal peak in the chromatogram obtained with reference solution (b) (2.0 per cent);
- *disregard limit*: 0.5 times the area of the principal peak in the chromatogram obtained with reference solution (b) (0.05 per cent).

Loss on drying (*2.2.32*): maximum 1.0 per cent, determined on 1.000 g by drying in an oven at 105 °C.

ASSAY

Dissolve 0.100 g in *ethanol (96 per cent) R* and dilute to 100.0 ml with the same solvent. Dilute 2.0 ml of this solution to 100.0 ml with *ethanol (96 per cent) R*. Measure the absorbance (*2.2.25*) at the absorption maximum at 241.5 nm.

Calculate the content of $C_{21}H_{30}O_5$ taking the specific absorbance to be 440.

STORAGE

Protected from light.

IMPURITIES

Specified impurities: A, B, C, D, E, F, G, H, I, N.

Other detectable impurities (the following substances would, if present at a sufficient level, be detected by one or other of the tests in the monograph. They are limited by the general acceptance criterion for other/unspecified impurities and/or by the general monograph *Substances for pharmaceutical use (2034)*. It is therefore not necessary to identify these impurities for demonstration of compliance. See also *5.10. Control of impurities in substances for pharmaceutical use*): J, K, L, M, O.

A. prednisolone,

B. 17,21-dihydroxypregn-4-ene-3,11,20-trione (cortisone),

C. hydrocortisone acetate (hydrocortisone-21-acetate),

D. R1 = R3 = OH, R2 = R4 = H, R5 = CH₂OH:
   6β,11β,17,21-tetrahydroxypregn-4-ene-3,20-dione
   (6β-hydroxyhydrocortisone),

F. R1 = R2 = R3 = R4 = H, R5 = CH₂OH:
   17,21-dihydroxypregn-4-ene-3,20-dione (Reichstein's
   substance S),

G. R1 = R2 = R4 = H, R3 = OH, R5 = CHO:
   11β,17-dihydroxy-3,20-dioxopregn-4-en-21-al
   (hydrocortisone-21-aldehyde),

H. R1 = R4 = H, R2 = R3 = OH, R5 = CH₂OH:
   7α,11β,17,21-tetrahydroxypregn-4-ene-3,20-dione
   (7α-hydroxyhydrocortisone),

I. R1 = R2 = H, R3 = R4 = OH, R5 = CH₂OH:
   11β,14,17,21-tetrahydroxypregn-4-ene-3,20-dione
   (14α-hydroxyhydrocortisone),

K. R1 = R2 = R3 = R4 = H, R5 = CH₂-O-CO-CH₃:
   17-hydroxy-3,20-dioxopregn-4-en-21-yl acetate
   (Reichstein's substance S-21-acetate),

E. 11β,17,21-trihydroxypregna-4,6-diene-3,20-dione
   (Δ6-hydrocortisone),

J. R1 = H, R2 = CO-CH₃, R3 = OH: 11β,21-dihydroxy-3,20-
   dioxopregn-4-en-17-yl acetate (hydrocortisone-17-acetate),

L. R1 = R2 = R3 = H: 11β,17-dihydroxypregn-4-ene-3,20-dione
   (oxenol),

O. R1 = R3 = OH, R2 = H: 11β,17,19,21-tetrahydroxypregn-4-
   ene-3,20-dione (19-hydroxyhydrocortisone),

M. 11α,17,21-trihydroxypregn-4-ene-3,20-dione
   (epi-hydrocortisone),

N. 11β,17,21-trihydroxy-21-(11β,17,21-trihydroxy-3,
   20-dioxopregn-4-en-21-yl)pregn-4-ene-3,20-dione
   (hydrocortisone dimer).

I

07/2008:0029
corrected 6.5

IMIPRAMINE HYDROCHLORIDE

Imipramini hydrochloridum

$C_{19}H_{25}ClN_2$ M_r 316.9
[113-52-0]

DEFINITION

3-(10,11-Dihydro-5H-dibenzo[b,f]azepin-5-yl)-N,N-dimethylpropan-1-amine hydrochloride.

Content: 98.5 per cent to 101.0 per cent (dried substance).

CHARACTERS

Appearance: white or slightly yellow, crystalline powder.

Solubility: freely soluble in water and in ethanol (96 per cent).

IDENTIFICATION

First identification: B, D.

Second identification: A, C, D.

A. Melting point (*2.2.14*): 170 °C to 174 °C.

B. Infrared absorption spectrophotometry (*2.2.24*).
   Comparison: imipramine hydrochloride CRS.

C. Dissolve about 5 mg in 2 ml of *nitric acid R*. An intense blue colour develops.

D. About 20 mg gives reaction (a) of chlorides (*2.3.1*).

TESTS

Solution S. To 3.0 g add 20 ml of *carbon dioxide-free water R*, dissolve rapidly by shaking and triturating with a glass rod and dilute to 30 ml with the same solvent.

Appearance of solution. Solution S is clear (*2.2.1*). Immediately after preparation, dilute solution S with an equal volume of *water R*. This solution is not more intensely coloured than reference solution BY_6 (*2.2.2, Method II*).

pH (*2.2.3*): 3.6 to 5.0 for solution S, measured immediately after preparation.

Related substances. Liquid chromatography (*2.2.29*).

Test solution. Dissolve 50.0 mg of the substance to be examined in the mobile phase and dilute to 50.0 ml with the mobile phase.

Reference solution (a). Dissolve 5.0 mg of *imipramine for system suitability CRS* (containing impurity B) in the mobile phase and dilute to 5.0 ml with the mobile phase.

Reference solution (b). Dilute 1.0 ml of the test solution to 100.0 ml with the mobile phase. Dilute 1.0 ml of this solution to 10.0 ml with the mobile phase.

Column:
- *size*: l = 0.15 m, Ø = 4.6 mm;
- *stationary phase*: *end-capped polar-embedded octadecylsilyl amorphous organosilica polymer R* (5 µm);

- *temperature*: 40 °C.

Mobile phase: mix 40 volumes of *acetonitrile R1* with 60 volumes of a 5.2 g/l solution of *dipotassium hydrogen phosphate R* previously adjusted to pH 7.0 with *phosphoric acid R*.

Flow rate: 1.0 ml/min.

Detection: spectrophotometer at 220 nm.

Injection: 10 µl.

Run time: 2.5 times the retention time of imipramine.

Relative retention with reference to imipramine (retention time = about 7 min): impurity B = about 0.7.

System suitability: reference solution (a):
- *resolution*: minimum 5.0 between the peaks due to impurity B and imipramine.

Limits:
- *impurity B*: not more than the area of the corresponding peak in the chromatogram obtained with reference solution (a) (0.1 per cent);
- *unspecified impurities*: for each impurity, not more than the area of the peak due to imipramine in the chromatogram obtained with reference solution (b) (0.10 per cent);
- *total*: not more than 3 times the area of the peak due to imipramine in the chromatogram obtained with reference solution (b) (0.3 per cent);
- *disregard limit*: 0.5 times the area of the peak due to imipramine in the chromatogram obtained with reference solution (b) (0.05 per cent).

Heavy metals (*2.4.8*): maximum 20 ppm.

Test solution. Dissolve 0.500 g of the substance to be examined in 20 ml of *water R*.

Reference solution. Dilute 10 ml of *lead standard solution (1 ppm Pb) R* to 20 ml with *water R*.

Blank solution. 20 ml of *water R*.

Monitor solution. Dissolve 0.500 g of the substance to be examined in 10 ml of *lead standard solution (1 ppm Pb) R* and dilute to 20 ml of *water R*.

To each solution add 2 ml of *buffer solution pH 3.5 R*. Mix and add to 1.2 ml of *thioacetamide reagent R*. Mix immediately. Filter the solutions through a suitable membrane filter (pore size 0.45 µm). Compare the spots on the filters obtained with the different solutions. The test is invalid if the reference solution and the monitor solution do not show a slight brown colour compared to the blank solution. The substance to be examined complies with the test if the brown colour of the spot resulting from the test solution is not more intense than that of the spot resulting from the reference solution.

Loss on drying (*2.2.32*): maximum 0.5 per cent, determined on 1.000 g by drying in an oven at 105 °C.

Sulphated ash (*2.4.14*): maximum 0.1 per cent, determined on 1.0 g.

ASSAY

Dissolve 0.250 g in 50 ml of *ethanol (96 per cent) R* and add 5.0 ml of *0.01 M hydrochloric acid*. Carry out a potentiometric titration (*2.2.20*), using *0.1 M sodium hydroxide*. Read the volume added between the 2 points of inflexion.

1 ml of *0.1 M sodium hydroxide* is equivalent to 31.69 mg of $C_{19}H_{25}ClN_2$.

STORAGE

Protected from light.

Monographs D-K

IMPURITIES

Specified impurities: B.

Other detectable impurities (the following substances would, if present at a sufficient level, be detected by one or other of the tests in the monograph. They are limited by the general acceptance criterion for other/unspecified impurities and/or by the general monograph Substances for pharmaceutical use (2034). It is therefore not necessary to identify these impurities for demonstration of compliance. See also 5.10. Control of impurities in substances for pharmaceutical use): A, C.

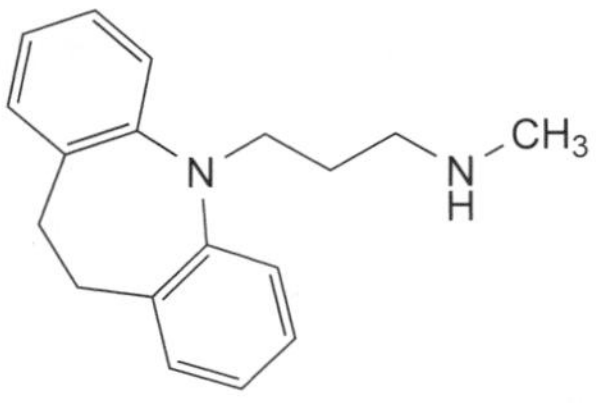

A. 3-(10,11-dihydro-5*H*-dibenzo[*b,f*]azepin-5-yl)-*N*-methylpropan-1-amine (desipramine),

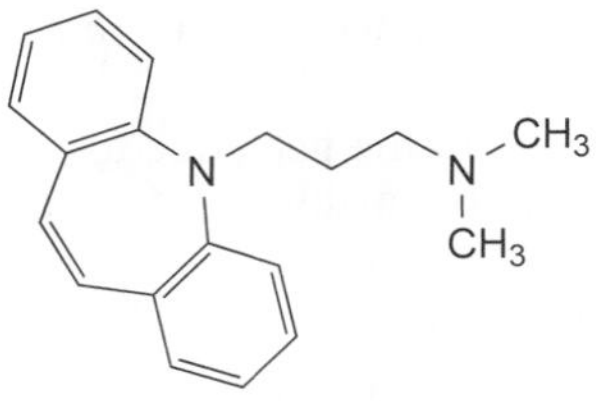

B. 3-(5*H*-dibenzo[*b,f*]azepin-5-yl)-*N,N*-dimethylpropan-1-amine (depramine),

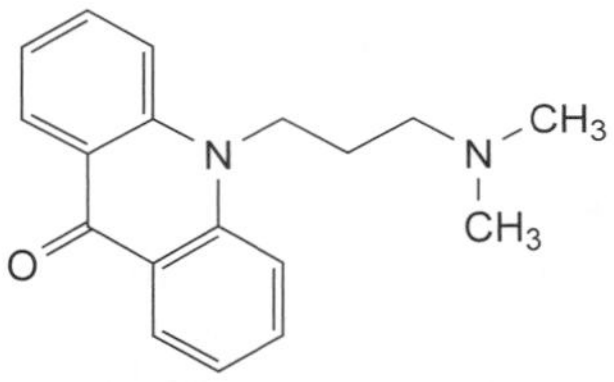

C. 10-[3-(dimethylamino)propyl]acridin-9(10*H*)-one.

01/2009:1639
corrected 6.5

INTERFERON BETA-1a CONCENTRATED SOLUTION

Interferoni beta-1a solutio concentrata

```
MSYNLLGFLQ  RSSNFQCQKL  LWQLNGRLEY  CLKDRMNFDI
PEEIKQLQQF  QKEDAALTIY  EMLQNIFAIF  RQDSSSTGWN*
ETIVENLLAN  VYHQINHLKT  VLEEKLEKED  FTRGKLMSSL
HLKRYYGRIL  HYLKAKEYSH  CAWTIVRVEI  LRNFYFINRL
TGYLRN
```

* glycosylation site

$C_{908}H_{1406}N_{246}O_{252}S_7$ M_r approx. 22 500

DEFINITION

Solution of a glycosylated protein having the same amino acid sequence and disulphide bridge and a similar glycosylation pattern as interferon beta produced by human diploid fibroblasts in response to viral infections and various other inducers. It exerts antiviral, antiproliferative and immunomodulatory activity.

Content: minimum 0.20 mg of protein per millilitre.

Potency: minimum 1.5×10^8 IU per milligram of protein.

It may contain buffer salts.

PRODUCTION

Interferon beta-1a concentrated solution is produced by a method based on recombinant DNA (rDNA) technology, using mammalian cells in culture.

Prior to release, the following tests are carried out on each batch of the final bulk product, unless exemption has been granted by the competent authority.

Host-cell-derived proteins. The limit is approved by the competent authority.

Host-cell or vector-derived DNA. The limit is approved by the competent authority.

***N*-terminal truncated forms**. Examination for specific *N*-terminal truncated forms should be performed using a suitable technique such as *N*-terminal sequence determination. The limits are approved by the competent authority.

Dimer and related substances of higher molecular mass: not more than the amount approved by the competent authority, using an appropriate validated liquid chromatography method.

CHARACTERS

Appearance: clear or slightly opalescent, colourless or slightly yellowish liquid.

IDENTIFICATION

A. It shows the expected biological activity (see Assay).

B. Isoform distribution. Mass spectrometry (*2.2.43*).

Introduction of the sample: direct inflow of a desalted preparation to be examined or liquid chromatography-mass spectrometry combination.

Mode of ionisation: electrospray.

Signal acquisition: complete spectrum mode from 1100 to 2400.

Calibration: use myoglobin in the *m/z* range of 600-2400; set the instrument within validated instrumental settings and analyse the sample; the deviation of the measured mass does not exceed 0.02 per cent of the reported mass.

Interpretation of results: a typical spectrum consists of 6 major glycoforms (A to F), which differ in their degree of sialylation and/or antennarity type as shown in Table 1639.-1.

Table 1639.-1.

MS peak	Glycoform*	Expected M_r	Sialylation level
A	2A2S1F	22 375	Disialylated
B	2A1S1F	22 084	Monosialylated
C	3A2S1F and/or 2A2S1F + 1 HexNacHex repeat	22 739	Disialylated
D	3A3S1F	23 031	Trisialylated
E	4A3S1F and/or 3A3S1F + 1 HexNacHex repeat	23 400	Trisialylated
F	2A0S1F	21 793	Non-sialylated

* 2A = biantennary complex type oligosaccharide; 3A = triantennary complex type oligosaccharide; 4A = tetraantennary complex type oligosaccharide; 0S = non-sialylated; 1S = monosialylated; 2S = disialylated; 3S = trisialylated; 1F = fucosylated.

Results: the mass spectrum obtained with the preparation to be examined corresponds, with respect to the 6 major peaks, to the mass spectrum obtained with *interferon beta-1a CRS*.

C. Peptide mapping (*2.2.55*) and liquid chromatography (*2.2.29*).

Test solution. Add 5 μl of a 242 g/l solution of *tris(hydroxymethyl)aminomethane R* and a volume of the preparation to be examined containing 20 μg of protein to a polypropylene tube of 0.5 ml capacity. Add 4 μl of a 1 mg/ml solution of *endoprotease LysC R* in *0.05 M tris-hydrochloride buffer solution pH 9.0 R*. Mix gently and incubate at 30 °C for 2 h. Add 10 μl of a 15.4 g/l solution of *dithiothreitol R*. Dilute the solution with the same volume of a 573 g/l solution of *guanidine hydrochloride R*. Incubate at 4 °C for 3-4 h.

Reference solution. Prepare at the same time and in the same manner as for the test solution but using *interferon beta-1a CRS* instead of the preparation to be examined.

Precolumn:
— *size*: l = 0.02 m, Ø = 2.1 mm;
— *stationary phase*: spherical *octadecylsilyl silica gel for chromatography R* (5 μm) with a pore size of 30 nm.

Column:
— *size*: l = 0.25 m, Ø = 2.1 mm;
— *stationary phase*: spherical *octadecylsilyl silica gel for chromatography R* (5 μm) with a pore size of 30 nm.

Mobile phase:
— *mobile phase A*: dilute 1 ml of *trifluoroacetic acid R* to 1000 ml with *water R*;
— *mobile phase B*: dilute 1 ml of *trifluoroacetic acid R* in 700 ml of *acetonitrile for chromatography R*, then dilute to 1000 ml with *water R*;

Time (min)	Mobile phase A (per cent V/V)	Mobile phase B (per cent V/V)
0 - 30	100 → 64	0 → 36
30 - 45	64 → 55	36 → 45
45 - 50	55 → 40	45 → 60
50 - 70	40 → 0	60 → 100
70 - 83	0	100
83 - 85	0 → 100	100 → 0

Flow rate: 0.2 ml/min.

Detection: spectrophotometer at 214 nm.

Injection: volume that contains 20 μg of digested protein.

System suitability: the chromatogram obtained with the reference solution is qualitatively similar to the chromatogram of interferon beta-1a digest supplied with *interferon beta-1a CRS*.

Results: the profile of the chromatogram obtained with the test solution corresponds to that of the chromatogram obtained with the reference solution.

TESTS

Impurities of molecular masses differing from that of interferon beta-1a. Polyacrylamide gel electrophoresis (*2.2.31*) under reducing conditions.

Resolving gel: 12 per cent acrylamide.

Concentrated sample buffer: concentrated SDS-PAGE sample buffer for reducing conditions R containing 2-mercaptoethanol as the reducing agent.

Sample buffer: mixture of equal volumes of *concentrated SDS-PAGE sample buffer for reducing conditions R* and *water R*.

Test solution (a). Concentrate the preparation to be examined using a suitable method to obtain a protein concentration of 1.5 mg/ml.

Test solution (b): mixture of equal volumes of test solution (a) and the concentrated sample buffer.

Test solution (c). Dilute test solution (a) to obtain a protein concentration of 0.6 mg/ml. Mix equal volumes of this solution and the concentrated sample buffer.

Test solution (d). Mix 8 μl of test solution (c) and 40 μl of the sample buffer.

Test solution (e). Mix 15 μl of test solution (d) and 35 μl of the sample buffer.

Test solution (f). Mix 18 μl of test solution (e) and 18 μl of the sample buffer.

Test solution (g). Mix 12 μl of test solution (f) and 12 μl of the sample buffer.

Reference solution (a). Solution of relative molecular mass markers suitable for calibrating SDS-PAGE gels in the range of 15-67 kDa. Dissolve in the sample buffer.

Reference solution (b): 0.75 mg/ml solution of *interferon beta-1a CRS* in sample buffer.

Sample treatment: boil for 3 min.

Application: 20 μl of test solutions (b) to (g) and reference solutions (a) and (b).

Detection: Coomassie staining, carried out as follows: immerse the gel in *Coomassie staining solution R1* at 33-37 °C for 90 min with gentle shaking, then remove the staining solution; destain the gel with a large excess of a mixture of 1 volume of *glacial acetic acid R*, 1 volume of *2-propanol R* and 8 volumes of *water R*.

Apparent molecular masses: interferon beta-1a = about 23 000; underglycosylated interferon beta-1a = about 21 000; deglycosylated interferon beta-1a = about 20 000; interferon beta-1a dimer = about 46 000.

Identification of bands: use the electropherogram provided with *interferon beta-1a CRS*.

System suitability:
— the validation criteria are met (*2.2.31*);
— a band is seen in the electropherogram obtained with test solution (g);
— a gradation of intensity of staining is seen in the electropherograms obtained with test solutions (b) to (g).

Limits:

— in the electropherogram obtained with test solution (c), the band corresponding to underglycosylated interferon beta-1a is not more intense than the principal band in the electropherogram obtained with test solution (e) (5 per cent);

— in the electropherogram obtained with test solution (b), the band corresponding to deglycosylated interferon beta-1a is not more intense than the principal band in the electropherogram obtained with test solution (e) (2 per cent); any other band corresponding to an impurity of a molecular mass lower than that of interferon beta-1a, apart from the band corresponding to underglycosylated interferon beta-1a is not more intense than the principal band in the electropherogram obtained with test solution (f) (1 per cent).

Oxidised interferon beta-1a: maximum 6 per cent.

Use the chromatogram obtained with the test solution in identification C. Locate the peaks due to the peptide fragment comprising amino acids 34-45 and its oxidised form using the chromatogram of oxidised interferon beta-1a digest supplied with *interferon beta-1a CRS*.

Calculate the percentage of oxidation of interferon beta-1a using the following expression:

$$\frac{A_{34-45ox}}{A_{34-45} + A_{34-45ox}} \times 100$$

$A_{34-45ox}$ = area of the peak corresponding to the oxidised peptide fragment 34-45;

A_{34-45} = area of the peak corresponding to the peptide fragment 34-45.

Bacterial endotoxins (*2.6.14*): less than 0.7 IU in the volume that contains 1×10^6 IU of interferon beta-1a, if intended for use in the manufacture of parenteral preparations without a further appropriate procedure for removal of bacterial endotoxins.

ASSAY

Protein. Liquid chromatography (*2.2.29*). Prepare 3 independent dilutions for each solution.

Test solution. Dilute the preparation to be examined to obtain a concentration of 100 µg/ml.

Reference solution. Dissolve the contents of a vial of *interferon beta-1a CRS* to obtain a concentration of 100 µg/ml.

Precolumn:

— *size*: *l* = 0.02 m, Ø = 2.1 mm;

— *stationary phase*: *butylsilyl silica gel for chromatography R* (5 µm) with a pore size of 30 nm.

Column:

— *size*: *l* = 0.25 m, Ø = 2.1 mm;

— *stationary phase*: *butylsilyl silica gel for chromatography R* (5 µm) with a pore size of 30 nm.

Mobile phase:

— *mobile phase A*: 0.1 per cent *V/V* solution of *trifluoroacetic acid R*;

— *mobile phase B*: to 300 ml of *water R*, add 1 ml of *trifluoroacetic acid R* and dilute to 1000 ml with *acetonitrile for chromatography R*;

Time (min)	Mobile phase A (per cent V/V)	Mobile phase B (per cent V/V)
0 - 20	100 → 0	0 → 100
20 - 25	0	100
25 - 26	0 → 100	100 → 0
26 - 40	100	0

Flow rate: 0.2 ml/min.

Detection: spectrophotometer at 214 nm.

Injection: 50 µl.

Retention time: interferon beta-1a = about 20 min.

System suitability: reference solution:

— *symmetry factor*: 0.8 to 2.0 for the peak due to interferon beta-1a;

— *repeatability*: maximum relative standard deviation of 3.0 per cent between the peak areas obtained after injection of the 3 independent dilutions.

Calculate the content of interferon beta-1a ($C_{908}H_{1406}N_{246}O_{252}S_7$) from the declared content of $C_{908}H_{1406}N_{246}O_{252}S_7$ in *interferon beta-1a CRS*.

Potency

The potency of interferon beta-1a is estimated by comparing its ability to protect cells against a viral cytopathic effect with the same ability of the appropriate International Standard of human recombinant interferon beta-1a or of a reference preparation calibrated in International Units.

The International Unit is the activity contained in a stated amount of the appropriate International Standard. The equivalence in International Units of the International Standard is stated by the World Health Organisation.

Carry out the assay using a suitable method, based on the following design.

Use, in standard culture conditions, an established cell line sensitive to the cytopathic effect of a suitable virus and responsive to interferon. The cell cultures and viruses that have been shown to be suitable include the following:

— WISH cells (ATCC No. CCL-25) and vesicular stomatitis virus VSV, Indiana strain (ATCC No. VR-158) as infective agent;

— A549 cells (ATCC No. CCL-185) and encephalomyocarditis virus EMC (ATCC No. VR-129B) as infective agent.

Incubate in at least 4 series, cells with 3 or more different concentrations of the preparation to be examined and the reference preparation in a microtitre plate and include in each series appropriate controls of untreated cells. Choose the concentrations of the preparations such that the lowest concentration produces some protection and the largest concentration produces less than maximal protection against the viral cytopathic effect. Add at a suitable time the cytopathic virus to all wells with the exception of a sufficient number of wells in all series, which are left with uninfected control cells. Determine the cytopathic effect of the virus quantitatively with a suitable method. Calculate the potency of the preparation to be examined by the usual statistical methods (for example, *5.3*).

The estimated potency is not less than 80 per cent and not more than 125 per cent of the stated potency. The confidence limits (*P* = 0.95) are not less than 64 per cent and not more than 156 per cent of the estimated potency.

STORAGE

In an airtight container, protected from light, at a temperature below – 70 °C. If the substance is sterile, store in a sterile, airtight, tamper-proof container.

LABELLING

The label states:

- the interferon beta-1a content, in milligrams per millilitre;
- the antiviral activity, in International Units per millilitre;
- where applicable, that the substance is suitable for use in the manufacture of parenteral preparations.

07/2009:1753

IOPROMIDE

Iopromidum

$C_{18}H_{24}I_3N_3O_8$ M_r 791
[73334-07-3]

DEFINITION

N,N'-Bis(2,3-dihydroxypropyl)-2,4,6-triiodo-5-
[(methoxyacetyl)amino]-*N*-methylbenzene-1,3-dicarboxamide.

Mixture of diastereoisomers and atropisomers.

Content: 97.0 per cent to 102.0 per cent (anhydrous substance).

CHARACTERS

Appearance: white or slightly yellowish powder.

Solubility: freely soluble in water and in dimethyl sulphoxide, practically insoluble in ethanol (96 per cent) and in acetone.

IDENTIFICATION

Infrared absorption spectrophotometry (*2.2.24*).

Comparison: iopromide CRS.

TESTS

Appearance of solution. The solution is clear (*2.2.1*) and not more intensely coloured than reference solutions BY_6, B_6 and Y_6 (*2.2.2, Method I*).

Dissolve 16.5 g in 20 ml of *carbon dioxide-free water R* while heating on a water-bath at a temperature not exceeding 70 °C. Allow to cool to room temperature.

Conductivity (*2.2.38*): maximum 50 µS·cm⁻¹.

Dissolve 1.000 g in *water R* and dilute to 50.0 ml with the same solvent.

Impurity A and related primary aromatic amines: maximum 0.01 per cent.

Protect the solutions from light throughout the test. All given times are critical for the test results. The test solution, reference solution and blank solution must be processed in parallel.

Test solution. Dissolve 0.500 g of the substance to be examined in 20.0 ml of *water R* in a 25 ml volumetric flask.

Reference solution. Dissolve the contents of a vial of *iopromide impurity A CRS* in 5.0 ml of *water R*. Transfer 2.0 ml of this solution to a 25 ml volumetric flask and add 18.0 ml of *water R*.

Blank solution. Place 20.0 ml of *water R* in a 25 ml volumetric flask.

Cool the test solution, reference solution and blank solution in a bath of iced water for 5 min. Add 1.0 ml of *hydrochloric acid R1* to each solution and cool again for 5 min in a bath of iced water. Add 1.0 ml of a 20 g/l solution of *sodium nitrite R*, shake vigorously and cool for another 5 min in a bath of iced water. To each solution add 0.50 ml of an 80 g/l solution of *sulphamic acid R*. Over the next 5 min, shake vigorously several times, raising the stoppers to vent the gas that evolves. Afterwards, add to each solution 1.0 ml of a 1 g/l solution of *naphthylethylenediamine dihydrochloride R* in a mixture of 300 volumes of *water R* and 700 volumes of *propylene glycol R*, shake, allow to cool to room temperature for 10 min and dilute to 25.0 ml with *water R*. Degas the solutions in an ultrasonic bath for 1 min and measure the absorbance (*2.2.25*) of the test solution and the reference solution at 495 nm against the blank, within 5 min. The test is not valid unless the absorbance of the reference solution is at least 0.08. The absorbance of the test solution is not greater than the absorbance of the reference solution.

Impurity B. Liquid chromatography (*2.2.29*).

Solvent mixture: methanol R, water R (50:50 V/V).

Test solution. Dissolve 40.0 mg of the substance to be examined in the solvent mixture and dilute to 25.0 ml with the solvent mixture.

Reference solution (a). Dissolve 40.0 mg of *iopromide CRS* in the solvent mixture and dilute to 25.0 ml with the solvent mixture.

Reference solution (b). Introduce several millilitres of reference solution (a) into a vial sealed with a crimp-top. Heat at 121 °C for 15 min.

Reference solution (c). Dilute 1.5 ml of the test solution to 100.0 ml with the solvent mixture.

Column:

- *size*: *l* = 0.25 m, Ø = 4.6 mm;
- *stationary phase*: end-capped octadecylsilyl silica gel for chromatography R (5 µm);
- *temperature*: 20 °C.

Mobile phase: mix 6 g of *chloroform R* with 59 g of *methanol R*. Add 900 g of *water for chromatography R* in small portions to the chloroform/methanol mixture and stir for at least 2 h to obtain a homogeneous solution.

Flow rate: 1.2 ml/min.

Detection: spectrophotometer at 254 nm.

Injection: 10 µl of the test solution and reference solutions (a) and (c).

Run time: 50 min.

Identification of impurities: use the chromatogram supplied with *iopromide CRS* and the chromatogram obtained with reference solution (a) to identify the peaks due to impurity B isomers Y_1 and Y_2.

Relative retention with reference to iopromide isomer Z_2 (retention time = about 34 min): impurity B isomer Y_1 = about 0.28; impurity B isomer Y_2 = about 0.31.

System suitability: reference solution (a):

- the chromatogram obtained shows 2 peaks due to impurity B isomers Y_1 and Y_2.

Limit:

- *sum of impurity B isomers Y_1 and Y_2*: not more than the sum of the areas of the 2 principal peaks due to the iopromide in the chromatogram obtained with reference solution (c) (1.5 per cent).

Related substances. Thin-layer chromatography (*2.2.27*).

Solvent mixture: methanol R, water R (50:50 V/V).

Monographs
D-K

Test solution. Dissolve 1.0 g of the substance to be examined in the solvent mixture and dilute to 10.0 ml with the solvent mixture.

Reference solution (a). Dilute 1.0 ml of the test solution to 100.0 ml with the solvent mixture.

Reference solution (b). Dilute 5.0 ml of reference solution (a) to 10.0 ml with the solvent mixture.

Reference solution (c). Dilute 2.0 ml of reference solution (a) to 10.0 ml with the solvent mixture.

Reference solution (d). Dilute 1.0 ml of reference solution (a) to 10.0 ml with the solvent mixture.

Reference solution (e). Dissolve the contents of a vial of *iopromide for system suitability 1 CRS* (containing impurities B and E) in 50 µl of the solvent mixture.

Reference solution (f). Dissolve the contents of a vial of *iopromide for system suitability 2 CRS* (containing impurities B, C, D and F) in 50 µl of the solvent mixture.

Plates: *TLC silica gel F$_{254}$ plate R* (2 plates).

A. *Mobile phase*: *concentrated ammonia R, water R, dioxan R* (4:15:85 *V/V/V*).

Application: 2 µl of the test solution and reference solutions (b), (d) and (e).

Development: over 3/4 of the plate.

Drying: in a current of air, until complete evaporation of the solvents, then at 120 °C for 30 min.

Detection: examine immediately in ultraviolet light at 254 nm; expose to ultraviolet light for 2-5 min until the principal spots appear clearly as yellow spots, then spray with *ferric chloride-ferricyanide-arsenite reagent R* and examine immediately in daylight.

Retardation factors: impurity B = about 0.26; iopromide = about 0.34; impurity E = about 0.41.

System suitability: reference solution (e):

— the chromatogram shows 3 clearly separated spots.

Limits:

— *impurity E*: any spot due to impurity E is not more intense than the principal spot in the chromatogram obtained with reference solution (b) (0.5 per cent);

— *unspecified impurities*: any other spot is not more intense than the principal spot in the chromatogram obtained with reference solution (d) (0.10 per cent); disregard any spot due to impurity B.

B. *Mobile phase*: *anhydrous formic acid R, water R, methanol R, chloroform R* (2:6:32:62 *V/V/V/V*).

Application: 2 µl of the test solution and reference solutions (a), (b) ,(c), (d) and (f).

Development: over 3/4 of the plate.

Drying: in a current of air, until complete evaporation of the solvents, then at 120 °C for 30 min.

Detection: examine immediately in ultraviolet light at 254 nm; expose to an ammonia vapour for 30 min, dry in a current of air for 10 min, then expose to ultraviolet light for 2-5 min until the principal spots appear clearly as yellow spots, then spray with *ferric chloride-ferricyanide-arsenite reagent R* and examine immediately in daylight.

Retardation factors: impurity C = about 0.23; impurity D = about 0.29; impurity B = about 0.36; iopromide = about 0.43; impurity F = about 0.71.

System suitability: reference solution (f):

— the chromatogram shows 5 clearly separated spots.

Limits:

— *impurity D*: any spot due to impurity D is not more intense than the principal spot in the chromatogram obtained with reference solution (a) (1.0 per cent);

— *impurity C*: any spot due to impurity C is not more intense than the principal spot in the chromatogram obtained with reference solution (b) (0.5 per cent);

— *impurity F*: any spot due to impurity F is not more intense than the principal spot in the chromatogram obtained with reference solution (c) (0.2 per cent);

— *unspecified impurities*: any other spot is not more intense than the principal spot in the chromatogram obtained with reference solution (d) (0.10 per cent); disregard any spot due to impurity B.

Isomer distribution. Liquid chromatography (*2.2.29*) as described in the test for impurity B with the following modifications.

Calculate the percentage content of the isomer groups with reference to the total area of all the peaks due to the 4 iopromide isomers, using the chromatogram obtained with the test solution.

Limits:

— *sum of iopromide isomers E_1 and Z_1*: 40.0 per cent to 51.0 per cent;

— *sum of iopromide isomers E_2 and Z_2*: 49.0 per cent to 60.0 per cent.

Free iodine. Dissolve 2.0 g in 20 ml of *water R* in a glass-stoppered test tube. Add 2 ml of *dilute sulphuric acid R* and 2 ml of *toluene R*, close and shake vigorously. The upper layer remains colourless (*2.2.2, Method II*).

Iodide: maximum 2 ppm.

Dissolve 10.0 g in 50 ml of *carbon dioxide-free water R*. Adjust to pH 3-4 adding about 0.15 ml of *0.1 M sulphuric acid*. Titrate with *0.001 M silver nitrate*. Determine the end-point potentiometrically (*2.2.20*) using a combined metal electrode. Not more than 0.15 ml of *0.001 M silver nitrate* is required to reach the end-point.

Heavy metals (*2.4.8*): maximum 10 ppm.

Dissolve 2.0 g in *water R* and dilute to 20 ml with the same solvent. 12 ml of the solution complies with test A. Prepare the reference solution using *lead standard solution (1 ppm Pb) R*.

Water (*2.5.12*): maximum 1.5 per cent, determined on 1.00 g.

Sulphated ash (*2.4.14*): maximum 0.1 per cent, determined on 1.0 g.

Bacterial endotoxins (*2.6.14*): less than 1.0 IU/g.

ASSAY

Liquid chromatography (*2.2.29*) as described in the test for impurity B with the following modifications.

Injection: test solution and reference solutions (a) and (b).

Identification of the isomers: the 2 principal peaks in the chromatogram obtained with reference solution (a) are due to iopromide isomers Z_1 and Z_2. The 2 peaks that have an increased size in the chromatogram obtained with reference solution (b) in comparison to the chromatogram obtained with reference solution (a), are due to iopromide isomers E_1 and E_2.

Relative retention with reference to iopromide isomer Z_2 (retention time = about 34 min): iopromide isomer E_1 = about 0.70; iopromide isomer E_2 = about 0.75; iopromide isomer Z_1 = about 0.85.

System suitability: reference solution (a):

- *resolution*: minimum 2.0 between the peaks due to iopromide isomers Z_1 and Z_2.

Calculate the percentage content of iopromide from the declared content of *iopromide CRS* and from the sum of the areas of all of the peaks due to isomer groups E and Z.

STORAGE

Protected from light.

IMPURITIES

Specified impurities: A, B, C, D, E, F.

Other detectable impurities (the following substances would, if present at a sufficient level, be detected by one or other of the tests in the monograph. They are limited by the general acceptance criterion for other/unspecified impurities and/or by the general monograph *Substances for pharmaceutical use (2034)*. It is therefore not necessary to identify these impurities for demonstration of compliance. See also *5.10. Control of impurities in substances for pharmaceutical use*): G, H.

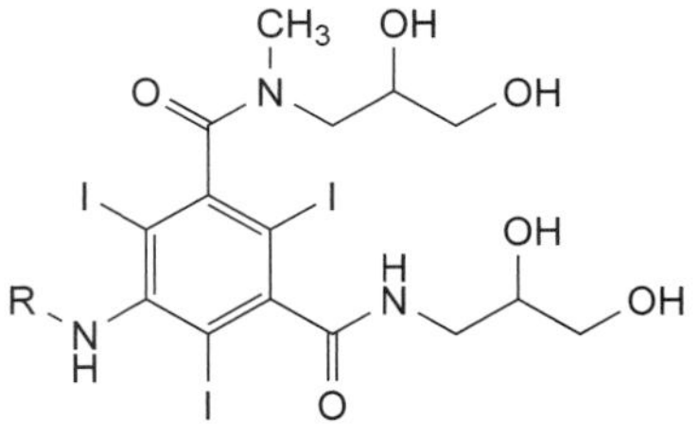

A. R = H: 5-amino-*N,N'*-bis(2,3-dihydroxypropyl)-2,4,6-triiodo-*N*-methylbenzene-1,3-dicarboxamide,

B. R = CO-CH₃: 5-(acetylamino)-*N,N'*-bis(2,3-dihydroxypropyl)-2,4,6-triiodo-*N*-methylbenzene-1,3-dicarboxamide,

C. R = CO-CH₂OH: *N,N'*-bis(2,3-dihydroxypropyl)-5-[(hydroxyacetyl)amino]-2,4,6-triiodo-*N*-methylbenzene-1,3-dicarboxamide,

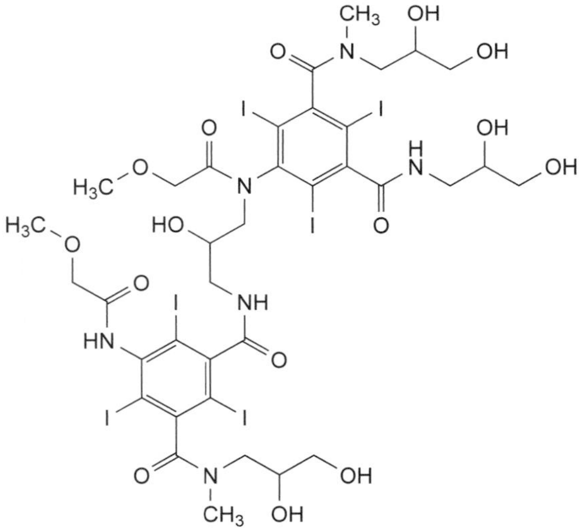

D. *N*-(2,3-dihydroxypropyl)-*N'*-[3-[[3-[(2,3-dihydroxypropyl)carbamoyl]-5-[(2,3-dihydroxypropyl)methylcarbamoyl]-2,4,6-triiodophenyl](methoxyacetyl)amino]-2-hydroxypropyl]-2,4,6-triiodo-5-[(methoxyacetyl)amino]-*N*-methyl-benzene-1,3-dicarboxamide,

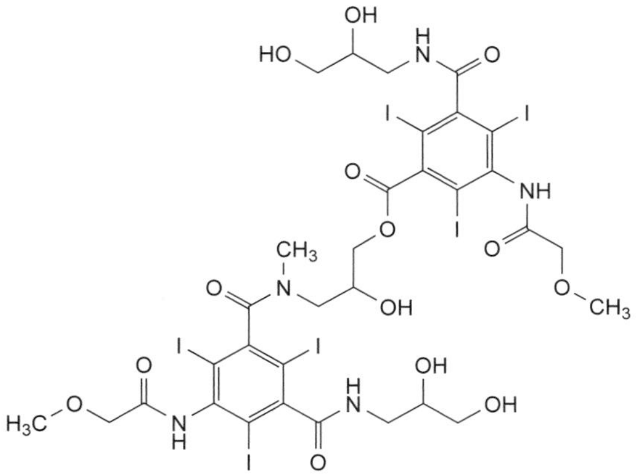

E. 3-[[3-[(2,3-dihydroxypropyl)carbamoyl]-2,4,6-triiodo-5-[(methoxyacetyl)amino]benzoyl]methylamino]-2-hydroxypropyl 3-[(2,3-dihydroxypropyl)carbamoyl]-2,4,6-triiodo-5-[(methoxyacetyl)amino]benzoate,

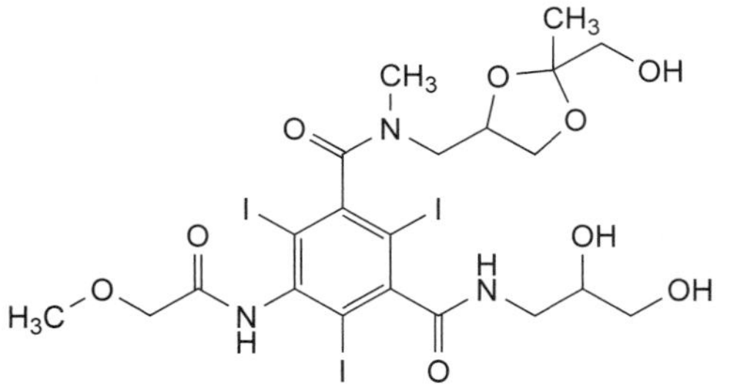

F. *N'*-(2,3-dihydroxypropyl)-*N*-[[2-(hydroxymethyl)-2-methyl-1,3-dioxolan-4-yl]methyl]-2,4,6-triiodo-5-[(methoxyacetyl)amino]-*N*-methylbenzene-1,3-dicarboxamide,

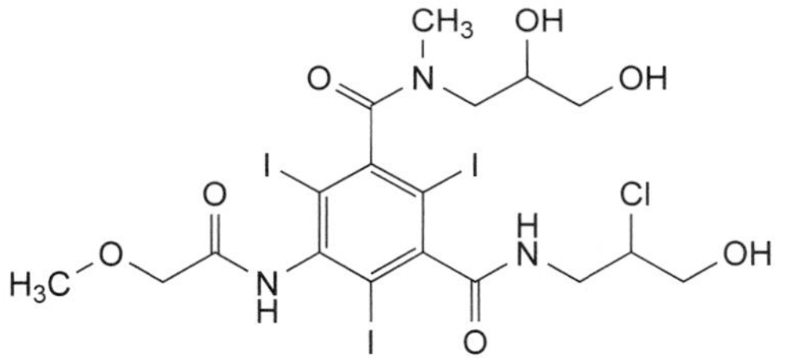

G. *N'*-(2-chloro-3-hydroxypropyl)-*N*-(2,3-dihydroxypropyl)-2,4,6-triiodo-5-[(methoxyacetyl)amino]-*N*-methylbenzene-1,3-dicarboxamide,

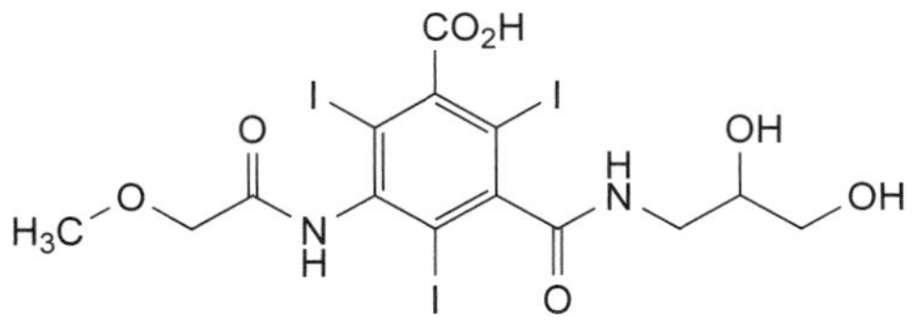

H. 3-[(2,3-dihydroxypropyl)carbamoyl]-2,4,6-triiodo-5-[(methoxyacetyl)amino]benzoic acid.

See the information section on general monographs (cover pages)

L

Monographs
L-P

See the information section on general monographs (cover pages)

01/2009:1337
corrected 6.5

LACTITOL MONOHYDRATE

Lactitolum monohydricum

$C_{12}H_{24}O_{11},H_2O$ M_r 362.3
[81025-04-9]

DEFINITION

4-O-(β-D-Galactopyranosyl)-D-glucitol monohydrate.

Content: 96.5 per cent to 102.0 per cent (anhydrous substance).

CHARACTERS

Appearance: white or almost white, crystalline powder.

Solubility: very soluble in water, slightly soluble in ethanol (96 per cent), practically insoluble in methylene chloride

IDENTIFICATION

First identification: B.

Second identification: A, C.

A. Specific optical rotation (see Tests).

B. Infrared absorption spectrophotometry (*2.2.24*).

   Comparison: lactitol monohydrate CRS.

C. Thin-layer chromatography (*2.2.27*).

   Test solution. Dissolve 50 mg of the substance to be examined in *methanol R* and dilute to 20 ml with the same solvent.

   Reference solution (a). Dissolve 5 mg of *lactitol monohydrate CRS* in *methanol R* and dilute to 2 ml with the same solvent.

   Reference solution (b). Dissolve 2.5 mg of *sorbitol CRS* (impurity E) in 1 ml of reference solution (a) and dilute to 10 ml with *methanol R*.

   Plate: TLC silica gel G plate R.

   Mobile phase: water R, acetonitrile R (25:75 V/V).

   Application: 2 μl.

   Development: over 2/3 of the plate.

   Drying: in air.

   Detection: spray with *4-aminobenzoic acid solution R* and dry in a current of cold air until the solvent is removed; heat at 100 °C for 15 min and allow to cool; spray with a 2 g/l solution of *sodium periodate R* and dry in a current of cold air; heat at 100 °C for 15 min.

   System suitability: the chromatogram obtained with reference solution (b) shows 2 clearly separated spots.

   Results: the principal spot in the chromatogram obtained with the test solution is similar in position, colour and size to the principal spot in the chromatogram obtained with reference solution (a).

TESTS

Solution S. Dissolve 5.000 g in *carbon dioxide-free water R* and dilute to 50.0 ml with the same solvent.

Appearance of solution. Solution S is clear (*2.2.1*) and not more intensely coloured than reference solution BY_7 (*2.2.2*, Method II).

Acidity or alkalinity. To 10 ml of solution S add 10 ml of *carbon dioxide-free water R*. To 10 ml of this solution add 0.05 ml of *phenolphthalein solution R*. Not more than 0.2 ml of *0.01 M sodium hydroxide* is required to change the colour of the indicator to pink. To a further 10 ml of the solution add 0.05 ml of *methyl red solution R*. Not more than 0.3 ml of *0.01 M hydrochloric acid* is required to change the colour of the indicator to red.

Specific optical rotation (*2.2.7*): + 13.5 to + 15.5 (anhydrous substance), determined on solution S.

Related substances. Liquid chromatography (*2.2.29*).

Test solution (a). Dissolve 50.0 mg of the substance to be examined in *water R* and dilute to 10.0 ml with the same solvent.

Test solution (b). Dilute 2.0 ml of test solution (a) to 50.0 ml with *water R*.

Reference solution (a). Dissolve 5.0 mg of *lactitol monohydrate CRS* and 5 mg of *glycerol R* in *water R* and dilute to 25.0 ml with the same solvent.

Reference solution (b). Dilute 1.0 ml of test solution (a) to 100.0 ml with *water R*. Dilute 5.0 ml of this solution to 100.0 ml with *water R*.

Reference solution (c). Dilute 2.5 ml of reference solution (a) to 10.0 ml with *water R*.

Column:

— *size*: l = 0.30 m, Ø = 7.8 mm;

— *stationary phase*: strong cation exchange resin (calcium form) R;

— *temperature*: 60 °C.

Mobile phase: water R.

Flow rate: 0.6 ml/min.

Detection: refractive index detector maintained at a constant temperature.

Injection: 100 μl; inject test solution (a) and reference solutions (b) and (c).

Run time: 2.5 times the retention time of lactitol.

Relative retention with reference to lactitol (retention time = about 13 min): impurity A = about 0.7; impurity B = about 0.8; glycerol = about 1.3; impurity C = about 1.5; impurity D = about 1.8; impurity E = about 1.9.

System suitability: reference solution (c):

— *resolution*: minimum 5 between the peaks due to lactitol and glycerol.

Limits:

— *impurity B*: not more than the area of the peak due to lactitol in the chromatogram obtained with reference solution (c) (1.0 per cent);

— *total of other impurities*: not more than the area of the peak due to lactitol in the chromatogram obtained with reference solution (c) (1.0 per cent);

— *disregard limit*: the area of the principal peak in the chromatogram obtained with reference solution (b) (0.05 per cent); disregard any peak due to the solvent.

Reducing sugars: maximum 0.2 per cent.

Dissolve 5.0 g in 3 ml of *water R* with gentle heating. Cool and add 20 ml of *cupri-citric solution R* and a few glass beads. Heat so that boiling begins after 4 min and maintain boiling for 3 min. Cool rapidly and add 100 ml of a 2.4 per cent *V/V* solution of *glacial acetic acid R* and 20.0 ml of *0.025 M iodine*. With continuous shaking, add 25 ml of a mixture of 6 volumes of *hydrochloric acid R* and 94 volumes of *water R*. When the precipitate has dissolved, titrate the excess of iodine with *0.05 M sodium thiosulphate* using 1 ml of *starch solution R* added towards the end of the titration, as indicator. Not less than 12.8 ml of *0.05 M sodium thiosulphate* is required.

Lead (*2.4.10*): maximum 0.5 ppm.

Nickel (*2.4.15*): maximum 1 ppm.

Water (*2.5.12*): 4.5 per cent to 5.5 per cent, determined on 0.30 g.

Sulphated ash (*2.4.14*): maximum 0.1 per cent, determined on 1.0 g.

Microbial contamination

TAMC: acceptance criterion 10^3 CFU/g (*2.6.12*).

TYMC: acceptance criterion 10^2 CFU/g (*2.6.12*).

Absence of *Escherichia coli* (*2.6.13*).

Absence of *Salmonella* (*2.6.13*).

Absence of *Pseudomonas aeruginosa* (*2.6.13*).

ASSAY

Liquid chromatography (*2.2.29*) as described in the test for related substances with the following modification.

Injection: test solution (b) and reference solution (a).

Calculate the percentage content of $C_{12}H_{24}O_{11}$ using the chromatograms obtained with test solution (b) and reference solution (a) and the declared content of *lactitol monohydrate CRS*.

IMPURITIES

Specified impurities: A, B, C, D, E.

A. lactose,

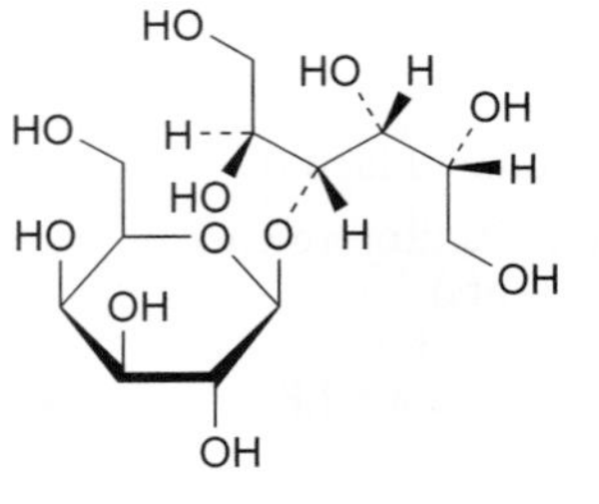

B. 3-*O*-(β-D-galactopyranosyl)-D-glucitol (lactulitol),

C. mannitol,

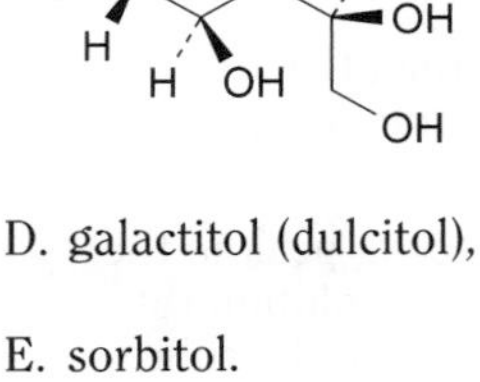

D. galactitol (dulcitol),

E. sorbitol.

See the information section on general monographs (cover pages)

07/2009:1061

LACTOSE, ANHYDROUS

Lactosum anhydricum

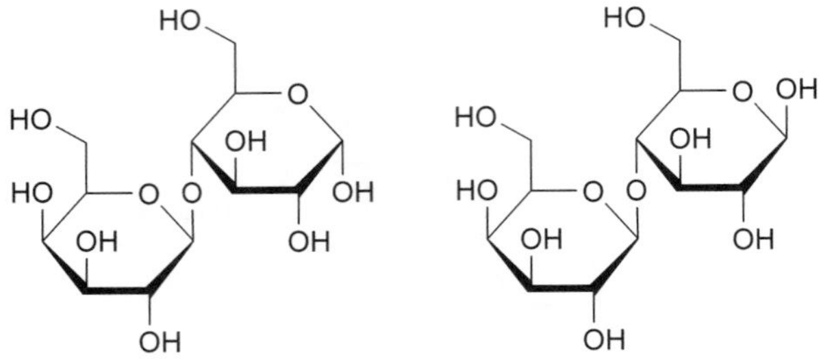

α-lactose   β-lactose

$C_{12}H_{22}O_{11}$ M_r 342.3

DEFINITION

O-β-D-Galactopyranosyl-(1→4)-β-D-glucopyranose or mixture of *O*-β-D-galactopyranosyl-(1→4)-α-D-glucopyranose and *O*-β-D-galactopyranosyl-(1→4)-β-D-glucopyranose.

CHARACTERS

Appearance: white or almost white, crystalline powder.

Solubility: freely but slowly soluble in water, practically insoluble in ethanol (96 per cent).

IDENTIFICATION

First identification: A, D.

Second identification: B, C, D.

A. Infrared absorption spectrophotometry (*2.2.24*).

   Comparison: anhydrous lactose CRS.

B. Thin-layer chromatography (*2.2.27*).

   Solvent mixture: water R, methanol R (2:3 V/V).

   Test solution. Dissolve 10 mg of the substance to be examined in the solvent mixture and dilute to 20 ml with the solvent mixture.

   Reference solution (a). Dissolve 10 mg of *anhydrous lactose CRS* in the solvent mixture and dilute to 20 ml with the solvent mixture.

   Reference solution (b). Dissolve 10 mg of *anhydrous lactose CRS*, 10 mg of *fructose CRS*, 10 mg of *glucose CRS* and 10 mg of *sucrose CRS* in the solvent mixture and dilute to 20 ml with the solvent mixture.

   Plate: TLC silica gel G plate R.

   Mobile phase: water R, methanol R, glacial acetic acid R, ethylene chloride R (10:15:25:50 *V/V/V/V*); measure the volumes accurately, as a slight excess of water produces cloudiness.

   Application: 2 µl; thoroughly dry the starting points.

   Development A: over a path of 15 cm.

   Drying A: in a current of warm air.

   Development B: immediately, over a path of 15 cm, after renewing the mobile phase.

   Drying B: in a current of warm air.

   Detection: spray with a solution of 0.5 g of *thymol R* in a mixture of 5 ml of *sulphuric acid R* and 95 ml of *ethanol (96 per cent) R*; heat at 130 °C for 10 min.

   System suitability: reference solution (b):

   – the chromatogram shows 4 clearly separated spots.

Results: the principal spot in the chromatogram obtained with the test solution is similar in position, colour and size to the principal spot in the chromatogram obtained with reference solution (a).

C. Dissolve 0.25 g in 5 ml of *water R*. Add 5 ml of *ammonia R* and heat in a water-bath at 80 °C for 10 min. A red colour develops.

D. Water (see Tests).

TESTS

Appearance of solution. The solution is clear (*2.2.1*) and not more intensely coloured than reference solution BY₇ (*2.2.2, Method II*).

Dissolve 1.0 g in boiling *water R* and dilute to 10 ml with the same solvent.

Acidity or alkalinity. Dissolve 6.0 g by heating in 25 ml of *carbon dioxide-free water R*, cool and add 0.3 ml of *phenolphthalein solution R1*. The solution is colourless. Not more than 0.4 ml of *0.1 M sodium hydroxide* is required to change the colour of the indicator to pink or red.

Specific optical rotation (*2.2.7*): + 54.4 to + 55.9 (anhydrous substance).

Dissolve 10.0 g in 80 ml of *water R*, heating to 50 °C. Allow to cool and add 0.2 ml of *dilute ammonia R1*. Allow to stand for 30 min and dilute to 100.0 ml with *water R*.

Absorbance (*2.2.25*).

Test solution (a). Dissolve 1.0 g in boiling *water R* and dilute to 10.0 ml with the same solvent.

Test solution (b). Dilute 1.0 ml of test solution (a) to 10.0 ml with *water R*.

Spectral range: 400 nm for test solution (a) and 210-300 nm for test solution (b).

Results:

— at 400 nm: maximum 0.04 for test solution (a);

— from 210 nm to 220 nm: maximum 0.25 for test solution (b);

— from 270 nm to 300 nm: maximum 0.07 for test solution (b).

Heavy metals (*2.4.8*): maximum 5 ppm.

2.0 g complies with test C. Prepare the reference solution using 1.0 ml of *lead standard solution (10 ppm Pb) R*.

Water (*2.5.12*): maximum 1.0 per cent, determined on 0.50 g, using a mixture of 1 volume of *formamide R* and 2 volumes of *methanol R* as the solvent.

Sulphated ash (*2.4.14*): maximum 0.1 per cent, determined on 1.0 g.

Microbial contamination

TAMC: acceptance criterion 10^2 CFU/g (*2.6.12*).

Absence of *Escherichia coli* (*2.6.13*).

FUNCTIONALITY-RELATED CHARACTERISTICS

This section provides information on characteristics that are recognised as being relevant control parameters for one or more functions of the substance when used as an excipient (see chapter 5.15). This section is a non-mandatory part of the monograph and it is not necessary to verify the characteristics to demonstrate compliance. Control of these characteristics can however contribute to the quality of a medicinal product by improving the consistency of the manufacturing process and the performance of the medicinal product during use. Where control methods are cited, they are recognised as

being suitable for the purpose, but other methods can also be used. Wherever results for a particular characteristic are reported, the control method must be indicated.

The following characteristics may be relevant for anhydrous lactose used as a filler/diluent in solid dosage forms (compressed and powder).

Particle size distribution (*2.9.31* or *2.9.38*).

Bulk and tapped density (*2.9.34*). Determine the bulk density and the tapped density. Calculate the Hausner index using the following expression:

$$\frac{V_0}{V_f}$$

V_0 = volume of bulk substance;

V_f = volume of tapped substance.

α-Lactose and β-lactose. Gas chromatography (*2.2.28*).

Silylation reagent. Mix 28 volumes of N-trimethylsilyl-imidazole R and 72 volumes of *pyridine R*.

Test solution. Dissolve about 1 mg of the substance to be examined in 0.45 ml of *dimethyl sulphoxide R*. Add 1.8 ml of the silylation reagent. Mix gently and allow to stand for 20 min.

Reference solution. Prepare a mixture of α-lactose monohydrate R and β-lactose R having an anomeric ratio of about 1:1 based on the labelled anomeric contents of the α-lactose monohydrate and β-lactose. Dissolve about 1 mg of this mixture in 0.45 ml of *dimethyl sulphoxide R*. Add 1.8 ml of the silylation reagent. Mix gently and allow to stand for 20 min.

Column:

— *material*: glass;

— *size*: l = 0.9 m, Ø = 4 mm;

— *stationary phase*: silanised diatomaceous earth for gas chromatography R impregnated with 3 per cent m/m of poly[(cyanopropyl)(methyl)][(phenyl)(methyl)] siloxane R.

Carrier gas: helium for chromatography R.

Flow rate: 40 ml/min.

Temperature:

— *column*: 215 °C;

— *injection port and detector*: 275 °C.

Detection: flame ionisation.

Injection: 2 µl.

System suitability: reference solution:

— *relative retention* with reference to β-lactose: α-lactose = about 0.7;

— *resolution*: minimum 3.0 between the peaks due to α-lactose and β-lactose.

Calculate the percentage content of α-lactose from the following expression:

$$\frac{100 S_a}{S_a + S_b}$$

Calculate the percentage content of β-lactose from the following expression:

$$\frac{100 S_b}{S_a + S_b}$$

S_a = area of the peak due to α-lactose;

S_b = area of the peak due to β-lactose.

Loss on drying (*2.2.32*). Determine on 1.000 g by drying in an oven at 80 °C for 2 h.

07/2009:0187

LACTOSE MONOHYDRATE

Lactosum monohydricum

$C_{12}H_{22}O_{11},H_2O$ M_r 360.3

DEFINITION

O-β-D-Galactopyranosyl-(1→4)-α-D-glucopyranose monohydrate.

CHARACTERS

Appearance: white or almost white, crystalline powder.

Solubility: freely but slowly soluble in water, practically insoluble in ethanol (96 per cent).

IDENTIFICATION

First identification: A, D.

Second identification: B, C, D.

A. Infrared absorption spectrophotometry (*2.2.24*).
   Comparison: lactose CRS.

B. Thin-layer chromatography (*2.2.27*).
   Solvent mixture: water R, methanol R (2:3 *V/V*).
   Test solution. Dissolve 10 mg of the substance to be examined in the solvent mixture and dilute to 20 ml with the solvent mixture.
   Reference solution (a). Dissolve 10 mg of *lactose CRS* in the solvent mixture and dilute to 20 ml with the solvent mixture.
   Reference solution (b). Dissolve 10 mg of *fructose CRS*, 10 mg of *glucose CRS*, 10 mg of *lactose CRS* and 10 mg of *sucrose CRS* in the solvent mixture and dilute to 20 ml with the solvent mixture.
   Plate: TLC silica gel G plate R.
   Mobile phase: water R, methanol R, glacial acetic acid R, ethylene chloride R (10:15:25:50 *V/V/V/V*); measure the volumes accurately, as a slight excess of water produces cloudiness.
   Application: 2 µl; thoroughly dry the starting points.
   Development A: over a path of 15 cm.
   Drying A: in a current of warm air.
   Development B: immediately, over a path of 15 cm, after renewing the mobile phase.
   Drying B: in a current of warm air.
   Detection: spray with a solution of 0.5 g of *thymol R* in a mixture of 5 ml of *sulphuric acid R* and 95 ml of *ethanol (96 per cent) R*; heat at 130 °C for 10 min.
   System suitability: reference solution (b):
   — the chromatogram shows 4 clearly separated spots.

Results: the principal spot in the chromatogram obtained with the test solution is similar in position, colour and size to the principal spot in the chromatogram obtained with reference solution (a).

C. Dissolve 0.25 g in 5 ml of *water R*. Add 5 ml of *ammonia R* and heat in a water-bath at 80 °C for 10 min. A red colour develops.

D. Water (see Tests).

TESTS

Appearance of solution. The solution is clear (*2.2.1*) and not more intensely coloured than reference solution BY_7 (*2.2.2, Method II*).

Dissolve 1.0 g in boiling *water R* and dilute to 10 ml with the same solvent.

Acidity or alkalinity. Dissolve 6.0 g by heating in 25 ml of *carbon dioxide-free water R*, cool and add 0.3 ml of *phenolphthalein solution R1*. The solution is colourless. Not more than 0.4 ml of *0.1 M sodium hydroxide* is required to change the colour of the indicator to pink or red.

Specific optical rotation (*2.2.7*): + 54.4 to + 55.9 (anhydrous substance).

Dissolve 10.0 g in 80 ml of *water R*, heating to 50 °C. Allow to cool and add 0.2 ml of *dilute ammonia R1*. Allow to stand for 30 min and dilute to 100.0 ml with *water R*.

Absorbance (*2.2.25*).

Test solution (a). Dissolve 1.0 g in boiling *water R* and dilute to 10.0 ml with the same solvent.

Test solution (b). Dilute 1.0 ml of test solution (a) to 10.0 ml with *water R*.

Spectral range: 400 nm for test solution (a) and 210-300 nm for test solution (b).

Results:

— at 400 nm: maximum 0.04 for test solution (a);

— from 210 nm to 220 nm: maximum 0.25 for test solution (b);

— from 270 nm to 300 nm: maximum 0.07 for test solution (b).

Heavy metals (*2.4.8*): maximum 5 ppm.

Dissolve 4.0 g in *water R* with warming, add 1 ml of *0.1 M hydrochloric acid* and dilute to 20 ml with *water R*. 12 ml of the solution complies with test A. Prepare the reference solution using *lead standard solution (1 ppm Pb) R*.

Water (*2.5.12*): 4.5 per cent to 5.5 per cent, determined on 0.50 g, using a mixture of 1 volume of *formamide R* and 2 volumes of *methanol R* as the solvent.

Sulphated ash (*2.4.14*): maximum 0.1 per cent, determined on 1.0 g.

Microbial contamination

TAMC: acceptance criterion 10^2 CFU/g (*2.6.12*).

Absence of *Escherichia coli* (*2.6.13*).

STORAGE

In an airtight container.

FUNCTIONALITY-RELATED CHARACTERISTICS

This section provides information on characteristics that are recognised as being relevant control parameters for one or more functions of the substance when used as an excipient (see chapter 5.15). This section is a non-mandatory part of the monograph and it is not necessary to verify the characteristics to demonstrate compliance. Control of these characteristics can however contribute to the quality of a medicinal product by improving the consistency of the manufacturing process and the performance of the medicinal product during use. Where control methods are cited, they are recognised as being suitable for the purpose, but other methods can also be used. Wherever results for a particular characteristic are reported, the control method must be indicated.

The following characteristics may be relevant for lactose monohydrate used as a filler/diluent in solid dosage forms (compressed and powder).

Particle size distribution (*2.9.31* or *2.9.38*).

Bulk and tapped density (*2.9.34*). Determine the bulk density and the tapped density. Calculate the Hausner Index using the following expression:

$$\frac{V_0}{V_f}$$

V_0 = volume of bulk substance;

V_f = volume of tapped substance.

01/2008:1787
corrected 6.5

LEVOMETHADONE HYDROCHLORIDE

Levomethadoni hydrochloridum

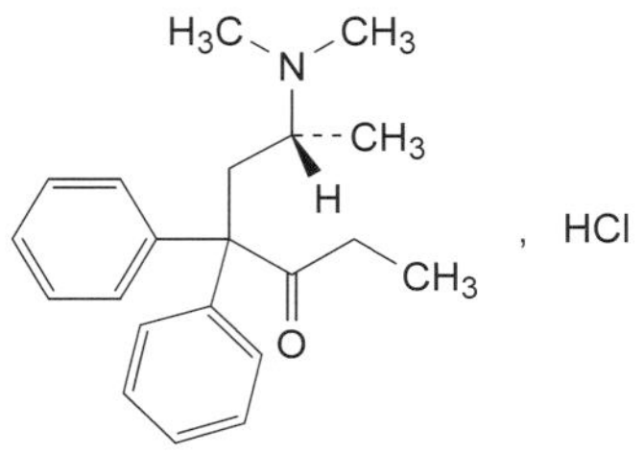

C$_{21}$H$_{28}$ClNO M_r 345.9
[5967-73-7]

DEFINITION

(6*R*)-6-(Dimethylamino)-4,4-diphenylheptan-3-one hydrochloride.

Content: 99.0 per cent to 101.0 per cent (dried substance).

CHARACTERS

Appearance: white or almost white, crystalline powder.

Solubility: soluble in water, freely soluble in ethanol (96 per cent).

IDENTIFICATION

First identification: A, C, D.

Second identification: A, B, D.

A. Specific optical rotation (see Tests).

B. Melting point (*2.2.14*): 239 °C to 242 °C.

C. Infrared absorption spectrophotometry (*2.2.24*).

    Comparison: *Ph. Eur. reference spectrum of methadone hydrochloride.*

D. Dilute 1 ml of solution S (see Tests) to 5 ml with *water R* and add 1 ml of *dilute ammonia R1*. Mix, allow to stand for 5 min and filter. The filtrate gives reaction (a) of chlorides (*2.3.1*).

TESTS

Solution S. Dissolve 2.50 g in *carbon dioxide-free water R* and dilute to 50.0 ml with the same solvent.

Appearance of solution. Solution S is clear (*2.2.1*) and colourless (*2.2.2, Method II*).

Acidity or alkalinity. Dilute 10 ml of solution S to 25 ml with *carbon dioxide-free water R*. To 10 ml of the solution add 0.2 ml of *methyl red solution R* and 0.2 ml of *0.01 M sodium hydroxide*. The solution is yellow. Add 0.4 ml of *0.01 M hydrochloric acid*. The solution is red.

Specific optical rotation (*2.2.7*): − 125 to − 135 (dried substance), determined on solution S.

Related substances. Liquid chromatography (*2.2.29*).

Test solution. Dissolve 25.0 mg of the substance to be examined in the mobile phase and dilute to 100.0 ml with the mobile phase.

Reference solution (a). Dilute 1.0 ml of the test solution to 50.0 ml with the mobile phase. Dilute 1.0 ml of the solution to 10.0 ml with the mobile phase.

Reference solution (b). Dissolve 12.0 mg of *imipramine hydrochloride CRS* in the mobile phase and dilute to 10 ml with the mobile phase. To 1 ml of the solution add 5 ml of the test solution and dilute to 10 ml with the mobile phase.

Column:

— *size*: *l* = 0.125 m, Ø = 4.6 mm;

— *stationary phase*: *octadecylsilyl silica gel for chromatography R* (5 µm);

— *temperature*: 25 °C.

Mobile phase: mix 35 volumes of *acetonitrile R* and 65 volumes of an 11.5 g/l solution of *phosphoric acid R* adjusted to pH 3.6 with *tetraethylammonium hydroxide solution R*.

Flow rate: 1.0 ml/min.

Detection: spectrophotometer at 210 nm.

Equilibration: about 30 min.

Injection: 10 µl.

Run time: 7 times the retention time of levomethadone.

Retention time: levomethadone = about 5 min.

System suitability: reference solution (b):

— *resolution*: minimum 2.5 between the peaks due to imipramine and levomethadone.

Limits:

— *any impurity*: not more than 0.5 times the area of the principal peak in the chromatogram obtained with reference solution (a) (0.1 per cent);

— *total*: not more than 2.5 times the area of the principal peak in the chromatogram obtained with reference solution (a) (0.5 per cent);

— *disregard limit*: 0.25 times the area of the principal peak in the chromatogram obtained with reference solution (a) (0.05 per cent).

Dextromethadone. Liquid chromatography (*2.2.29*).

Test solution. Dissolve 40.0 mg of the substance to be examined in the mobile phase and dilute to 100.0 ml with the mobile phase.

Reference solution. Dilute 1.0 ml of the test solution to 10.0 ml with the mobile phase. Dilute 1.0 ml of this solution to 20.0 ml with the mobile phase.

Column:

— *size*: *l* = 0.25 m, Ø = 4.6 mm;

— *stationary phase*: *2-hydroxypropylbetadex for chromatography R* (5 µm);

— *temperature*: 10 °C.

Mobile phase: mix 1 volume of *triethylamine R* adjusted to pH 4.0 with *phosphoric acid R*, 15 volumes of *acetonitrile R* and 85 volumes of a 13.6 g/l solution of *potassium dihydrogen phosphate R*.

Flow rate: 0.7 ml/min.

Detection: spectrophotometer at 210 nm.

Equilibration: about 30 min.

Injection: 10 µl.

Relative retention with reference to levomethadone: dextromethadone = about 1.4.

System suitability: test solution:

— *number of theoretical plates*: minimum 2000, calculated for the peak due to levomethadone;

— *tailing factor*: maximum 3 for the peak due to levomethadone.

Limit:

— *dextromethadone*: not more than the area of the principal peak in the chromatogram obtained with the reference solution (0.5 per cent).

Loss on drying (*2.2.32*): maximum 0.5 per cent, determined on 1.000 g by drying in an oven at 105 °C.

Sulphated ash (*2.4.14*): maximum 0.1 per cent, determined on 1.0 g.

ASSAY

Dissolve 0.300 g in a mixture of 40 ml of *water R* and 5 ml of *acetic acid R*. Titrate with *0.1 M silver nitrate*. Determine the end-point potentiometrically (*2.2.20*), using a silver electrode.

1 ml of *0.1 M silver nitrate* is equivalent to 34.59 mg of $C_{21}H_{28}ClNO$.

STORAGE

Protected from light.

IMPURITIES

Specified impurities: A, B, C, D, E, F.

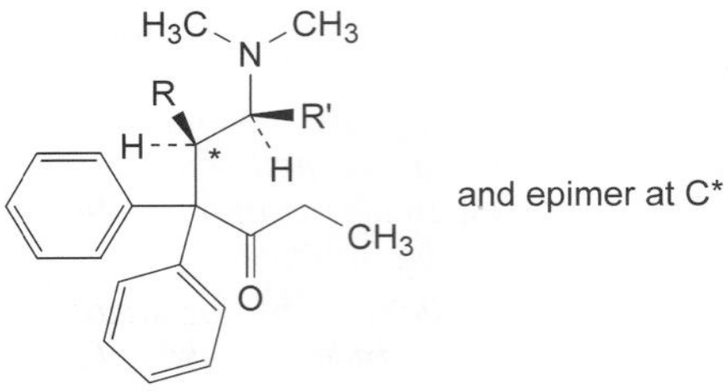

and epimer at C*

A. R = H, R′ = CH_3: (6*S*)-6-(dimethylamino)-4,4-diphenylheptan-3-one,

D. R = CH_3, R′ = H: (5*RS*)-6-(dimethylamino)-5-methyl-4,4-diphenylhexan-3-one,

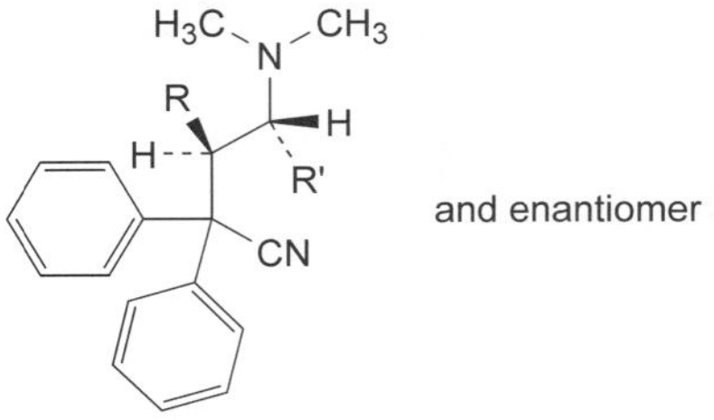

and enantiomer

B. R = H, R′ = CH_3: (4*RS*)-4-(dimethylamino)-2,2-diphenylpentanenitrile,

C. R = CH_3,R′ = H: (3*RS*)-4-(dimethylamino)-3-methyl-2,2-diphenylbutanenitrile,

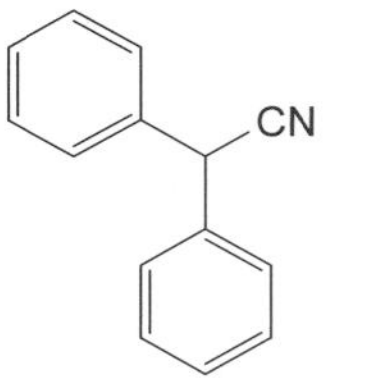

E. diphenylacetonitrile,

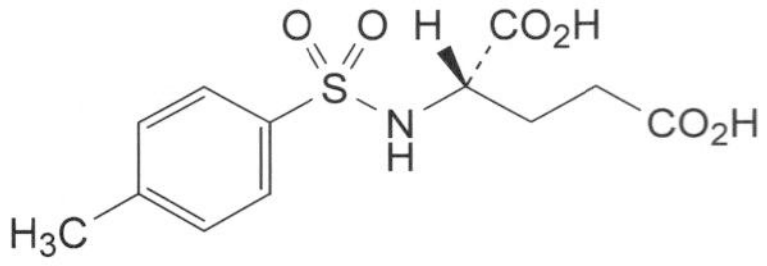

F. (2*S*)-2-[[(4-methylphenyl)sulphonyl]amino]pentanedioic acid (*N-p*-tosyl-L-glutamic acid).

M

See the information section on general monographs (cover pages)

07/2008:0043
corrected 6.5

MAGNESIUM CARBONATE, HEAVY

Magnesii subcarbonas ponderosus

DEFINITION
Hydrated basic magnesium carbonate.

Content: 40.0 per cent to 45.0 per cent, calculated as MgO (M_r 40.30).

CHARACTERS
Appearance: white or almost white powder.

Solubility: practically insoluble in water. It dissolves in dilute acids with effervescence.

IDENTIFICATION
A. Bulk density (*2.9.34*): minimum 0.25 g/ml.

B. It gives the reaction of carbonates (*2.3.1*).

C. Dissolve about 15 mg in 2 ml of *dilute nitric acid R* and neutralise with *dilute sodium hydroxide solution R*. The solution gives the reaction of magnesium (*2.3.1*).

TESTS
Solution S. Dissolve 5.0 g in 100 ml of *dilute acetic acid R*. When the effervescence has ceased, boil for 2 min, allow to cool and dilute to 100 ml with *dilute acetic acid R*. Filter, if necessary, through a previously ignited and tared porcelain or silica filter crucible of suitable porosity to give a clear filtrate.

Appearance of solution. Solution S is not more intensely coloured than reference solution B_4 (*2.2.2, Method II*).

Soluble substances: maximum 1.0 per cent.

Mix 2.00 g with 100 ml of *water R* and boil for 5 min. Filter whilst hot through a sintered-glass filter (40) (*2.1.2*), allow to cool and dilute to 100 ml with *water R*. Evaporate 50 ml of the filtrate to dryness and dry at 100-105 °C. The residue weighs not more than 10 mg.

Substances insoluble in acetic acid: maximum 0.05 per cent.

Any residue obtained during the preparation of solution S, washed, dried, and ignited at 600 ± 50 °C, weighs not more than 2.5 mg.

Chlorides (*2.4.4*): maximum 700 ppm.

Dilute 1.5 ml of solution S to 15 ml with *water R*.

Sulphates (*2.4.13*): maximum 0.6 per cent.

Dilute 0.5 ml of solution S to 15 ml with *distilled water R*.

Arsenic (*2.4.2, Method A*): maximum 2 ppm, determined on 10 ml of solution S.

Calcium (*2.4.3*): maximum 0.75 per cent.

Dilute 2.6 ml of solution S to 150 ml with *distilled water R*. 15 ml of the solution complies with the test.

Iron (*2.4.9*): maximum 400 ppm.

Dissolve 0.1 g in 3 ml of *dilute hydrochloric acid R* and dilute to 10 ml with *water R*. Dilute 2.5 ml of the solution to 10 ml with *water R*.

Heavy metals (*2.4.8*): maximum 20 ppm.

To 20 ml of solution S add 15 ml of *hydrochloric acid R1* and shake with 25 ml of *methyl isobutyl ketone R* for 2 min. Allow to stand, separate the aqueous lower layer and evaporate to dryness. Dissolve the residue in 1 ml of

acetic acid R and dilute to 20 ml with *water R*. 12 ml of the solution complies with test A. Prepare the reference solution using *lead standard solution (1 ppm Pb) R*.

ASSAY
Dissolve 0.150 g in a mixture of 2 ml of *dilute hydrochloric acid R* and 20 ml of *water R*. Carry out the complexometric titration of magnesium (*2.5.11*).

1 ml of *0.1 M sodium edetate* is equivalent to 4.030 mg of MgO.

FUNCTIONALITY-RELATED CHARACTERISTICS
This section provides information on characteristics that are recognised as being relevant control parameters for one or more functions of the substance when used as an excipient (see chapter 5.15). This section is a non-mandatory part of the monograph and it is not necessary to verify the characteristics to demonstrate compliance. Control of these characteristics can however contribute to the quality of a medicinal product by improving the consistency of the manufacturing process and the performance of the medicinal product during use. Where control methods are cited, they are recognised as being suitable for the purpose, but other methods can also be used. Wherever results for a particular characteristic are reported, the control method must be indicated.

The following characteristics may be relevant for heavy magnesium carbonate used as filler in tablets.

Particle-size distribution (*2.9.31* or *2.9.38*).

Bulk and tapped density (*2.9.34*).

07/2009:0229

MAGNESIUM STEARATE

Magnesii stearas

DEFINITION
Compound of magnesium with a mixture of solid organic acids and consisting mainly of variable proportions of magnesium stearate and magnesium palmitate obtained from sources of vegetable or animal origin.

Content:
- *magnesium* (Mg; A_r 24.305): 4.0 per cent to 5.0 per cent (dried substance);
- *stearic acid in the fatty acid fraction*: minimum 40.0 per cent;
- *sum of stearic acid and palmitic acid in the fatty acid fraction*: minimum 90.0 per cent.

CHARACTERS
Appearance: a white, very fine, light powder, greasy to the touch.

Solubility: practically insoluble in water and in anhydrous ethanol.

IDENTIFICATION
First identification: C, D.

Second identification: A, B, D.

A. Freezing point (*2.2.18*): minimum 53 °C, determined on the residue obtained in the preparation of solution S (see Tests).

B. Acid value (*2.5.1*): 195 to 210.

Dissolve 0.200 g of the residue obtained in the preparation of solution S in 25 ml of the prescribed mixture of solvents.

C. Examine the chromatograms obtained in the assay of stearic acid and palmitic acid.

Results: the 2 principal peaks in the chromatogram obtained with the test solution are similar in retention time to the 2 principal peaks in the chromatogram obtained with the reference solution.

D. To 1 ml of solution S add 1 ml of *dilute ammonia R1*; a white precipitate is formed that dissolves on addition of 1 ml of *ammonium chloride solution R*. Add 1 ml of a 1.2 g/l solution of *disodium hydrogen phosphate R*; a white crystalline precipitate is formed.

TESTS

Solution S. To 5.0 g add 50 ml of *peroxide-free ether R*, 20 ml of *dilute nitric acid R* and 20 ml of *water R* and heat under a reflux condenser until dissolution is complete. Allow to cool. In a separating funnel, separate the aqueous layer and shake the ether layer with 2 quantities, each of 4 ml, of *water R*. Combine the aqueous layers, wash with 15 ml of *peroxide-free ether R* and dilute to 50.0 ml with *water R* (solution S). Evaporate the organic layer to dryness and dry the residue at 100-105 °C. Keep the residue for identification tests A and B.

Acidity or alkalinity. To 1.0 g add 20 ml of *carbon dioxide-free water R* and boil for 1 min with continuous shaking. Cool and filter. To 10 ml of the filtrate add 0.05 ml of *bromothymol blue solution R4*. Not more than 0.05 ml of *0.1 M hydrochloric acid* or *0.1 M sodium hydroxide* is required to change the colour of the indicator.

Chlorides: maximum 0.1 per cent.

Dilute 10.0 ml of solution S to 40 ml with *water R*. Neutralise if necessary with *nitric acid R* using *litmus R* as indicator. Add 1 ml of *nitric acid R* and 1 ml of *0.1 M silver nitrate* and dilute to 50 ml with *water R*. Mix and allow to stand for 5 min protected from light. The turbidity, if any, is not greater than that produced in a solution containing 1.4 ml of *0.02 M hydrochloric acid*.

Sulphates: maximum 1.0 per cent.

Dilute 6.0 ml of solution S to 40 ml with *water R*. Neutralise if necessary with *hydrochloric acid R* using *litmus R* as indicator. Add 1 ml of *3 M hydrochloric acid* and 3 ml of a 120 g/l solution of *barium chloride R* and dilute to 50 ml with *water R*. Mix and allow to stand for 10 min. The turbidity, if any, is not greater than that produced in a solution containing 3.0 ml of *0.02 M sulphuric acid*.

Cadmium: maximum 3 ppm.

Atomic absorption spectrometry (*2.2.23, Method II*).

For the preparation of all aqueous solutions and for the rinsing of glassware before use, employ water that has been passed through a strong-acid, strong-base, mixed-bed ion-exchange resin before use. Select all reagents to have as low a content of cadmium, lead and nickel as practicable and store all reagent solutions in containers of borosilicate glass. Clean glassware before use by soaking in warm 8 M nitric acid for 30 min and by rinsing with deionised water.

Blank solution. Dilute 25 ml of *cadmium- and lead-free nitric acid R* to 100.0 ml with *water R*.

Modifier solution. Dissolve 20 g of *ammonium dihydrogen phosphate R* and 1 g of *magnesium nitrate R* in *water R* and dilute to 100 ml with the same solvent. Alternatively, use an appropriate matrix modifier as recommended by the graphite furnace atomic absorption (GFAA) spectrometer manufacturer.

Test solution. Place 0.100 g of the substance to be examined in a polytetrafluoroethylene digestion bomb and add 2.5 ml of *cadmium- and lead-free nitric acid R*. Close and seal the bomb according to the manufacturer's operating instructions *(when using a digestion bomb, be thoroughly familiar with the safety and operating instructions. Carefully follow the bomb manufacturer's instructions regarding care and maintenance of these digestion bombs. Do not use metal jacketed bombs or liners which have been used with hydrochloric acid due to contamination from corrosion of the metal jacket by hydrochloric acid).* Heat the bomb in an oven at 170 °C for 3 h. Cool the bomb slowly in air to room temperature according to the bomb manufacturer's instructions. Place the bomb in a hood and open carefully as corrosive gases may be expelled. Dissolve the residue in *water R* and dilute to 10.0 ml with the same solvent.

Reference solution. Prepare a solution of 0.0030 µg/ml of Cd by suitable dilutions of a 0.00825 µg/ml solution of *cadmium nitrate tetrahydrate R* in the blank solution. Dilute 1.0 ml of the test solution to 10.0 ml with the blank solution. Prepare mixtures of this solution, the reference solution and the blank solution in the following proportions: (1.0:0:1.0 *V/V/V*), (1.0:0.5:0.5 *V/V/V*), (1.0:1.0:0 *V/V/V*). To each mixture add 50 µl of modifier solution and mix. These solutions contain respectively 0 µg, 0.00075 µg and 0.0015 µg of cadmium per millilitre from the reference solution (keep the remaining test solution for use in the test for lead and nickel).

Source: cadmium hollow-cathode lamp.

Wavelength: 228.8 nm.

Atomisation device: furnace.

Platform: pyrolytically coated with integrated tube.

Operating conditions: use the temperature programme recommended for cadmium by the GFAA manufacturer. An example of temperature parameters for GFAA analysis of cadmium is shown below.

Stage	Final temperature (°C)	Ramp time (s)	Hold time (s)
Drying	110	10	20
Ashing	600	10	30
Atomisation	1800	0	5

Lead: maximum 10 ppm.

Atomic absorption spectrometry (*2.2.23, Method II*).

For the preparation of all aqueous solutions and for the rinsing of glassware before use, employ water that has been passed through a strong-acid, strong-base, mixed-bed ion-exchange resin before use. Select all reagents to have as low a content of cadmium, lead and nickel as practicable and store all reagent solutions in containers of borosilicate glass. Clean glassware before use by soaking in warm 8 M nitric acid for 30 min and by rinsing with deionised water.

Blank solution. Use the solution described in the test for cadmium.

Modifier solution. Use the solution described in the test for cadmium.

Test solution. Use the solution described in the test for cadmium.

Reference solution. Prepare a solution of 0.100 µg/ml of Pb by suitable dilutions of *lead standard solution (100 ppm Pb) R* with the blank solution.

Prepare mixtures of the test solution, the reference solution and the blank solution in the following proportions: (1.0:0:1.0 *V/V/V*), (1.0:0.5:0.5 *V/V/V*), (1.0:1.0:0 *V/V/V*). To each mixture add 50 µl of modifier solution and mix. These solutions contain respectively 0 µg, 0.025 µg and 0.05 µg of lead per millilitre from the reference solution.

Source: lead hollow-cathode lamp.

Wavelength: 283.3 nm.

Atomisation device: furnace.

Platform: pyrolytically coated with integrated tube.

Operating conditions: use the temperature programme recommended for lead by the GFAA manufacturer. An example of temperature parameters for GFAA analysis of lead is shown below.

Stage	Final temperature (°C)	Ramp time (s)	Hold time (s)
Drying	110	10	20
Ashing	450	10	30
Atomisation	2000	0	5

Nickel: maximum 5 ppm.

Atomic absorption spectrometry (*2.2.23, Method II*).

For the preparation of all aqueous solutions and for the rinsing of glassware before use, employ water that has been passed through a strong-acid, strong-base, mixed-bed ion-exchange resin before use. Select all reagents to have as low a content of cadmium, lead and nickel as practicable and store all reagent solutions in containers of borosilicate glass. Clean glassware before use by soaking in warm 8 M nitric acid for 30 min and by rinsing with deionised water.

Blank solution. Use the solution described in the test for cadmium.

Modifier solution. Dissolve 20 g of *ammonium dihydrogen phosphate R* in *water R* and dilute to 100 ml with the same solvent. Alternatively, use an appropriate matrix modifier as recommended by the GFAA spectrometer manufacturer.

Test solution. Use the solution described in the test for cadmium.

Reference solution. Prepare a solution of 0.050 μg/ml of Ni by suitable dilutions of a 0.2477 μg/ml solution of *nickel nitrate hexahydrate R* in the blank solution.

Prepare mixtures of the test solution, the reference solution and the blank solution in the following proportions: (1.0:0:1.0 *V/V/V*), (1.0:0.5:0.5 *V/V/V*), (1.0:1.0:0 *V/V/V*). To each mixture add 50 μl of matrix modifier solution and mix. These reference solutions contain respectively 0 μg, 0.0125 μg and 0.025 μg of nickel per millilitre from the reference solution.

Source: nickel hollow-cathode lamp.

Wavelength: 232.0 nm.

Atomisation device: furnace.

Platform: pyrolytically coated with integrated tube.

Operating conditions: use the temperature programme recommended for nickel by the GFAA manufacturer. An example of temperature parameters for GFAA analysis of nickel is shown below.

Stage	Final temperature (°C)	Ramp time (s)	Hold time (s)
Drying	110	10	20
Ashing	1000	20	30
Atomisation	2300	0	5

Loss on drying (*2.2.32*): maximum 6.0 per cent, determined on 1.000 g by drying in an oven at 105 °C.

Microbial contamination.

TAMC: acceptance criterion 10^3 CFU/g (*2.6.12*).

TYMC: acceptance criterion 10^2 CFU/g (*2.6.12*).

Absence of *Escherichia coli* (*2.6.13*).

Absence of *Salmonella* (*2.6.13*).

ASSAY

Magnesium. To 0.500 g in a 250 ml conical flask add 50 ml of a mixture of equal volumes of *butanol R* and *anhydrous ethanol R*, 5 ml of *concentrated ammonia R*, 3 ml of *ammonium chloride buffer solution pH 10.0 R*, 30.0 ml of *0.1 M sodium edetate* and 15 mg of *mordant black 11 triturate R*. Heat at 45-50 °C until the solution is clear and titrate with *0.1 M zinc sulphate* until the colour changes from blue to violet. Carry out a blank titration.

1 ml of *0.1 M sodium edetate* is equivalent to 2.431 mg of Mg.

Stearic acid and palmitic acid. Gas chromatography (*2.2.28*): use the normalisation procedure.

Test solution. In a conical flask fitted with a reflux condenser, dissolve 0.10 g of the substance to be examined in 5 ml of *boron trifluoride-methanol solution R*. Boil under a reflux condenser for 10 min. Add 4 ml of *heptane R* through the condenser and boil again under a reflux condenser for 10 min. Allow to cool. Add 20 ml of *saturated sodium chloride solution R*. Shake and allow the layers to separate. Dry the organic layer over 0.1 g of *anhydrous sodium sulphate R* (previously washed with *heptane R*). Dilute 1.0 ml of the solution to 10.0 ml with *heptane R*.

Reference solution. Prepare the reference solution in the same manner as the test solution using 50.0 mg of *palmitic acid CRS* and 50.0 mg of *stearic acid CRS* instead of the substance to be examined.

Column:

— *material*: fused silica;

— *size*: *l* = 30 m, Ø = 0.32 mm;

— *stationary phase*: macrogol 20 000 R (film thickness 0.5 μm).

Carrier gas: *helium for chromatography R*.

Flow rate: 2.4 ml/min.

Temperature:

	Time (min)	Temperature (°C)
Column	0 - 2	70
	2 - 36	70 → 240
	36 - 41	240
Injection port		220
Detector		260

Detection: flame ionisation.

Injection: 1 μl.

Relative retention with reference to methyl stearate: methyl palmitate = about 0.9.

System suitability: reference solution:

— *resolution*: minimum 5.0 between the peaks due to methyl palmitate and methyl stearate;

— *relative standard deviation*: maximum 3.0 per cent for the areas of the peaks due to methyl palmitate and methyl stearate, determined on 6 injections; maximum 1.0 per cent for the ratio of the areas of the peaks due to methyl palmitate to the areas of the peaks due to methyl stearate, determined on 6 injections.

FUNCTIONALITY-RELATED CHARACTERISTICS

This section provides information on characteristics that are recognised as being relevant control parameters for one or more functions of the substance when used as an excipient (see chapter 5.15). This section is a non-mandatory part of the monograph and it is not necessary to verify the characteristics to demonstrate compliance. Control of these characteristics can however

Monographs L-P

contribute to the quality of a medicinal product by improving the consistency of the manufacturing process and the performance of the medicinal product during use. Where control methods are cited, they are recognised as being suitable for the purpose, but other methods can also be used. Wherever results for a particular characteristic are reported, the control method must be indicated.

The following characteristic may be relevant for magnesium stearate used as lubricant in solid dosage forms (compressed and powder).

Specific surface area (*2.9.26, Method I*). Determine the specific surface area in the P/P_o range of 0.05 to 0.15.

Sample outgassing: 2 h at 40 °C.

07/2009:1542

MALTODEXTRIN

Maltodextrinum

DEFINITION

Mixture of glucose, disaccharides and polysaccharides, obtained by the partial hydrolysis of starch.

The degree of hydrolysis, expressed as dextrose equivalent (DE), is less than 20 (nominal value).

CHARACTERS

Appearance: white or almost white, slightly hygroscopic powder or granules.

Solubility: freely soluble in water.

IDENTIFICATION

A. Dissolve 0.1 g in 2.5 ml of *water R* and heat with 2.5 ml of *cupri-tartaric solution R*. A red precipitate is formed.

B. Dip, for 1 s, a suitable stick with a reactive pad containing glucose-oxidase, peroxidase and a hydrogen-donating substance, such as tetramethylbenzidine, in a 100 g/l solution of the substance to be examined. Observe the colour of the reactive pad; within 60 s the colour changes from yellow to green or blue.

C. It is a powder or granules.

D. Dextrose equivalent (see Tests).

TESTS

Solution S. Dissolve 12.5 g in *carbon dioxide-free water R* and dilute to 50.0 ml with the same solvent.

pH (*2.2.3*): 4.0 to 7.0.

Mix 1 ml of a 223.6 g/l solution of *potassium chloride R* and 30 ml of solution S.

Sulphur dioxide (*2.5.29*): maximum 20 ppm.

Heavy metals (*2.4.8*): maximum 10 ppm.

Dilute 4 ml of solution S to 30 ml with *water R*. The solution complies with test E. Prepare the reference solution using 10 ml of *lead standard solution (1 ppm Pb) R*.

Loss on drying (*2.2.32*): maximum 6.0 per cent, determined on 10.00 g by drying in an oven at 105 °C.

Sulphated ash (*2.4.14*): maximum 0.5 per cent, determined on 1.0 g.

Dextrose equivalent (DE): within 2 DE units of the nominal value.

Weigh an amount of the substance to be examined equivalent to 2.85-3.15 g of reducing carbohydrates, calculated as dextrose equivalent, into a 500 ml volumetric flask. Dissolve in *water R* and dilute to 500.0 ml with the same solvent. Transfer the solution to a 50 ml burette.

Pipette 25.0 ml of *cupri-tartaric solution R* into a 250 ml flask and add 18.5 ml of the test solution from the burette, mix and add a few glass beads. Place the flask on a hot plate, previously adjusted so that the solution begins to boil within 2 min ± 15 s. Allow to boil for exactly 120 s, add 1 ml of a 1 g/l solution of *methylene blue R* and titrate with the test solution (V_1) until the blue colour disappears. Maintain the solution at boiling throughout the titration.

Standardise the cupri-tartaric solution using a 6.00 g/l solution of *glucose R* (V_0).

Calculate the dextrose equivalent using the following expression:

$$\frac{300 \times V_0 \times 100}{V_1 \times M \times D}$$

V_0 = total volume of glucose standard solution, in millilitres;

V_1 = total volume of test solution, in millilitres;

M = sample mass, in grams;

D = percentage content of dry matter in the substance.

Microbial contamination

TAMC: acceptance criterion 10^3 CFU/g (*2.6.12*).

TYMC: acceptance criterion 10^2 CFU/g (*2.6.12*).

Absence of *Escherichia coli* (*2.6.13*).

Absence of *Salmonella* (*2.6.13*).

LABELLING

The label states the dextrose equivalent (DE) (= nominal value).

FUNCTIONALITY-RELATED CHARACTERISTICS

This section provides information on characteristics that are recognised as being relevant control parameters for one or more functions of the substance when used as an excipient (see chapter 5.15). This section is a non-mandatory part of the monograph and it is not necessary to verify the characteristics to demonstrate compliance. Control of these characteristics can however contribute to the quality of a medicinal product by improving the consistency of the manufacturing process and the performance of the medicinal product during use. Where control methods are cited, they are recognised as being suitable for the purpose, but other methods can also be used. Wherever results for a particular characteristic are reported, the control method must be indicated.

The following characteristics may be relevant for maltodextrin used as filler and binder in tablets and capsules.

Dextrose equivalent (see Tests).

Particle-size distribution (*2.9.31* or *2.9.38*).

Powder flow (*2.9.36*).

07/2009:0045

METHYLDOPA

Methyldopum

$C_{10}H_{13}NO_4,1^1/_2H_2O$ M_r 238.2
[41372-08-1]

DEFINITION

(2S)-2-Amino-3-(3,4-dihydroxyphenyl)-2-methylpropanoic acid.

Content: 98.5 per cent to 101.0 per cent (anhydrous substance).

CHARACTERS

Appearance: white or yellowish white, crystalline powder or colourless or almost colourless crystals.

Solubility: slightly soluble in water, very slightly soluble in ethanol (96 per cent). It is freely soluble in dilute mineral acids.

IDENTIFICATION

Carry out either Tests A, B or Tests A, C

A. Infrared absorption spectrophotometry (*2.2.24*).

   Comparison: methyldopa CRS.

B. Enantiomeric purity (see Tests).

C. Specific optical rotation (*2.2.7*): − 25.0 to − 28.0.

   Dissolve a quantity equivalent to 2.20 g of the anhydrous substance in *aluminium chloride solution R* and dilute to 50.0 ml with the same solution.

TESTS

Appearance of solution. Dissolve 1.0 g in *1 M hydrochloric acid* and dilute to 25 ml with the same solvent. The solution is not more intensely coloured than reference solution BY_6 or B_6 (*2.2.2, Method II*).

Acidity. Dissolve 1.0 g with heating in 100 ml of *carbon dioxide-free water R*. Add 0.1 ml of *methyl red solution R*. Not more than 0.5 ml of *0.1 M sodium hydroxide* is required to produce the pure yellow colour of the indicator.

Absorbance (*2.2.25*).

Test solution. Dissolve 40.0 mg in *0.1 M hydrochloric acid* and dilute to 100.0 ml with the same acid. Dilute 10.0 ml of this solution to 100.0 ml with *0.1 M hydrochloric acid*.

Spectral range: 230-350 nm.

Absorption maximum: at 280 nm.

Specific absorbance at the absorption maximum: 122 to 137 (anhydrous substance).

Related substances. Liquid chromatography (*2.2.29*). *Prepare the solutions immediately before use*.

Test solution. Dissolve 0.100 g of the substance to be examined in *0.1 M hydrochloric acid* and dilute to 25.0 ml with the same acid.

Reference solution (a). Dilute 1.0 ml of the test solution to 50.0 ml with *0.1 M hydrochloric acid*. Dilute 5.0 ml of this solution to 100.0 ml with *0.1 M hydrochloric acid*.

Reference solution (b). Dissolve the contents of a vial of *methyldopa for system suitability CRS* (containing impurities A, B and C) in 1.0 ml of *0.1 M hydrochloric acid*.

Column:

— *size*: l = 0.25 m, Ø = 4.6 mm;

— *stationary phase*: spherical *di-isobutyloctadecylsilyl silica gel for chromatography R* (5 μm) with a pore size of 8 nm.

Mobile phase: methanol R, 0.1 M phosphate buffer solution pH 3.0 R (15:85 V/V).

Flow rate: 1 ml/min.

Detection: spectrophotometer at 280 nm.

Injection: 20 μl.

Run time: 6 times the retention time of methyldopa.

Identification of impurities: use the chromatogram supplied with *methyldopa for system suitability CRS* and the chromatogram obtained with reference solution (b) to identify the peaks due to impurities A, B and C.

Relative retention with reference to methyldopa (retention time = about 5 min): impurity A = about 1.9; impurity B = about 4.3; impurity C = about 4.9.

System suitability: reference solution (b):

— *resolution*: minimum 2.0 between the peaks due to impurities B and C.

Limits:

— *correction factors*: for the calculation of content, multiply the peak areas of the following impurities by the corresponding correction factor: impurity B = 2.6; impurity C = 1.3;

— *impurities A, B, C*: for each impurity, not more than 1.5 times the area of the principal peak in the chromatogram obtained with reference solution (a) (0.15 per cent);

— *unspecified impurities*: for each impurity, not more than 0.5 times the area of the principal peak in the chromatogram obtained with reference solution (a) (0.05 per cent);

— *total*: not more than 5 times the area of the principal peak in the chromatogram obtained with reference solution (a) (0.5 per cent);

— *disregard limit*: 0.3 times the area of the principal peak in the chromatogram obtained with reference solution (a) (0.03 per cent).

Enantiomeric purity. Liquid chromatography (*2.2.29*).

Test solution. Dissolve 25 mg of the substance to be examined in the mobile phase and dilute to 25.0 ml with the mobile phase.

Reference solution (a). Dilute 5.0 ml of the test solution to 20.0 ml with the mobile phase. Dilute 1.0 ml of this solution to 50.0 ml with the mobile phase.

Reference solution (b). Dissolve 2 mg of *racemic methyldopa R* in the mobile phase and dilute to 10.0 ml with the mobile phase.

Column:

— *size*: l = 0.15 m, Ø = 3.9 mm;

— *stationary phase*: spherical *end-capped octadecylsilyl silica gel for chromatography R* (5 μm).

Mobile phase: dissolve separately 0.200 g of *copper acetate R* and 0.387 g of *N,N-dimethyl-L-phenylalanine R* in *water R*; mix the 2 solutions and adjust immediately to pH 4.3 with *acetic acid R*; add 50 ml of *methanol R* and dilute to 1000 ml with *water R*; mix and filter.

Equilibrate the column with the mobile phase for about 2 h.

If necessary, decrease the concentration of *methanol R* so the peak corresponding to D-methyldopa is clearly separated from the negative system peak that appears at about 6 min.

Flow rate: 1 ml/min.

Detection: spectrophotometer at 280 nm.

Injection: 20 µl.

Run time: twice the retention time of L-methyldopa.

Relative retention with reference to L-methyldopa (retention time = about 14 min): D-methyldopa = about 0.7.

System suitability: reference solution (b):

— *resolution*: minimum 5.0 between the peaks due to D-methyldopa and L-methyldopa.

Limits:

— *D-methyldopa*: not more than the area of the principal peak in the chromatogram obtained with reference solution (a) (0.5 per cent).

Heavy metals (*2.4.8*): maximum 20 ppm.

1.0 g complies with test C. Prepare the reference solution using 2 ml of *lead standard solution (10 ppm Pb) R*.

Water (*2.5.12*): 10.0 per cent to 13.0 per cent, determined on 0.20 g.

Sulphated ash (*2.4.14*): maximum 0.1 per cent, determined on 1.0 g.

ASSAY

Dissolve 0.180 g, heating if necessary, in 50 ml of *glacial acetic acid R*. Titrate with *0.1 M perchloric acid*, determining the end-point potentiometrically (*2.2.20*).

1 ml of *0.1 M perchloric acid* is equivalent to 21.12 mg of $C_{10}H_{13}NO_4$.

STORAGE

Protected from light.

IMPURITIES

Specified impurities: A, B, C, D.

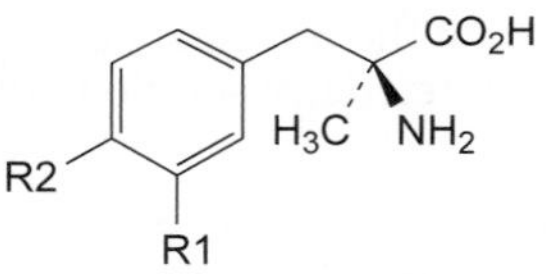

A. R1 = OCH_3, R2 = OH: (2S)-2-amino-3-(4-hydroxy-3-methoxyphenyl)-2-methylpropanoic acid (3-methoxymethyldopa),

B. R1 = H, R2 = OCH_3: (2S)-2-amino-3-(4-methoxyphenyl)-2-methylpropanoic acid,

C. R1 = R2 = OCH_3: (2S)-2-amino-3-(3,4-dimethoxyphenyl)-2-methylpropanoic acid,

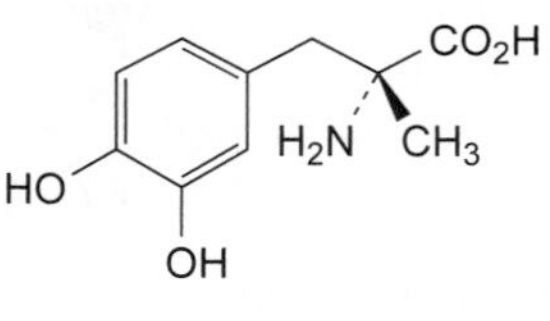

D. (2R)-2-amino-3-(3,4-dihydroxyphenyl)-2-methylpropanoic acid (D-methyldopa).

07/2009:1788

METHYLERGOMETRINE MALEATE

Methylergometrini maleas

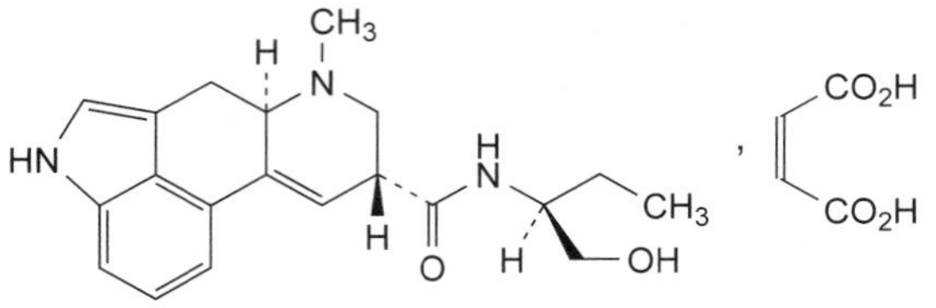

$C_{24}H_{29}N_3O_6$
[57432-61-8]

M_r 455.5

DEFINITION

(6a*R*,9*R*)-*N*-[(1*S*)-1-(Hydroxymethyl)propyl]-7-methyl-4,6,6a,7,8,9-hexahydroindolo[4,3-*fg*]quinoline-9-carboxamide (*Z*)-butenedioate.

Content: 99.0 per cent to 101.0 per cent (dried substance).

CHARACTERS

Appearance: white or almost white, hygroscopic, crystalline powder.

Solubility: soluble in water, slightly soluble in anhydrous ethanol.

IDENTIFICATION

A. Specific optical rotation (see Tests).

B. Infrared absorption spectrophotometry (*2.2.24*).

Comparison: *methylergometrine maleate CRS*.

TESTS

Solution S. Dissolve 0.100 g in *carbon dioxide-free water R* and dilute to 20.0 ml with the same solvent.

pH (*2.2.3*): 4.4 to 5.2.

Dilute 2.0 ml of solution S to 50.0 ml with *carbon dioxide-free water R*.

Specific optical rotation (*2.2.7*): + 44.0 to + 50.0 (dried substance), determined on solution S.

Related substances. Liquid chromatography (*2.2.29*). *Carry out the test protected from light.*

Test solution. Dissolve 25 mg of the substance to be examined in 15 ml of mobile phase B and dilute to 50.0 ml with *water R*.

Reference solution (a). Dilute 1.0 ml of the test solution to 100.0 ml with *water R*. Dilute 1.0 ml of this solution to 10.0 ml with *water R*.

Reference solution (b). Dissolve the contents of a vial of *methylergometrine for system suitability CRS* (containing impurities A, B, C, D, E, F, G, H and I) in 1.0 ml of a mixture of 30 volumes of mobile phase B and 70 volumes of *water R*.

Column:

— *size*: *l* = 0.10 m, Ø = 4.6 mm;

— *stationary phase*: *end-capped octadecylsilyl silica gel for chromatography R* (3.5 µm).

Mobile phase:

— *mobile phase A*: 2 g/l solution of *ammonium carbamate R*;

— *mobile phase B*: *acetonitrile R*, *water R* (50:50 *V/V*);

Time (min)	Mobile phase A (per cent V/V)	Mobile phase B (per cent V/V)
0 - 2	85	15
2 - 7	85 → 65	15 → 35
7 - 12	65	35
12 - 17	65 → 20	35 → 80
17 - 19	20	80

Flow rate: 2.0 ml/min.

Detection: spectrophotometer at 310 nm.

Injection: 20 µl.

Identification of impurities: use the chromatogram supplied with *methylergometrine for system suitability CRS* and the chromatogram obtained with reference solution (b) to identify the peaks due to impurities A, B, C, D, E, F, G, H and I.

Relative retention with reference to methylergometrine (retention time = about 12 min): impurity A = about 0.2; impurity B = about 0.5; impurity C = about 0.6; impurity D = about 0.7; impurity I = about 1.10; impurity E = about 1.14; impurity F = about 1.2; impurity G = about 1.3; impurity H = about 1.4.

System suitability: reference solution (b):

— *resolution*: minimum 3.0 between the peaks due to methylergometrine and impurity I; minimum 1.5 between the peaks due to impurities I and E.

Limits:

— *impurity I*: not more than 3 times the area of the principal peak in the chromatogram obtained with reference solution (a) (0.3 per cent);

— *impurity C*: not more than twice the area of the principal peak in the chromatogram obtained with reference solution (a) (0.2 per cent);

— *impurities A, B, D, E, F, G, H*: for each impurity, not more than 1.5 times the area of the principal peak in the chromatogram obtained with reference solution (a) (0.15 per cent);

— *unspecified impurities*: for each impurity, not more than the area of the principal peak in the chromatogram obtained with reference solution (a) (0.10 per cent);

— *total*: not more than 6 times the area of the principal peak in the chromatogram obtained with reference solution (a) (0.6 per cent);

— *disregard limit*: 0.5 times the area of the principal peak in the chromatogram obtained with reference solution (a) (0.05 per cent).

Loss on drying (*2.2.32*): maximum 2.0 per cent, determined on 1.000 g by drying in an oven at 105 °C.

Sulphated ash (*2.4.14*): maximum 0.1 per cent, determined on 1.0 g.

ASSAY

Dissolve 0.300 g in 60 ml of *anhydrous acetic acid R*. Titrate with *0.1 M perchloric acid*, determining the end-point potentiometrically (*2.2.20*).

1 ml of *0.1 M perchloric acid* is equivalent to 45.55 mg of $C_{24}H_{29}N_3O_6$.

STORAGE

In an airtight container, protected from light.

IMPURITIES

Specified impurities: A, B, C, D, E, F, G, H, I.

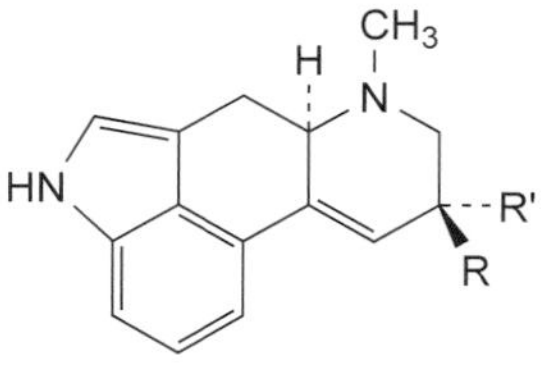

A. R = H, R′ = CO_2H: (6a*R*,9*R*)-7-methyl-4,6,6a,7,8,9-hexahydroindolo[4,3-*fg*]quinoline-9-carboxylic acid,

B. R = CO_2H, R′ = H: (6a*R*,9*S*)-7-methyl-4,6,6a,7,8,9-hexahydroindolo[4,3-*fg*]quinoline-9-carboxylic acid,

C. R = H, R′ = $CONH_2$: (6a*R*,9*R*)-7-methyl-4,6,6a,7,8,9-hexahydroindolo[4,3-*fg*]quinoline-9-carboxamide,

E. R = $CONH_2$, R′ = H: (6a*R*,9*S*)-7-methyl-4,6,6a,7,8,9-hexahydroindolo[4,3-*fg*]quinoline-9-carboxamide,

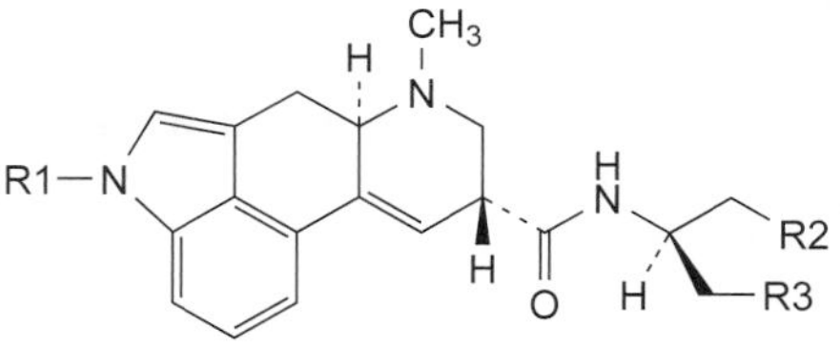

D. R1 = R2 = H, R3 = OH: (6a*R*,9*R*)-*N*-[(1*S*)-2-hydroxy-1-methylethyl]-7-methyl-4,6,6a,7,8,9-hexahydroindolo[4,3-*fg*]quinoline-9-carboxamide (ergometrine),

G. R1 = R2 = CH_3, R3 = OH: (6a*R*,9*R*)-*N*-[(1*S*)-1-(hydroxymethyl)propyl]-4,7-dimethyl-4,6,6a,7,8,9-hexahydroindolo[4,3-*fg*]quinoline-9-carboxamide (methysergide),

I. R1 = H, R2 = OH, R3 = CH_3: (6a*R*,9*R*)-*N*-[(1*R*)-1-(hydroxymethyl)propyl]-7-methyl-4,6,6a,7,8,9-hexahydroindolo[4,3-*fg*]quinoline-9-carboxamide (1′-*epi*-methylergometrine),

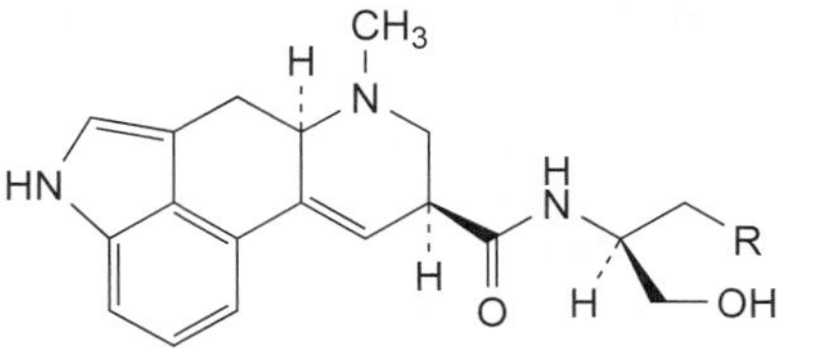

F. R = H: (6a*R*,9*S*)-*N*-[(1*S*)-2-hydroxy-1-methylethyl]-7-methyl-4,6,6a,7,8,9-hexahydroindolo[4,3-*fg*]quinoline-9-carboxamide (ergometrinine),

H. R = CH_3: (6a*R*,9*S*)-*N*-[(1*S*)-1-(hydroxymethyl)propyl]-7-methyl-4,6,6a,7,8,9-hexahydroindolo[4,3-*fg*]quinoline-9-carboxamide (methylergometrinine).

07/2009:2338

MIRTAZAPINE

Mirtazapinum

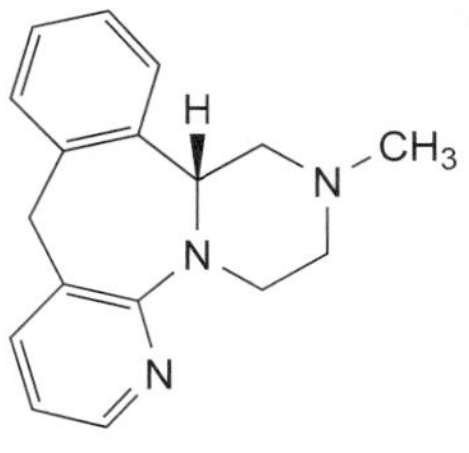

and enantiomer

$C_{17}H_{19}N_3$ M_r 265.4
[61337-67-5]

DEFINITION

(14bRS)-2-Methyl-1,2,3,4,10,14b-hexahydropyrazino[2,1-a]pyrido[2,3-c][2]benzazepine.

Content: 99.0 per cent to 101.0 per cent (anhydrous substance).

CHARACTERS

Appearance: white or almost white powder, slightly hygroscopic to hygroscopic.

Solubility: practically insoluble in water, freely soluble in anhydrous ethanol.

It shows polymorphism (5.9).

IDENTIFICATION

Infrared absorption spectrophotometry (2.2.24).

Comparison: mirtazapine CRS.

If the spectra obtained in the solid state show differences, dissolve the substance to be examined and the reference substance separately in anhydrous ethanol R, evaporate to dryness and record new spectra using the residues.

TESTS

Optical rotation (2.2.7): − 0.10° to + 0.10° (anhydrous substance).

Dissolve 0.250 g in anhydrous ethanol R and dilute to 25.0 ml with the same solvent.

Related substances. Liquid chromatography (2.2.29).

Solvent mixture: acetonitrile R, water R (50:50 V/V).

Buffer solution. Dissolve 18.0 g of tetramethylammonium hydroxide R in 950 ml of water R. While stirring, adjust to pH 7.4 with phosphoric acid R, then dilute to 1000 ml with water R and mix.

Test solution. Dissolve 30 mg of the substance to be examined in the solvent mixture and dilute to 20 ml with the solvent mixture.

Reference solution (a). Dissolve 3 mg of mirtazapine for system suitability CRS (containing impurities A, B, C, D, E and F) in 2 ml of the solvent mixture.

Reference solution (b). Dilute 1.0 ml of the test solution to 100.0 ml with the solvent mixture. Dilute 1.0 ml of this solution to 10.0 ml with the solvent mixture.

Column:
— size: l = 0.25 m, Ø = 4.6 mm;
— stationary phase: end-capped octadecylsilyl silica gel for chromatography R (5 μm);
— temperature: 40 °C.

Mobile phase: tetrahydrofuran for chromatography R, methanol R, acetonitrile R, buffer solution (7.5:12.5:15:65 V/V/V/V).

Flow rate: 1.5 ml/min.

Detection: spectrophotometer at 240 nm.

Injection: 10 μl.

Run time: twice the retention time of mirtazapine.

Identification of impurities: use the chromatogram supplied with mirtazapine for system suitability CRS and the chromatogram obtained with reference solution (a) to identify the peaks due to impurities A, B, C, D, E and F.

Relative retention with reference to mirtazapine (retention time = about 25 min): impurity A = about 0.2; impurity B = about 0.3; impurity C = about 0.35; impurity D = about 0.4; impurity E = about 1.3; impurity F = about 1.35.

System suitability:
— resolution: minimum 1.5 between the peaks due to impurities E and F in the chromatogram obtained with reference solution (a);
— symmetry factor: 0.8 to 2.0 for the principal peak in the chromatogram obtained with reference solution (b).

Limits:
— correction factors: for the calculation of content, multiply the peak areas of the following impurities by the corresponding correction factor: impurity A = 1.3; impurity B = 1.3; impurity F = 0.2;
— impurities A, B, C, D, E, F: for each impurity, not more than the area of the principal peak in the chromatogram obtained with reference solution (b) (0.1 per cent);
— unspecified impurities: for each impurity, not more than the area of the principal peak in the chromatogram obtained with reference solution (b) (0.10 per cent);
— total: not more than twice the area of the principal peak in the chromatogram obtained with reference solution (b) (0.2 per cent);
— disregard limit: 0.5 times the area of the principal peak in the chromatogram obtained with reference solution (b) (0.05 per cent).

Water (2.5.12): maximum 3.5 per cent, determined on 1.00 g.

Sulphated ash (2.4.14): maximum 0.1 per cent, determined on 1.0 g.

ASSAY

Dissolve 0.100 g in 35 ml of glacial acetic acid R. Titrate with 0.1 M perchloric acid, determining the end-point potentiometrically (2.2.20).

1 ml of 0.1 M perchloric acid is equivalent to 13.27 mg of $C_{17}H_{19}N_3$.

STORAGE

In an airtight container.

IMPURITIES

Specified impurities: A, B, C, D, E, F.

its epimer at N* and their enantiomers

A. (14bRS)-2-methyl-1,2,3,4,10,14b-hexahydropyrazino[2,1-a]pyrido[2,3-c][2]benzazepine 2-oxide,

and enantiomer

B. R = OH: [2-[(2RS)-4-methyl-2-phenylpiperazin-1-yl]pyridin-3-yl]methanol,

E. R = H: (2RS)-4-methyl-1-(3-methylpyridin-2-yl)-2-phenylpiperazine,

See the information section on general monographs (cover pages)

and enantiomer

C. R = CH₃, X = H₂, X′ = O: (14bRS)-2-methyl-3,4,10,14b-tetrahydropyrazino[2,1-a]pyrido[2,3-c][2]benzazepin-1(2H)-one,

D. R = H, X = X′ = H₂: (14bRS)-1,2,3,4,10,14b-hexahydropyrazino[2,1-a]pyrido[2,3-c][2]benzazepine,

F. R = CH₃, X = O, X′ = H₂: (14bRS)-2-methyl-1,3,4,14b-tetrahydropyrazino[2,1-a]pyrido[2,3-c][2]benzazepin-10(2H)-one.

04/2008:1701
corrected 6.5

MOLSIDOMINE

Molsidominum

$C_9H_{14}N_4O_4$ M_r 242.2
[25717-80-0]

DEFINITION

N-(Ethoxycarbonyl)-3-(morpholin-4-yl)sydnonimine.

Content: 99.0 per cent to 101.0 per cent (dried substance).

CHARACTERS

Appearance: white or almost white, crystalline powder.

Solubility: sparingly soluble in water, soluble in anhydrous ethanol and in methylene chloride.

mp: about 142 °C.

IDENTIFICATION

Infrared absorption spectrophotometry (*2.2.24*).

Comparison: molsidomine CRS.

TESTS

Appearance of solution. The solution is clear (*2.2.1*) and not more intensely coloured than reference solution B₇ (*2.2.2, Method II*).

Dissolve 1.0 g in *anhydrous ethanol R* and dilute to 20.0 ml with the same solvent.

pH (*2.2.3*): 5.5 to 7.5.

Dissolve 0.50 g in *carbon dioxide-free water R* and dilute to 50.0 ml with the same solvent.

Impurity B. Liquid chromatography (*2.2.29*) as described in the test for related substances with the following modifications.

Detection: spectrophotometer at 240 nm.

Injection: 20 μl of test solution (a) and reference solution (b).

Relative retention with reference to molsidomine (retention time = about 9 min): impurity B = about 0.43.

System suitability: reference solution (b):

— *signal-to-noise ratio*: minimum 20 for the principal peak.

Limit:

— *impurity B*: not more than the area of the corresponding peak in the chromatogram obtained with reference solution (b) (3 ppm).

Impurity E. Liquid chromatography (*2.2.29*).

Test solution. Dissolve 0.200 g of the substance to be examined in the mobile phase and dilute to 100.0 ml with the mobile phase.

Reference solution (a). Dissolve 50.0 mg of *morpholine for chromatography R* in 500.0 ml of *water for chromatography R*. Dilute 20.0 ml of the solution to 500.0 ml with *water for chromatography R*. Dilute 5.0 ml of this solution to 100.0 ml with *water for chromatography R*.

Reference solution (b). Mix 10.0 ml of the test solution with 10.0 ml of reference solution (a).

Column:

— *size*: l = 0.25 m, Ø = 4.0 mm;

— *stationary phase*: resin for reversed-phase ion chromatography R;

— *temperature*: 25 °C.

Mobile phase: mix 3.0 ml of *methanesulphonic acid R* and 75 ml of *acetonitrile R* in *water for chromatography R* and dilute to 5000 ml with *water for chromatography R*.

Suppressor regenerant: water for chromatography R.

Flow rate: 1.0 ml/min.

Expected background conductivity: less than 0.5 μS.

Detection: conductivity detector at 10 μS.

Injection: 50 μl.

Run time: 20 min.

Relative retention with reference to molsidomine (retention time = about 3 min): impurity E = about 2.4.

System suitability: reference solution (b):

— *signal-to-noise ratio*: minimum 6 for the peak due to impurity E.

Limit:

— *impurity E*: not more than the area of the principal peak in the chromatogram obtained with reference solution (a) (0.01 per cent).

Related substances. Liquid chromatography (*2.2.29*).
Protect the solutions from light.

Solvent mixture: methanol R, mobile phase A (10:90 V/V).

Test solution (a). Dissolve 0.200 g of the substance to be examined in 2.5 ml of *methanol R* and dilute to 5.0 ml with mobile phase A.

Test solution (b). Dilute 1.0 ml of test solution (a) to 20.0 ml with the solvent mixture.

Reference solution (a). Dilute 1.0 ml of test solution (b) to 100.0 ml with the solvent mixture. Dilute 1.0 ml of this solution to 10.0 ml with the solvent mixture.

Reference solution (b). Dissolve 2.4 mg of *molsidomine impurity B CRS* in 80 ml of *methanol R* and dilute to 100.0 ml with *methanol R*. Dilute 2.0 ml of the solution to 100.0 ml with the solvent mixture. Dilute 5.0 ml of this solution to 20.0 ml with the solvent mixture.

Reference solution (c). Dissolve 10 mg of *linsidomine hydrochloride R* (impurity A) and 5 mg of *molsidomine impurity D CRS* in 10 ml of *methanol R* and dilute to 50.0 ml with the solvent mixture. Dilute 5.0 ml of this solution to 50.0 ml with the solvent mixture.

Column:

— *size*: $l = 0.15$ m, $\emptyset = 4.6$ mm;

— *stationary phase*: *end-capped octadecylsilyl silica gel for chromatography R* (5 μm);

— *temperature*: 30 °C.

Mobile phase:

— *mobile phase A*: dissolve 4.0 g of *potassium dihydrogen phosphate R* in *water for chromatography R* and dilute to 1000 ml with the same solvent;

— *mobile phase B*: *methanol R1*;

Time (min)	Mobile phase A (per cent *V/V*)	Mobile phase B (per cent *V/V*)
0 - 3	90	10
3 - 10	90 → 20	10 → 80
10 - 13	20	80

Flow rate: 1.3 ml/min.

Detection: spectrophotometer at 210 nm.

Injection: 20 μl of test solution (b) and reference solutions (a) and (c).

Relative retention with reference to molsidomine (retention time = about 9 min): impurity A = about 0.2; impurity D = about 0.3.

System suitability: reference solution (c):

— *resolution*: minimum 3.5 between the peaks due to impurities A and D.

Limits:

— *unspecified impurities*: for each impurity, not more than the area of the peak due to molsidomine in the chromatogram obtained with reference solution (a) (0.10 per cent);

— *total*: not more than 3 times the area of the peak due to molsidomine in the chromatogram obtained with reference solution (a) (0.3 per cent);

— *disregard limit*: 0.5 times the area of the peak due to molsidomine in the chromatogram obtained with reference solution (a) (0.05 per cent).

Heavy metals: maximum 20 ppm.

Prescribed solution. Dissolve 0.5 g in 20 ml of *ethanol (96 per cent) R*.

Test solution. 12 ml of the prescribed solution.

Reference solution. Mix 6 ml of lead standard solution (1 ppm Pb) (obtained by diluting *lead standard solution (100 ppm Pb) R* with *ethanol (96 per cent) R*) with 2 ml of the prescribed solution and 4 ml of *water R*.

Blank solution. Mix 10 ml of *ethanol (96 per cent) R* and 2 ml of the prescribed solution.

To each solution, add 2 ml of *buffer solution pH 3.5 R*. Mix and add to 1.2 ml of *thioacetamide reagent R*. Mix immediately. Filter the solutions through a membrane filter (pore size 0.45 μm) (*2.4.8*). Carry out the filtration slowly and uniformly, applying moderate and constant pressure to the piston. Compare the spots on the filters obtained with the different solutions. The test is invalid if the reference solution does not show a slight brown colour compared to the blank solution. The substance to be examined complies with the test if the brown colour of the spot resulting from the test solution is not more intense than that of the spot resulting from the reference solution.

Loss on drying (*2.2.32*): maximum 0.5 per cent, determined on 1.000 g by drying in an oven at 105 °C.

Sulphated ash (*2.4.14*): maximum 0.1 per cent, determined on 1.0 g.

ASSAY

Dissolve 0.200 g in a mixture of 5 ml of *acetic anhydride R* and 50 ml of *anhydrous acetic acid R*. Titrate with *0.1 M perchloric acid*, determining the end-point potentiometrically (*2.2.20*).

1 ml of *0.1 M perchloric acid* is equivalent to 24.22 mg of $C_9H_{14}N_4O_4$.

STORAGE

Protected from light.

IMPURITIES

Specified impurities: B, E.

Other detectable impurities (the following substances would, if present at a sufficient level, be detected by one or other of the tests in the monograph. They are limited by the general acceptance criterion for other/unspecified impurities and/or by the general monograph *Substances for pharmaceutical use (2034)*. It is therefore not necessary to identify these impurities for demonstration of compliance. See also *5.10. Control of impurities in substances for pharmaceutical use): A, C, D.*

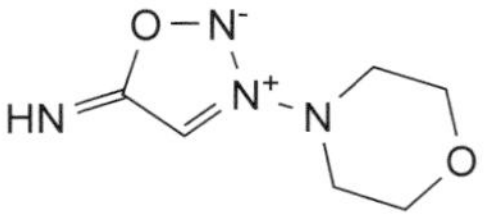

A. 3-(morpholin-4-yl)sydnonimine (linsidomine),

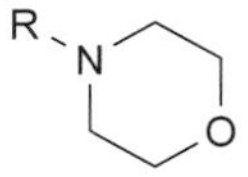

B. R = NO: 4-nitrosomorpholine,

D. R = CHO: morpholine-4-carbaldehyde,

E. R = H: morpholine,

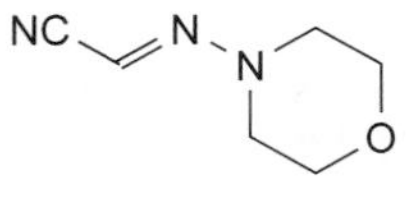

C. (2*E*)-(morpholin-4-ylimino)acetonitrile.

01/2008:1656
corrected 6.5

MOXIDECTIN FOR VETERINARY USE

Moxidectinum ad usum veterinarium

C$_{37}$H$_{53}$NO$_8$ M$_r$ 640
[113507-06-5]

DEFINITION

(2a*E*,2'*R*,4*E*,4'*E*,5'*S*,6*R*,6'*S*,8*E*,11*R*,15*S*,17a*R*,20*R*,20a*R*, 20b*S*)-6'-[(1*E*)-1,3-Dimethylbut-1-enyl]-20,20b-dihydroxy-4'-(methoxyimino)-5',6,8,19-tetramethyl-3',4',5',6,6',7,10,- 11,14,15,17a,20,20a,20b-tetradecahydrospiro[2*H*,17*H*-11,- 15-methanofuro[4,3,2-*pq*][2,6]benzodioxacyclooctadecine-13,2'-pyran]-17-one ((6*R*,23*E*,25*S*)-5*O*-demethyl-28-deoxy-25-[(1*E*)-1,3-dimethylbut-1-enyl]-6,28-epoxy-23-(methoxyimino)milbemycin B).

Semi-synthetic product derived from a fermentation product.

It may contain suitable stabilisers such as antioxidants.

Content: 92.0 per cent to 102.0 per cent (anhydrous substance).

CHARACTERS

Appearance: white or pale yellow, amorphous powder.

Solubility: practically insoluble in water, very soluble in ethanol (96 per cent), slightly soluble in hexane.

IDENTIFICATION

Infrared absorption spectrophotometry (*2.2.24*).

Comparison: moxidectin CRS.

TESTS

Appearance of solution. The solution is clear (*2.2.1*) and not more intensely coloured than reference solution GY$_5$ (*2.2.2, Method II*).

Dissolve 0.40 g in *benzyl alcohol R* and dilute to 20 ml with the same solvent.

Related substances. Liquid chromatography (*2.2.29*).

A. *Test solution*. Dissolve 25.0 mg of the substance to be examined in *acetonitrile R* and dilute to 25.0 ml with the same solvent.

Reference solution (a). Dilute 1.0 ml of the test solution to 100.0 ml *acetonitrile R*.

Reference solution (b). Dissolve 5 mg of *moxidectin for system suitability CRS* (containing impurities A, B, C, D, E, F, G, H, I, J and K) in 5 ml of *acetonitrile R*.

Reference solution (c). Dissolve 25.0 mg of *moxidectin CRS* in *acetonitrile R* and dilute to 25.0 ml with the same solvent.

Column:
— *size*: *l* = 0.15 m, Ø = 3.9 mm;
— *stationary phase*: end-capped octadecylsilyl silica gel for chromatography *R* (4 µm);
— *temperature*: 50 °C.

Mobile phase: dissolve 7.7 g of *ammonium acetate R* in 400 ml of *water R*, adjust to pH 4.8 with *glacial acetic acid R* and add 600 ml of *acetonitrile R*.

Flow rate: 2.5 ml/min.

Detection: spectrophotometer at 242 nm.

Injection: 10 µl of the test solution and reference solutions (a) and (b).

Run time: 2 times the retention time of moxidectin.

Identification of impurities: use the chromatogram supplied with *moxidectin for system suitability CRS* and the chromatogram obtained with reference solution (b) to identify the peaks due to impurities A, B, C, D, E + F and G.

Relative retention with reference to moxidectin (retention time = about 12 min): impurity A = about 0.5; impurity B = about 0.7; impurity C = about 0.75; impurity D = about 0.94; impurities E and F = about 1.3-1.5; impurity G = about 1.6.

System suitability: reference solution (b):
— *peak-to-valley ratio*: minimum 3.0, where H$_p$ = height above the baseline of the peak due to impurity D and H$_v$ = height above the baseline of the lowest point of the curve separating this peak from the peak due to moxidectin.

Limits:
— *impurity D*: not more than 2.5 times the area of the principal peak in the chromatogram obtained with reference solution (a) (2.5 per cent);
— *sum of impurities E and F*: not more than 1.7 times the area of the principal peak in the chromatogram obtained with reference solution (a) (1.7 per cent);
— *impurities A, C, G*: for each impurity, not more than 1.5 times the area of the principal peak in the chromatogram obtained with reference solution (a) (1.5 per cent);
— *impurity B*: not more than 0.5 times the area of the principal peak in the chromatogram obtained with reference solution (a) (0.5 per cent);
— *any other impurity eluting before impurity G*: for each impurity, not more than 0.5 times the area of the principal peak in the chromatogram obtained with reference solution (a) (0.5 per cent);
— *disregard limit*: 0.1 times the area of the principal peak in the chromatogram obtained with reference solution (a) (0.1 per cent); disregard the peak due to the stabiliser (identify this peak, where applicable, by injecting a suitable reference solution).

B. *Test solution*. Dissolve 75.0 mg of the substance to be examined in *acetonitrile R* and dilute to 25.0 ml with the same solvent.

Reference solution (a). Dilute 1.0 ml of the test solution to 100.0 ml with *acetonitrile R*.

Reference solution (b). Dissolve 5 mg of *moxidectin for system suitability CRS* (containing impurities A, B, C, D, E, F, G, H, I, J and K) in 5 ml of *acetonitrile R*.

Column:
- *size*: l = 0.15 m, Ø = 3.9 mm;
- *stationary phase*: end-capped octadecylsilyl silica gel for chromatography R (4 μm);
- *temperature*: 35 °C.

Mobile phase: dissolve 3.8 g of *ammonium acetate R* in 250 ml of *water R*, adjust to pH 4.2 with *acetic acid R* and add 750 ml of *acetonitrile R*.

Flow rate: 2.0 ml/min.

Detection: spectrophotometer at 242 nm.

Injection: 10 μl.

Run time: 10 times the retention time of moxidectin.

Identification of impurities: use the chromatogram supplied with *moxidectin for system suitability CRS* and the chromatogram obtained with reference solution (b) to identify the peaks due to impurities H + I, J and K.

Relative retention with reference to moxidectin (retention time = about 4 min): impurity G = about 1.4; impurities H and I = about 2.0; impurity J = about 2.2; impurity K = about 3.4.

System suitability: reference solution (b):
- *resolution*: baseline separation between the peaks due to impurities H + I and J.

Limits:
- *sum of impurities H and I*: not more than the area of the principal peak in the chromatogram obtained with reference solution (a) (1.0 per cent);
- *impurities J, K*: for each impurity, not more than 0.5 times the area of the principal peak in the chromatogram obtained with reference solution (a) (0.5 per cent);
- *any other impurity eluting after impurity G*: for each impurity, not more than 0.5 times the area of the principal peak in the chromatogram obtained with reference solution (a) (0.5 per cent);
- *disregard limit*: 0.1 times the area of the principal peak in the chromatogram obtained with reference solution (a) (0.1 per cent); disregard the peak due to the stabiliser (identify this peak, where applicable, by injecting a suitable reference solution).

Total of all impurities. Calculate the sum of the impurities eluting from the start of the run to impurity G in test A, and from impurities H + I to the end of the run in test B. The total of all impurities is not more than 7.0 per cent.

Heavy metals (*2.4.8*): maximum 20 ppm.

It complies with test A with the following modifications.

Prescribed solution. Dissolve 0.50 g in 20 ml of *ethanol (96 per cent) R*.

Test solution. 12 ml of the prescribed solution.

Reference solution. A mixture of 2 ml of the prescribed solution, 4 ml of *water R* and 6 ml of *lead standard solution (1 ppm Pb) R*.

Blank solution. A mixture of 2 ml of the prescribed solution and 10 ml of *ethanol (96 per cent) R*.

Use a membrane filter (nominal pore size 0.45 μm).

Water (*2.5.12*): maximum 1.3 per cent, determined on 0.50 g.

Sulphated ash (*2.4.14*): maximum 0.2 per cent, determined on 1.0 g.

ASSAY

Liquid chromatography (*2.2.29*) as described in test A for related substances with the following modification.

Injection: test solution and reference solution (c).

Calculate the percentage content of $C_{37}H_{53}NO_8$ using the declared content of *moxidectin CRS*.

IMPURITIES

Specified impurities: A, B, C, D, E, F, G, H, I, J, K.

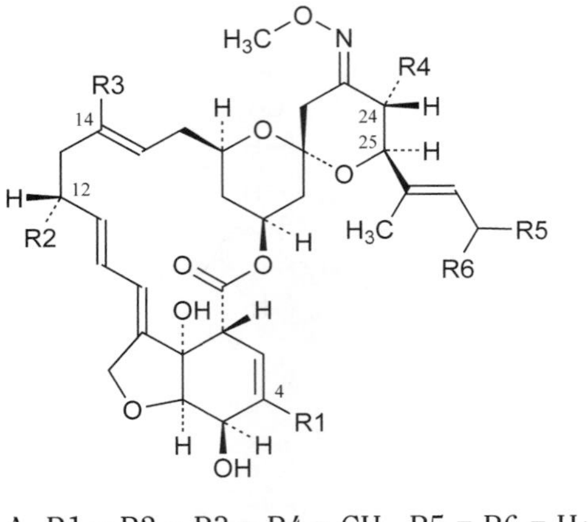

A. R1 = R2 = R3 = R4 = CH$_3$, R5 = R6 = H: 25-des[(1E)-1,3-dimethylbut-1-enyl]-25-[(1E)-1-methylprop-1-enyl]moxidectin,

B. R1 = R2 = R3 = R5 = R6 = CH$_3$, R4 = H: 24-desmethylmoxidectin,

C. R1 = R2 = R3 = R4 = R5 = CH$_3$, R6 = H: 25-des[(1E)-1,3-dimethylbut-1-enyl]-25-[(1E)-1-methylbut-1-enyl]moxidectin,

F. one of groups R1 to R6 is C$_2$H$_5$, the others are CH$_3$: x-desmethyl-x-ethylmoxidectin,

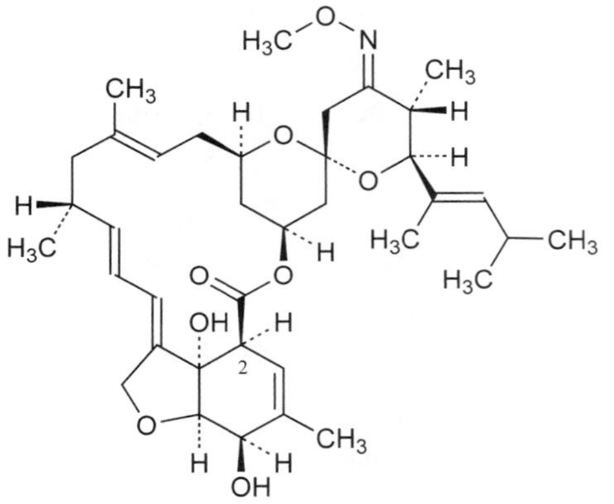

D. 2-*epi*-moxidectin,

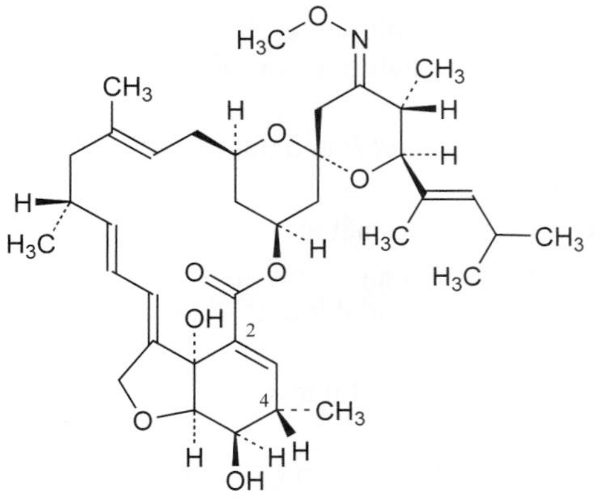

E. (4S)-2-dehydro-4-hydromoxidectin,

G. (23*E*,25*S*)-5*O*-desmethyl-28-deoxy-25-[(1*E*)-1,3-dimethylbut-1-enyl]-23-(methoxyimino)milbemycin B,

H. 2,5-didehydro-5-deoxymoxidectin,

I. (23*S*)-23-des(methoxyimino)-23-[(methylsulphanyl)meth-oxy]moxidectin,

J. R = CH$_2$-S-CH$_3$, R′ = H: 7-*O*-[(methylsulphanyl)methyl]-moxidectin,

K. R = H, R′ = CO-C$_6$H$_4$-*p*NO$_2$: 5-*O*-(4-nitrobenzoyl)moxidectin,

L. (23*Z*)-moxidectin.

O

Monographs
L-P

See the information section on general monographs (cover pages)

07/2009:1353

OXOLINIC ACID

Acidum oxolinicum

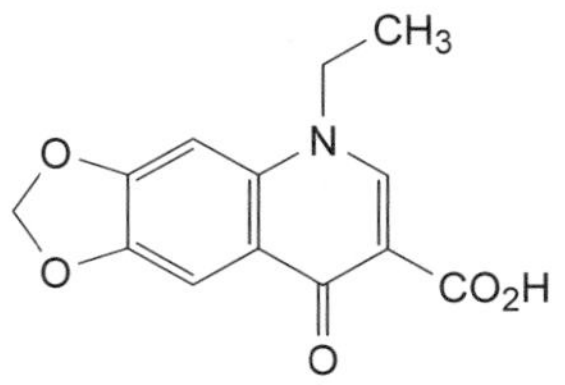

$C_{13}H_{11}NO_5$ M_r 261.2
[14698-29-4]

DEFINITION

5-Ethyl-8-oxo-5,8-dihydro-1,3-dioxolo[4,5-*g*]quinoline-7-carboxylic acid.

Content: 98.0 per cent to 102.0 per cent (dried substance).

CHARACTERS

Appearance: almost white or pale yellow, crystalline powder.

Solubility: practically insoluble in water, very slightly soluble in methylene chloride, practically insoluble in ethanol (96 per cent). It dissolves in dilute solutions of alkali hydroxides.

IDENTIFICATION

First identification: B.

Second identification: A, C.

A. Ultraviolet and visible absorption spectrophotometry (*2.2.25*).

   Test solution. Dissolve 25.0 mg in 5 ml of *0.1 M sodium hydroxide*, heating on a water-bath. Allow to cool and dilute to 100.0 ml with *methanol R*. Dilute 2.0 ml of this solution to 100.0 ml with *0.1 M hydrochloric acid*.

   Spectral range: 220-350 nm.

   Absorption maxima: at 260 nm, 322 nm and 336 nm.

   Absorbance ratio: A_{260}/A_{336} = 4.9 to 5.2.

B. Infrared absorption spectrophotometry (*2.2.24*).

   Preparation: discs.

   Comparison: *oxolinic acid CRS*.

C. Thin-layer chromatography (*2.2.27*).

   Test solution. Dissolve 10 mg of the substance to be examined in 3 ml of *dilute sodium hydroxide solution R* and dilute to 20 ml with *ethanol (96 per cent) R*.

   Reference solution (a). Dissolve 10 mg of *oxolinic acid CRS* in 3 ml of *dilute sodium hydroxide solution R* and dilute to 20 ml with *ethanol (96 per cent) R*.

   Reference solution (b). Dissolve 5 mg of *ciprofloxacin hydrochloride CRS* in *methanol R* and dilute to 10 ml with the same solvent. Dilute 1 ml of this solution to 2 ml with reference solution (a).

   Plate: *TLC silica gel plate R*.

   Mobile phase: acetonitrile R, concentrated ammonia R, methanol R, methylene chloride R (10:20:40:40 *V/V/V/V*).

   Application: 10 µl.

   Development: at the bottom of a chromatographic tank, place an evaporating disk containing 50 ml of *concentrated ammonia R* and expose the plate to the

ammonia vapour for 15 min in the closed tank; withdraw the plate, transfer to a second chromatographic tank and proceed with development over a path of 15 cm.

   Drying: in air.

   Detection: examine in ultraviolet light at 254 nm.

   System suitability: reference solution (b):

   — the chromatogram shows 2 clearly separated principal spots.

   Results: the principal spot in the chromatogram obtained with the test solution is similar in position, colour and size to the principal spot in the chromatogram obtained with reference solution (a).

TESTS

Solution S. Dissolve 0.6 g in 20 ml of a 40 g/l solution of *sodium hydroxide R*.

Appearance of solution. Solution S is clear (*2.2.1*) and not more intensely coloured than reference solution B_7 (*2.2.2*, *Method II*).

Related substances. Thin-layer chromatography (*2.2.27*).

Test solution. Dissolve 0.10 g of the substance to be examined in 3 ml of *dilute sodium hydroxide solution R* and dilute to 10 ml with *ethanol (96 per cent) R*.

Reference solution (a). Dilute 1 ml of the test solution to 50.0 ml with *ethanol (96 per cent) R*. Dilute 1.0 ml of this solution to 5.0 ml with *ethanol (96 per cent) R*.

Reference solution (b). Dissolve 2 mg of *oxolinic acid impurity B CRS* in *ethanol (96 per cent) R* and dilute to 10 ml with the same solvent. Dilute 1.0 ml of this solution to 10 ml with *ethanol (96 per cent) R*.

Reference solution (c). Dissolve 5 mg of the substance to be examined and 5 mg of *oxolinic acid impurity A CRS* in 2 ml of *dilute sodium hydroxide solution R* and dilute to 40 ml with *ethanol (96 per cent) R*.

Plate: *cellulose for chromatography R* as the coating substance.

Mobile phase: ammonia R, water R, propanol R (15:30:55 *V/V/V*).

Application: 5 µl, in sufficiently small portions to obtain small spots.

Development: over 2/3 of the plate.

Drying: in air.

Detection: examine in ultraviolet light at 254 nm.

System suitability: reference solution (c):

   — the chromatogram shows 2 clearly separated principal spots.

Limits:

   — *impurity B*: any spot due to impurity B is not more intense than the corresponding spot in the chromatogram obtained with reference solution (b) (0.2 per cent);

   — *impurities A, C*: any spot due to impurities A or C is not more intense than the principal spot in the chromatogram obtained with reference solution (a) (0.4 per cent).

Heavy metals (*2.4.8*): maximum 10 ppm.

2.0 g complies with test D. Prepare the reference solution using 2 ml of *lead standard solution (10 ppm Pb) R*.

Loss on drying (*2.2.32*): maximum 0.5 per cent, determined on 1.000 g by heating in an oven at 105 °C.

Sulphated ash (*2.4.14*): maximum 0.1 per cent, determined on 1.0 g.

ASSAY

Dissolve 0.200 g in 150 ml of *dimethylformamide R*. Titrate with *0.1 M tetrabutylammonium hydroxide*, determining the end-point potentiometrically (*2.2.20*). Use a glass indicator electrode and a calomel reference electrode containing, as the electrolyte, a saturated solution of *potassium chloride R* in *methanol R*. Carry out a blank titration.

1 ml of *0.1 M tetrabutylammonium hydroxide* is equivalent to 26.12 mg of $C_{13}H_{11}NO_5$.

STORAGE

Protected from light.

IMPURITIES

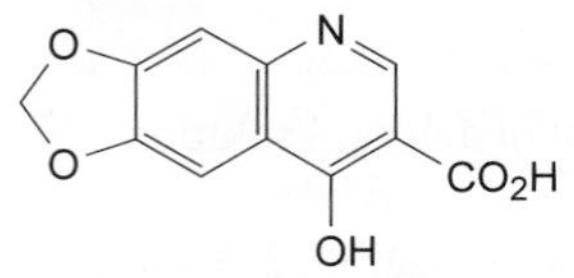

A. 8-hydroxy-1,3-dioxolo[4,5-*g*]quinoline-7-carboxylic acid,

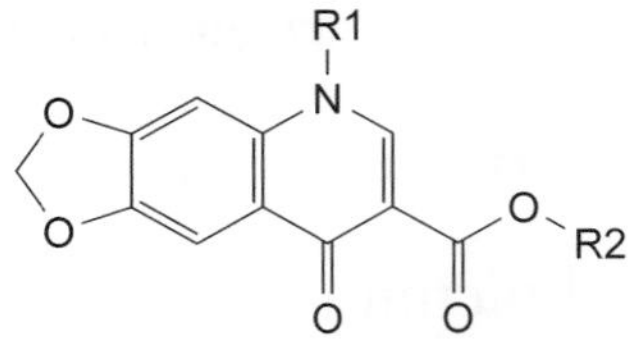

B. R1 = R2 = C_2H_5: ethyl 5-ethyl-8-oxo-5,8-dihydro-1,3-dioxolo[4,5-*g*]quinoline-7-carboxylate,

C. R1 = CH_3, R2 = H: 5-methyl-8-oxo-5,8-dihydro-1,3-dioxolo[4,5-*g*]quinoline-7-carboxylic acid.

P

Monographs
L-P

See the information section on general monographs (cover pages)

07/2009:1799

PARAFFIN, WHITE SOFT

Vaselinum album

DEFINITION

Purified and wholly or nearly decolorised mixture of semi-solid hydrocarbons, obtained from petroleum. It may contain a suitable antioxidant. White soft paraffin described in this monograph is not suitable for oral use.

CHARACTERS

Appearance: white or almost white, translucent, soft unctuous mass, slightly fluorescent in daylight when melted.

Solubility: practically insoluble in water, slightly soluble in methylene chloride, practically insoluble in ethanol (96 per cent) and in glycerol.

IDENTIFICATION

First identification: A, B, D.

Second identification: A, C, D.

A. The drop point is between 35 °C and 70 °C and does not differ by more than 5 °C from the value stated on the label, according to method (*2.2.17*) with the following modification to fill the cup: heat the substance to be examined at a temperature not exceeding 80 °C, with stirring to ensure uniformity. Warm the metal cup at a temperature not exceeding 80 °C in an oven, remove it from the oven, place on a clean plate or ceramic tile and pour a sufficient quantity of the melted sample into the cup to fill it completely. Allow the filled cup to cool for 30 min on the plate or the ceramic tile and place it in a water bath at 24-26 °C for 30-40 min. Level the surface of the sample with a single stroke of a knife or razor blade, avoiding compression of the sample.

B. Infrared absorption spectrophotometry (*2.2.24*).

   Preparation: place about 2 mg on a *sodium chloride R* plate, spread the substance with another *sodium chloride R* plate and remove 1 of the plates.

   Comparison: repeat the operations using *white soft paraffin CRS*.

C. Melt 2 g and when a homogeneous phase is obtained, add 2 ml of *water R* and 0.2 ml of *0.05 M iodine*. Shake. Allow to cool. The solid upper layer is violet-pink or brown.

D. Appearance (see Tests).

TESTS

Appearance. The substance is white. Melt 12 g on a water-bath. The melted mass is not more intensely coloured than a mixture of 1 volume of yellow primary solution and 9 volumes of a 10 g/l solution of *hydrochloric acid R* (*2.2.2, Method II*).

Acidity or alkalinity. To 10 g add 20 ml of boiling *water R* and shake vigorously for 1 min. Allow to cool and decant. To 10 ml of the aqueous layer add 0.1 ml of *phenolphthalein solution R*. The solution is colourless. Not more than 0.5 ml of *0.01 M sodium hydroxide* is required to change the colour of the indicator to red.

Consistency (*2.9.9*): 60 to 300.

Polycyclic aromatic hydrocarbons. *Use reagents for ultraviolet spectrophotometry*. Dissolve 1.0 g in 50 ml of *hexane R* which has been previously shaken twice with 10 ml of *dimethyl sulphoxide R*. Transfer the solution to a 125 ml separating funnel with unlubricated ground-glass parts (stopper, stopcock). Add 20 ml of *dimethyl sulphoxide R*.

Shake vigorously for 1 min and allow to stand until 2 clear layers are formed. Transfer the lower layer to a second separating funnel. Repeat the extraction with a further 20 ml of *dimethyl sulphoxide R*. Shake vigorously the combined lower layers with 20 ml of *hexane R* for 1 min. Allow to stand until 2 clear layers are formed. Separate the lower layer and dilute to 50.0 ml with *dimethyl sulphoxide R*. Measure the absorbance (*2.2.25*) over the range 260 nm to 420 nm using a path length of 4 cm and as compensation liquid the clear lower layer obtained by vigorously shaking 10 ml of *dimethyl sulphoxide R* with 25 ml of *hexane R* for 1 min. Prepare a reference solution in *dimethyl sulphoxide R* containing 6.0 mg of *naphthalene R* per litre and measure the absorbance of the solution at the maximum at 278 nm using a path length of 4 cm and *dimethyl sulphoxide R* as compensation liquid. At no wavelength in the range 260 nm to 420 nm does the absorbance of the test solution exceed that of the reference solution at 278 nm.

Sulphated ash (*2.4.14*): maximum 0.05 per cent, determined on 2.0 g.

STORAGE

Protected from light.

LABELLING

The label states the nominal drop point.

07/2009:0566

PENICILLAMINE

Penicillaminum

$C_5H_{11}NO_2S$
[52-67-5]

M_r 149.2

DEFINITION

(2*S*)-2-Amino-3-methyl-3-sulphanylbutanoic acid.

Content: 98.0 per cent to 101.0 per cent (dried substance).

CHARACTERS

Appearance: white or almost white, crystalline powder.

Solubility: freely soluble in water, slightly soluble in ethanol (96 per cent).

IDENTIFICATION

First identification: A, B, D.

Second identification: A, C, D.

A. Dissolve 0.5 g in a mixture of 0.5 ml of *hydrochloric acid R* and 4 ml of warm *acetone R*, cool in iced water and initiate crystallisation by scratching the wall of the tube with a glass rod. A white precipitate is formed. Filter with the aid of vacuum, wash with *acetone R* and dry with suction. A 10 g/l solution of the precipitate is dextrorotatory.

B. Examine the chromatograms obtained in the test for impurity A.

   Results: the principal peak in the chromatogram obtained with the test solution is similar in retention time and approximate size to the principal peak in the chromatogram obtained with reference solution (a).

C. Thin-layer chromatography (*2.2.27*).

Test solution. Dissolve 10 mg of the substance to be examined in 4 ml of *water R*.

Reference solution. Dissolve 10 mg of *penicillamine CRS* in 4 ml of *water R*.

Plate: *TLC silica gel G plate R*.

Mobile phase: *glacial acetic acid R, water R, butanol R* (18:18:72 *V/V/V*).

Application: 2 µl.

Development: over a path of 10 cm.

Drying: at 100-105 °C for 5-10 min.

Detection: expose to iodine vapour for 5-10 min.

Results: the principal spot in the chromatogram obtained with the test solution is similar in position, colour and size to the principal spot in the chromatogram obtained with the reference solution.

D. Dissolve 40 mg in 4 ml of *water R* and add 2 ml of *phosphotungstic acid solution R*. Allow to stand for 5 min. A blue colour develops.

TESTS

Solution S. Dissolve 2.5 g in *carbon dioxide-free water R* and dilute to 25 ml with the same solvent.

Appearance of solution. Solution S is clear (*2.2.1*) and not more intensely coloured than intensity 6 of the range of reference solutions of the most appropriate colour (*2.2.2, Method II*).

pH (*2.2.3*): 4.5 to 5.5.

Dilute 1 ml of solution S to 10 ml with *carbon dioxide-free water R*.

Specific optical rotation (*2.2.7*): − 61.0 to − 65.0 (dried substance).

Dissolve 0.500 g in *1 M sodium hydroxide* and dilute to 10.0 ml with the same solvent.

Ultraviolet-absorbing substances: maximum 0.5 per cent of penilloic acid.

Dissolve 0.100 g in *water R* and dilute to 50.0 ml with the same solvent. The absorbance (*2.2.25*) of the solution at 268 nm is not greater than 0.07.

Impurity A. Liquid chromatography (*2.2.29*). *Prepare the solutions immediately before use.*

Test solution. Dissolve 40.0 mg of the substance to be examined in the mobile phase and dilute to 10.0 ml with the mobile phase.

Reference solution (a). Dissolve 40 mg of *penicillamine CRS* in the mobile phase and dilute to 10.0 ml with the mobile phase.

Reference solution (b). Dissolve 20.0 mg of *penicillamine disulphide CRS* (impurity A) in the mobile phase and dilute to 50.0 ml with the mobile phase. Dilute 1.0 ml of this solution to 10.0 ml with the mobile phase.

Column:
- *size*: l = 0.25 m, Ø = 4.6 mm;
- *stationary phase*: *octylsilyl silica gel for chromatography R* (10 µm).

Mobile phase: solution containing 0.1 g/l of *sodium edetate R* and 2 g/l of *methanesulphonic acid R*.

Flow rate: 1.7 ml/min.

Detection: spectrophotometer at 220 nm.

Injection: 20 µl.

Relative retention with reference to penicillamine (retention time = about 6 min): impurity A = about 1.8.

System suitability: reference solution (a):
- *resolution*: minimum 4.0 between the peaks due to penicillamine and impurity A.

Limit:
- *impurity A*: not more than the area of the corresponding peak in the chromatogram obtained with reference solution (b) (1 per cent).

Impurity B: maximum 0.1 ppm.

Carry out all the operations in a penicillin-free atmosphere and with equipment reserved for this test. Sterilise the equipment at 180 °C for 3 h and the buffer solutions at 121 °C for 20 min before use.

Test solution (a). Dissolve 1.000 g in 8 ml of *buffer solution pH 2.5 R* and add 8 ml of *ether R*. Shake vigorously for 1 min. Repeat the extraction and combine the ether layers. Add 8 ml of *buffer solution pH 2.5 R*. Shake for 1 min, allow to settle and quantitatively separate the upper layer, taking care to eliminate the aqueous phase completely (*penicillin is unstable at pH 2.5; carry out operations at this pH within 6-7 min*). Add 8 ml of *phosphate buffer solution pH 6.0 R2* to the ether phase, shake for 5 min, allow to settle, then separate the aqueous layer and check that the pH is 6.0.

Test solution (b). To 2 ml of test solution (a) add 20 µl of *penicillinase solution R* and incubate at 37 °C for 1 h.

Reference solution (a). Dissolve 5 mg of *benzylpenicillin sodium R* in 500 ml of *phosphate buffer solution pH 6.0 R2*. Dilute 0.25 ml of the solution to 200.0 ml with *buffer solution pH 2.5 R*. Carry out the extraction using 8 ml of this solution as described for test solution (a).

Reference solution (b). To 2 ml of reference solution (a) add 20 µl of *penicillinase solution R* and incubate at 37 °C for 1 h.

Blank solution. Prepare the solution as described for test solution (a) but omitting the substance to be examined.

Liquefy a suitable nutrient medium such as that described below and inoculate it at a suitable temperature with a culture of *Kocuria rhizophila* (ATCC 9341), to give 5×10^4 micro-organisms per millilitre or a different quantity if necessary to obtain the required sensitivity and formation of clearly defined inhibition zones of suitable diameter. Immediately pour the inoculated medium into 5 Petri dishes 10 cm in diameter to give uniform layers 2-5 mm deep. The medium may alternatively consist of 2 layers, only the upper layer being inoculated. Store the dishes so that no appreciable growth or death of the micro-organisms occurs before use and so that the surface of the agar is dry at the time of use. In each dish, place 5 stainless steel hollow cylinders 6 mm in diameter on the surface of the agar evenly spaced on a circle with a radius of about 25 mm and concentric with the dish. For each dish, place in separate cylinders 0.15 ml of test solutions (a) and (b), reference solutions (a) and (b) and the blank solution. Maintain at 30 °C for at least 24 h. Measure the diameters of the inhibition zones with a precision of at least 0.1 mm. The test is valid if reference solution (a) gives a clear inhibition zone and if reference solution (b) and the blank solution give no inhibition zone. If test solution (a) gives an inhibition zone, this is caused by penicillin if test solution (b) gives no inhibition zone. If this is so, the average diameter of the inhibition zones given by test solution (a) for the 5 Petri dishes is less than the average diameter of the inhibition zones given by reference solution (a) measured in the same conditions.

Nutrient medium (pH 6.0)

Peptone	5 g
Yeast extract	1.5 g
Meat extract	1.5 g
Sodium chloride	3.5 g
Agar	15 g
Distilled water R	1000 ml

Mercury: maximum 10.0 ppm.

Atomic absorption spectrometry (*2.2.23, Method I*).

Test solution. To 1.00 g add 10 ml of *water R* and 0.15 ml of *perchloric acid R* and swirl until dissolution is complete. Add 1.0 ml of a 10 g/l solution of *ammonium pyrrolidinedithiocarbamate R* which has been washed immediately before use 3 times, each time with an equal volume of *methyl isobutyl ketone R*. Mix and add 2.0 ml of *methyl isobutyl ketone R* and shake for 1 min. Dilute to 25.0 ml with *water R* and allow the 2 layers to separate; use the methyl isobutyl ketone layer.

Reference solutions. Dissolve a quantity of *mercuric oxide R* equivalent to 0.108 g of HgO in the smallest necessary volume of *dilute hydrochloric acid R* and dilute to 1000.0 ml with *water R* (100 ppm Hg). Prepare the reference solutions in the same manner as the test solution but using instead of the substance to be examined suitable volumes of the solution containing 100 ppm of Hg.

Source: mercury hollow-cathode lamp.

Wavelength: 254 nm.

Atomisation device: air-acetylene flame.

Set the zero of the instrument using a methyl isobutyl ketone layer obtained as described for the test solution but omitting the substance to be examined.

Heavy metals (*2.4.8*): maximum 20 ppm.

12 ml of solution S complies with test A. Prepare the reference solution using *lead standard solution (2 ppm Pb) R*.

Loss on drying (*2.2.32*): maximum 0.5 per cent, determined on 1.000 g by drying over *diphosphorus pentoxide R* at 60 °C at a pressure not exceeding 0.67 kPa.

Sulphated ash (*2.4.14*): maximum 0.1 per cent, determined on 1.0 g.

ASSAY

Dissolve 0.1000 g in 30 ml of *anhydrous acetic acid R*. Titrate with *0.1 M perchloric acid*, determining the end-point potentiometrically (*2.2.20*).

1 ml of *0.1 M perchloric acid* is equivalent to 14.92 mg of $C_5H_{11}NO_2S$.

IMPURITIES

Specified impurities: A, B.

A. 3,3'-(disulphanediyl)bis[(2S)-2-amino-3-methylbutanoic] acid (penicillamine disulphide),

B. penicillin.

07/2009:1355

PENTAERYTHRITYL TETRANITRATE, DILUTED

Pentaerythrityli tetranitras dilutus

$C_5H_8N_4O_{12}$ M_r 316.1

DEFINITION

Dry mixture of 2,2-bis(hydroxymethyl)propane-1,3-diol tetranitrate (pentaerythrityl tetranitrate) and *Lactose monohydrate (0187)* or *Mannitol (0559)*.

Content: 95.0 per cent *m/m* to 105.0 per cent *m/m* of the declared content of pentaerythrityl tetranitrate.

CAUTION: undiluted pentaerythrityl tetranitrate may explode if subjected to percussion or excessive heat. Appropriate precautions must be taken and only very small quantities handled.

CHARACTERS

Appearance of pentaerythrityl tetranitrate: white or slightly yellowish powder.

Solubility of pentaerythrityl tetranitrate: practically insoluble in water, soluble in acetone, slightly soluble in ethanol (96 per cent).

The solubility of diluted pentaerythrityl tetranitrate depends on the diluent and its concentration.

IDENTIFICATION

First identification: A, C.

Second identification: B, C.

A. Infrared absorption spectrophotometry (*2.2.24*).

    Preparation: separately shake a quantity of the substance to be examined and a quantity of the reference substance, each corresponding to 25 mg of pentaerythrityl tetranitrate, with 10 ml of *acetone R* for 5 min; filter, evaporate to dryness at a temperature below 40 °C, and dry the residue over *diphosphorus pentoxide R* at a pressure of 0.7 kPa for 16 h. Examine the residues prepared as discs.

    Comparison: *diluted pentaerythrityl tetranitrate CRS*.

B. Thin-layer chromatography (*2.2.27*).

    Test solution. Shake a quantity of the substance to be examined corresponding to 10 mg of pentaerythrityl tetranitrate with 10 ml of *ethanol (96 per cent) R* for 5 min and filter.

Monographs L-P

Reference solution. Shake a quantity of *diluted pentaerythrityl tetranitrate CRS* corresponding to 10 mg of pentaerythrityl tetranitrate with 10 ml of *ethanol (96 per cent) R* for 5 min and filter.

Plate: *TLC silica gel plate R.*

Mobile phase: *ethyl acetate R, toluene R* (20:80 *V/V*).

Application: 10 µl.

Development: over 2/3 of the plate.

Drying: in air.

Detection: spray with freshly prepared *potassium iodide and starch solution R*, expose to ultraviolet light at 254 nm for 15 min and examine in daylight.

Results: the principal spot in the chromatogram obtained with the test solution is similar in position, colour and size to the principal spot in the chromatogram obtained with the reference solution.

C. Thin-layer chromatography (*2.2.27*).

Test solution. Shake a quantity of the substance to be examined corresponding to 0.10 g of lactose or mannitol with 10 ml of *water R*. Filter if necessary.

Reference solution (a) Dissolve 0.10 g of *lactose R* in *water R* and dilute to 10 ml with the same solvent.

Reference solution (b). Dissolve 0.10 g of *mannitol R* in *water R* and dilute to 10 ml with the same solvent.

Reference solution (c). Mix equal volumes of reference solutions (a) and (b).

Plate: *TLC silica gel G plate R.*

Mobile phase: *water R, methanol R, anhydrous acetic acid R, ethylene chloride R* (10:15:25:50 *V/V/V/V*). Measure the volumes accurately since a slight excess of water produces cloudiness.

Application: 1 µl; thoroughly dry the starting points.

Development A: over 2/3 of the plate.

Drying A: in a current of warm air.

Development B: immediately, over 2/3 of the plate, after renewing the mobile phase.

Drying B: in a current of warm air.

Detection: spray with *4-aminobenzoic acid solution R*, dry in a current of cold air until the acetone is removed, then heat at 100 °C for 15 min; allow to cool, spray with a 2 g/l solution of *sodium periodate R*, dry in a current of cold air and heat at 100 °C for 15 min.

System suitability: reference solution (c):

— the chromatogram shows 2 clearly separated spots.

Results: the principal spot in the chromatogram obtained with the test solution is similar in position, colour and size to the principal spot in the chromatogram obtained with reference solution (a) for lactose or to the principal spot in the chromatogram obtained with reference solution (b) for mannitol.

TESTS

Impurity A. Thin-layer chromatography (*2.2.27*).

Test solution. Shake a quantity of the substance to be examined corresponding to 0.10 g of pentaerythrityl tetranitrate with 5 ml of *ethanol (96 per cent) R* and filter.

Reference solution. Dissolve 10 mg of *potassium nitrate R* in 1 ml of *water R* and dilute to 100 ml with *ethanol (96 per cent) R.*

Plate: *TLC silica gel plate R.*

Mobile phase: *glacial acetic acid R, acetone R, toluene R* (15:30:60 *V/V/V*).

Application: 10 µl.

Development: over 2/3 of the plate.

Drying: in a current of air until the acetic acid is completely removed.

Detection: spray copiously with freshly prepared *potassium iodide and starch solution R*, expose the plate to ultraviolet light at 254 nm for 15 min and examine in daylight.

Limit:

— *nitrate*: any spot due to nitrate is not more intense than the spot in the chromatogram obtained with the reference solution (0.5 per cent, calculated as potassium nitrate).

Related substances. Liquid chromatography (*2.2.29*).

Test solution (a). Sonicate for 15 min a quantity of the substance to be examined corresponding to 25.0 mg of pentaerythrityl tetranitrate in 20 ml of the mobile phase and dilute to 25.0 ml with the mobile phase. Filter.

Test solution (b). Dilute 1.0 ml of test solution (a) to 10.0 ml with the mobile phase.

Reference solution (a). Sonicate for 15 min a quantity of *diluted pentaerythrityl tetranitrate CRS* corresponding to 25.0 mg of pentaerythrityl tetranitrate in 20 ml of the mobile phase and dilute to 25.0 ml with the mobile phase. Filter.

Reference solution (b). Dilute 1.0 ml of reference solution (a) to 10.0 ml with the mobile phase.

Reference solution (c). Dilute 0.3 ml of reference solution (b) to 10.0 ml with the mobile phase.

Reference solution (d). Dilute 200 µl of *glyceryl trinitrate solution CRS* to 25.0 ml with the mobile phase.

Reference solution (e). To 1 ml of reference solution (b) add 1 ml of reference solution (d) and dilute to 10 ml with the mobile phase.

Reference solution (f). Dilute 1.0 ml of reference solution (a) to 20.0 ml with the mobile phase. Dilute 0.5 ml of this solution to 50.0 ml with the mobile phase.

Column:

— *size*: l = 0.15 m, Ø = 3.9 mm;

— *stationary phase*: *octylsilyl silica gel for chromatography R* (5 µm).

Mobile phase: *water R, acetonitrile R* (35:65 *V/V*).

Flow rate: 1.4 ml/min.

Detection: spectrophotometer at 220 nm.

Injection: 20 µl of test solution (a) and reference solutions (c), (e) and (f).

Run time: 5 times the retention time of pentaerythrityl tetranitrate.

Relative retention with reference to pentaerythrityl tetranitrate (retention time = about 2.4 min): impurity B = about 0.7; impurity C = about 3.0.

System suitability: reference solution (e):

— *resolution*: minimum 3.0 between the peaks due to glyceryl trinitrate and pentaerythrityl tetranitrate.

Limits:

— *impurities C, D*: for each impurity, not more than the area of the principal peak in the chromatogram obtained with reference solution (c) (0.3 per cent);

— *unspecified impurities*: for each impurity, not more than twice the area of the principal peak in the chromatogram obtained with reference solution (f) (0.10 per cent);

— *total*: not more than twice the area of the principal peak in the chromatogram obtained with reference solution (c) (0.6 per cent);

— *disregard limit*: the area of the principal peak in the chromatogram obtained with reference solution (f) (0.05 per cent).

ASSAY

Liquid chromatography (*2.2.29*) as described in the test for related substances with the following modification.

Injection: test solution (b) and reference solution (b).

Calculate the percentage content of $C_5H_8N_4O_{12}$ from the declared content of *diluted pentaerythrityl tetranitrate CRS*.

STORAGE

Protected from light and heat.

LABELLING

The label states:

— the percentage content of pentaerythrityl tetranitrate;

— the diluent used.

IMPURITIES

Specified impurities: *A, C, D.*

Other detectable impurities (the following substances would, if present at a sufficient level, be detected by one or other of the tests in the monograph. They are limited by the general acceptance criterion for other/unspecified impurities and/or by the general monograph *Substances for pharmaceutical use (2034)*. It is therefore not necessary to identify these impurities for demonstration of compliance. See also *5.10. Control of impurities in substances for pharmaceutical use*): *B.*

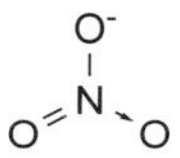

A. NO_3^-: inorganic nitrates,

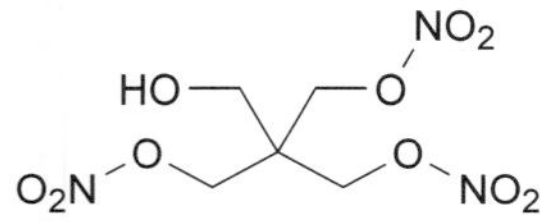

B. 2,2-bis(hydroxymethyl)propane-1,3-diol trinitrate (pentaerythritol trinitrate),

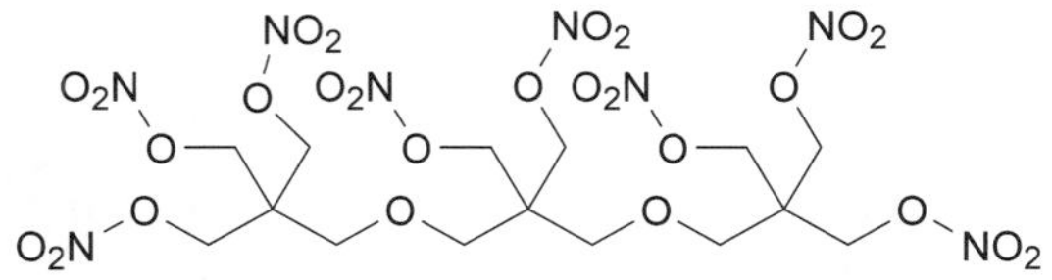

C. 2,2-bis[[3-hydroxy-2,2-bis(hydroxy-methyl)propoxy]methyl]propane-1,3-diol octanitrate (tripentaerythrityl octanitrate),

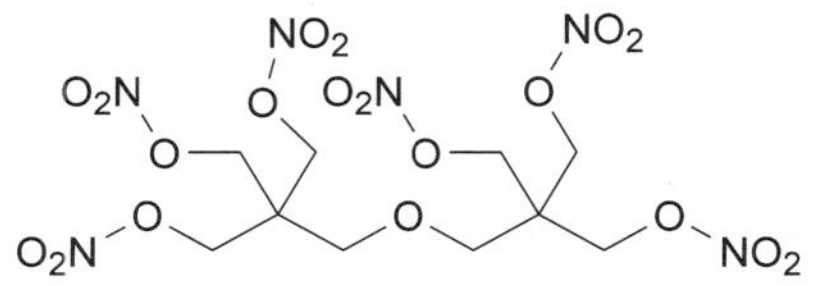

D. 2,2'-(oxybismethylene)bis[2-(hydroxymethyl)propane-1,3-diol] hexanitrate (dipentaerythrityl hexanitrate).

01/2008:0424
corrected 6.5

PIPERAZINE CITRATE

Piperazini citras

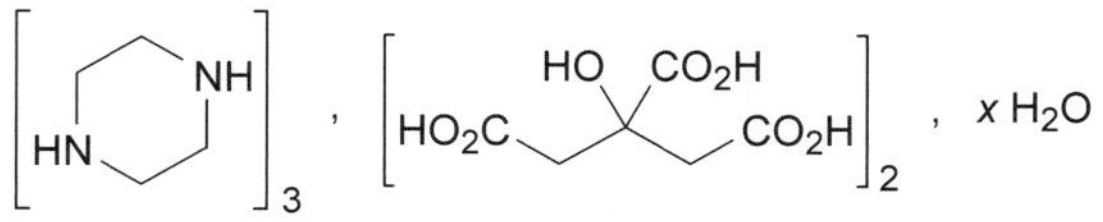

$C_{24}H_{46}N_6O_{14}\cdot xH_2O$ M_r 643 (anhydrous substance)

DEFINITION

Piperazine citrate contains not less than 98.0 per cent and not more than the equivalent of 101.0 per cent of tripiperazine bis(2-hydroxy-propane-1,2,3-tricarboxylate), calculated with reference to the anhydrous substance. It contains a variable quantity of water.

CHARACTERS

A white or almost white granular powder, freely soluble in water, practically insoluble in ethanol (96 per cent).

After drying at 100 °C to 105 °C, it melts at about 190 °C.

IDENTIFICATION

First identification: A.

Second identification: B, C.

A. Examine by infrared absorption spectrophotometry (*2.2.24*), comparing with the spectrum obtained with *piperazine citrate CRS*. Dry the substance to be examined and the reference substance at 120 °C for 5 h, powder the substances avoiding uptake of water, prepare discs and record the spectra without delay.

B. Examine the chromatograms obtained in the test for related substances after spraying with the ninhydrin solutions. The principal spot in the chromatogram obtained with test solution (b) is similar in position, colour and size to the principal spot in the chromatogram obtained with reference solution (a).

C. Dissolve 0.5 g in *water R* and dilute to 5 ml with the same solvent. The solution gives the reaction of citrates (*2.3.1*).

TESTS

Solution S. Dissolve 1.25 g in *water R* and dilute to 25 ml with the same solvent.

Appearance of solution. Solution S is clear (*2.2.1*) and not more intensely coloured than reference solution B_8 (*2.2.2, Method II*).

Related substances. Examine by thin-layer chromatography (*2.2.27*), using a suitable silica gel as the coating substance.

Test solution (a). Dissolve 1.0 g of the substance to be examined in 6 ml of *concentrated ammonia R* and dilute to 10 ml with *anhydrous ethanol R*.

Test solution (b). Dilute 1 ml of test solution (a) to 10 ml with a mixture of 2 volumes of *anhydrous ethanol R* and 3 volumes of *concentrated ammonia R*.

Reference solution (a). Dissolve 0.1 g of *piperazine citrate CRS* in a mixture of 2 volumes of *anhydrous ethanol R* and 3 volumes of *concentrated ammonia R* and dilute to 10 ml with the same mixture of solvents.

Reference solution (b). Dissolve 25 mg of *ethylenediamine R* in a mixture of 2 volumes of *anhydrous ethanol R* and 3 volumes of *concentrated ammonia R* and dilute to 100 ml with the same mixture of solvents.

Reference solution (c). Dissolve 25 mg of *triethylenediamine R* in a mixture of 2 volumes of *anhydrous ethanol R* and 3 volumes of *concentrated ammonia R* and dilute to 100 ml with the same mixture of solvents.

Reference solution (d). Dissolve 12.5 mg of *triethylenediamine R* in 5.0 ml of test solution (a) and dilute to 50 ml with a mixture of 2 volumes of *anhydrous ethanol R* and 3 volumes of *concentrated ammonia R.*

Apply separately to the plate 5 µl of each solution. Develop over a path of 15 cm using a freshly prepared mixture of 20 volumes of *concentrated ammonia R* and 80 volumes of *acetone R.* Dry the plate at 105 °C and spray successively with a 3 g/l solution of *ninhydrin R* in a mixture of 3 volumes of *anhydrous acetic acid R* and 100 volumes of *butanol R* and a 1.5 g/l solution of *ninhydrin R* in *anhydrous ethanol R.* Dry the plate at 105 °C for 10 min. Any spot in the chromatogram obtained with test solution (a), apart from the principal spot, is not more intense than the spot in the chromatogram obtained with reference solution (b) (0.25 per cent). Spray the plate with *0.05 M iodine* and allow to stand for about 10 min. Any spot corresponding to triethylenediamine in the chromatogram obtained with test solution (a) is not more intense than the spot in the chromatogram obtained with reference solution (c) (0.25 per cent). The test is not valid unless the chromatogram obtained with reference solution (d) shows 2 clearly separated spots. Disregard any spots remaining on the starting line.

Heavy metals (*2.4.8*). 12 ml of solution S complies with limit test A for heavy metals (20 ppm). Prepare the reference solution using *lead standard solution (1 ppm Pb) R.*

Water (*2.5.12*). 10.0 per cent to 14.0 per cent, determined on 0.300 g by the semi-micro determination of water.

Sulphated ash (*2.4.14*). Not more than 0.1 per cent, determined on 1.0 g.

ASSAY

Dissolve 0.100 g in 10 ml of *anhydrous acetic acid R* with gentle heating and dilute to 70 ml with the same acid. Titrate with *0.1 M perchloric acid* using 0.25 ml of *naphtholbenzein solution R* as indicator until the colour changes from brownish-yellow to green.

1 ml of *0.1 M perchloric acid* is equivalent to 10.71 mg of $C_{24}H_{46}N_6O_{14}.$

07/2009:0428

POLYSORBATE 80

Polysorbatum 80

DEFINITION

Mixture of partial esters of fatty acids, mainly *Oleic acid (0799)*, with sorbitol and its anhydrides ethoxylated with approximately 20 moles of ethylene oxide for each mole of sorbitol and sorbitol anhydrides.

CHARACTERS

Appearance: oily, colourless or brownish-yellow, clear or slightly opalescent liquid.

Solubility: dispersible in water, in anhydrous ethanol, in ethyl acetate and in methanol, practically insoluble in fatty oils and in liquid paraffin.

Relative density: about 1.10.

Viscosity: about 400 mPa·s at 25 °C.

IDENTIFICATION

First identication: A, D.

Second identification: B, C, D, E.

A. Infrared absorption spectrophotometry (*2.2.24*).

   Comparison: Ph. Eur. reference spectrum of polysorbate 80.

B. Hydroxyl value (see Tests).

C. Saponification value (see Tests).

D. Composition of fatty acids (see Tests).

E. Dissolve 0.1 g in 5 ml of *methylene chloride R.* Add 0.1 g of *potassium thiocyanate R* and 0.1 g of *cobalt nitrate R.* Stir with a glass rod. The solution becomes blue.

TESTS

Acid value (*2.5.1*): maximum 2.0.

Dissolve 5.0 g in 50 ml of the prescribed mixture of solvents.

Hydroxyl value (*2.5.3, Method A*): 65 to 80.

Peroxide value: maximum 10.0.

Introduce 10.0 g into a 100 ml beaker and dissolve with 20 ml of *glacial acetic acid R.* Add 1 ml of *saturated potassium iodide solution R* and allow to stand for 1 min. Add 50 ml of *carbon dioxide-free water R* and a magnetic stirring bar. Titrate with *0.01 M sodium thiosulphate*, determining the end-point potentiometrically (*2.2.20*). Carry out a blank titration.

Determine the peroxide value using the following expression:

$$\frac{(n_1 - n_2) \times M \times 1000}{m}$$

n_1 = volume of *0.01 M sodium thiosulphate* required for the substance to be examined, in millilitres;

n_2 = volume of *0.01 M sodium thiosulphate* required for the blank, in millilitres;

M = molarity of the sodium thiosulphate solution, in moles per litre;

m = mass of substance to be examined, in grams.

Saponification value (*2.5.6*): 45 to 55, determined on 4.0 g.

Use 30.0 ml of *0.5 M alcoholic potassium hydroxide*, heat under reflux for 60 min and add 50 ml of *anhydrous ethanol R* before carrying out the titration.

Composition of fatty acids. Gas chromatography (*2.4.22, Method C*). Use the mixture of calibrating substances in Table *2.4.22.-3.*

Column:

— *material*: fused silica;

— *size*: l = 30 m, Ø = 0.32 mm;

— *stationary phase*: *macrogol 20 000 R* (film thickness 0.5 µm).

Carrier gas: *helium for chromatography R.*

Linear velocity: 50 cm/s.

Temperature:

	Time (min)	Temperature (°C)
Column	0 - 14	80 → 220
	14 - 54	220
Injection port		250
Detector		250

Detection: flame ionisation.

Injection: 1 µl.

Composition of the fatty-acid fraction of the substance:

— *myristic acid*: maximum 5.0 per cent;

— *palmitic acid*: maximum 16.0 per cent;

— *palmitoleic acid*: maximum 8.0 per cent;

— *stearic acid*: maximum 6.0 per cent;

— *oleic acid*: minimum 58.0 per cent;

— *linoleic acid*: maximum 18.0 per cent;

— *linolenic acid*: maximum 4.0 per cent.

Ethylene oxide and dioxan: maximum 1 ppm of ethylene oxide and maximum 10 ppm of dioxan.

Head-space gas chromatography (*2.2.28*).

Ethylene oxide stock solution. Dilute 0.5 ml of a commercially available solution of ethylene oxide in methylene chloride (50 mg/ml) to 50.0 ml with *water R*. [NOTE: the solution is stable for 3 months, if stored in vials with a polytetrafluoroethylene coated silicone membrane crimped caps at – 20 °C]. Allow to reach room temperature. Dilute 1.0 ml of this solution to 250.0 ml with *water R*.

Dioxan stock solution. Dilute 1.0 ml of *dioxan R* to 200.0 ml with *water R*. Dilute 1.0 ml of this solution to 100.0 ml with *water R*.

Acetaldehyde stock solution. Weigh about 0.100 g of *acetaldehyde R* into a 100 ml volumetric flask and dilute to 100.0 ml with *water R*. Dilute 1.0 ml of this solution to 100.0 ml with *water R*.

Standard solution. To 6.0 ml of ethylene oxide stock solution add 2.5 ml of dioxan stock solution and dilute to 25.0 ml with *water R*.

Test solution (a). Weigh 1.00 g of the substance to be examined into a 10 ml headspace vial. Add 2.0 ml of *water R*, seal the vial immediately with a polytetrafluoromethylene coated silicon membrane and an aluminum cap. Mix carefully.

Test solution (b). Weigh 1.00 g of the substance to be examined into a 10 ml headspace vial. Add 2.0 ml of standard solution, seal the vial immediately with a polytetrafluoromethylene coated silicon membrane and an aluminum cap. Mix carefully.

Reference solution. Introduce 2.0 ml of acetaldehyde stock solution and 2.0 ml of ethylene oxide stock solution to a 10 ml headspace vial and seal the vial immediately with a polytetrafluoromethylene coated silicon membrane and an aluminum cap. Mix carefully.

Column:

— *material*: *fused silica R*;

— *size*: *l* = 50 m, Ø = 0.53 mm;

— *stationary phase*: *poly(dimethyl)(diphenyl)siloxane R* (5 µm).

Carrier gas: *helium for chromatography R*.

Flow rate: 4.0 ml/min.

Split ratio: 1:3.5.

Static head-space conditions that may be used:

— *equilibration temperature*: 80 °C;

— *equilibration time*: 30 min.

Temperature:

	Time (min)	Temperature (°C)
Column	0 - 18	70 → 250
	18 - 23	250
Injection port		85
Detector		250

Detection: flame ionisation.

Injection: 1.0 ml of test solution (a) and (b) and reference solution.

Relative retention with reference to ethylene oxide (retention time = about 6.5 min): acetaldehyde = about 0.9; dioxan = about 1.9.

System suitability: reference solution:

— *resolution*: mininum 2.0 between the peaks due to acetaldehyde and to ethylene oxide.

Calculate the content of ethylene oxide using the following expression:

$$\frac{2\,C_{EO} \times A_a}{A_b - A_a}$$

C_{EO} = concentration of ethylene oxide in test solution (a), in micrograms per millilitre;

A_a = peak area of ethylene oxide in the chromatogram obtained with test solution (a);

A_b = peak area of ethylene oxide in the chromatogram obtained with test solution (b).

Calculate the content of dioxan using the following expression:

$$\frac{2 \times 1.03 \times C_D \times A_{a'}}{A_{b'} - A_{a'}}$$

C_D = concentration of dioxan in test solution (a), in microlitres per millilitre;

1.03 = density of dioxan, in grams per millilitre;

$A_{a'}$ = peak area of dioxan in the chromatogram obtained with test solution (a);

$A_{b'}$ = peak area of dioxan in the chromatogram obtained with test solution (b).

Heavy metals (*2.4.8*): maximum 10 ppm.

2.0 g complies with test C. Prepare the reference solution using 2 ml of *lead standard solution (10 ppm Pb) R*.

Water (*2.5.12*): maximum 3.0 per cent, determined on 1.00 g.

Total ash (*2.4.16*): maximum 0.25 per cent, determined on 2.0 g.

STORAGE

In an airtight container, protected from light.

07/2009:0685

POVIDONE

Povidonum

$C_{6n}H_{9n+2}N_nO_n$
[9003-39-8]

DEFINITION

α-Hydro-ω-hydropoly[1-(2-oxopyrrolidin-1-yl)ethylene]. It consists of linear polymers of 1-ethenylpyrrolidin-2-one.

Content: 11.5 per cent to 12.8 per cent of nitrogen (N; A_r 14.01) (anhydrous substance).

The different types of povidone are characterised by their viscosity in solution expressed as a K-value.

CHARACTERS

Appearance: white or yellowish-white, hygroscopic powder or flakes.

Solubility: freely soluble in water, in ethanol (96 per cent) and in methanol, very slightly soluble in acetone.

IDENTIFICATION

First identification: A, E.

Second identification: B, C, D, E.

A. Infrared absorption spectrophotometry (*2.2.24*).

   Preparation: dry the substances beforehand at 105 °C for 6 h. Record the spectra using 4 mg of substance.

   Comparison: povidone CRS.

B. To 0.4 ml of solution S1 (see Tests) add 10 ml of *water R*, 5 ml of *dilute hydrochloric acid R* and 2 ml of *potassium dichromate solution R*. An orange-yellow precipitate is formed.

C. To 1 ml of solution S1 add 0.2 ml of *dimethylaminobenz-aldehyde solution R1* and 0.1 ml of *sulphuric acid R*. A pink colour is produced.

D. To 0.1 ml of solution S1 add 5 ml of *water R* and 0.2 ml of *0.05 M iodine*. A red colour is produced.

E. To 0.5 g add 10 ml of *water R* and shake. The substance dissolves.

TESTS

Solution S. Dissolve 1.0 g in *carbon dioxide-free water R* and dilute to 20 ml with the same solvent. Add the substance to be examined to the water in small portions, stirring using a magnetic stirrer.

Solution S1. Dissolve 2.5 g in *carbon dioxide-free water R* and dilute to 25 ml with the same solvent. Add the substance to be examined to the water in small portions, stirring using a magnetic stirrer.

Appearance of solution. Solution S is clear (*2.2.1*) and not more intensely coloured than reference solution B_6, BY_6 or R_6 (*2.2.2, Method II*).

pH (*2.2.3*): 3.0 to 5.0 for solution S, for povidone having a stated K-value of not more than 30; 4.0 to 7.0 for solution S, for povidone having a stated K-value of more than 30.

Viscosity, expressed as K-value. For povidone having a stated value of 18 or less, use a 50 g/l solution. For povidone having a stated value of more than 18 and not more than 95, use a 10 g/l solution. For povidone having a stated value of more than 95, use a 1.0 g/l solution. Allow to stand for 1 h and determine the viscosity (*2.2.9*) of the solution at 25 °C, using viscometer No.1 with a minimum flow time of 100 s. Calculate the K-value using the following expression:

$$\frac{1.5 \log \eta - 1}{0.15 + 0.003c} + \frac{\sqrt{300c \log\eta + (c + 1.5c \log\eta)^2}}{0.15c + 0.003c^2}$$

c = concentration of the substance to be examined, calculated with reference to the anhydrous substance, in grams per 100 ml;

η = kinematic viscosity of the solution relative to that of *water R*.

The K-value of povidone having a stated K-value of 15 or less is 85.0 per cent to 115.0 per cent of the stated value.

The K-value of povidone having a stated K-value or a stated K-value range with an average of more than 15 is 90.0 per cent to 108.0 per cent of the stated value or of the average of the stated range.

Aldehydes: maximum 5.00×10^2 ppm, expressed as acetaldehyde.

Test solution. Dissolve 1.0 g of the substance to be examined in *phosphate buffer solution pH 9.0 R* and dilute to 100.0 ml with the same solvent. Stopper the flask tightly and heat at 60 °C for 1 h. Allow to cool to room temperature.

Reference solution. Dissolve 0.140 g of *acetaldehyde ammonia trimer trihydrate R* in *water R* and dilute to 200.0 ml with the same solvent. Dilute 1.0 ml of this solution to 100.0 ml with *phosphate buffer solution pH 9.0 R*.

Into 3 identical spectrophotometric cells with a path length of 1 cm, introduce separately 0.5 ml of the test solution, 0.5 ml of the reference solution and 0.5 ml of *water R* (blank). To each cell, add 2.5 ml of *phosphate buffer solution pH 9.0 R* and 0.2 ml of *nicotinamide-adenine dinucleotide solution R*. Mix and stopper tightly. Allow to stand at 22 ± 2 °C for 2-3 min and measure the absorbance (*2.2.25*) of each solution at 340 nm, using *water R* as the compensation liquid. To each cell, add 0.05 ml of *aldehyde dehydrogenase solution R*, mix and stopper tightly. Allow to stand at 22 ± 2 °C for 5 min. Measure the absorbance of each solution at 340 nm using *water R* as the compensation liquid.

Calculate the content of aldehydes using the following expression:

$$\frac{(A_{t2} - A_{t1}) - (A_{b2} - A_{b1})}{(A_{s2} - A_{s1}) - (A_{b2} - A_{b1})} \times \frac{100\,000 \times C}{m}$$

A_{t1} = absorbance of the test solution before the addition of aldehyde dehydrogenase;

A_{t2} = absorbance of the test solution after the addition of aldehyde dehydrogenase;

A_{S1} = absorbance of the reference solution before the addition of aldehyde dehydrogenase;

A_{S2} = absorbance of the reference solution after the addition of aldehyde dehydrogenase;

A_{b1} = absorbance of the blank before the addition of aldehyde dehydrogenase;

A_{b2} = absorbance of the blank after the addition of aldehyde dehydrogenase;

m = mass of povidone calculated with reference to the anhydrous substance, in grams;

C = concentration of acetaldehyde in the reference solution, calculated from the weight of the acetaldehyde ammonia trimer trihydrate with the factor 0.72, in milligrams per millilitre.

Peroxides: maximum 400 ppm, expressed as H_2O_2.

Dissolve a quantity of the substance to be examined equivalent to 4.0 g of the anhydrous substance in *water R* and dilute to 100.0 ml with the same solvent (stock solution). To 25.0 ml of this solution, add 2.0 ml of *titanium trichloride-sulphuric acid reagent R*. Allow to stand for 30 min. The absorbance (*2.2.25*) of the solution, measured at 405 nm using a mixture of 25.0 ml of stock solution and 2.0 ml of a 13 per cent *V/V* solution of *sulphuric acid R* as the compensation liquid, is not greater than 0.35.

Formic acid. Liquid chromatography (*2.2.29*).

Test solution. Dissolve a quantity of the substance to be examined equivalent to 2.0 g of the anhydrous substance in *water R* and dilute to 100.0 ml with the same solvent (test stock solution). Transfer a suspension of *strongly acidic ion exchange resin R* for column chromatography in *water R* to a column of about 0.8 cm in internal diameter to give a packing of about 20 mm in length and keep the strongly acidic ion exchange resin layer constantly immersed in *water R*. Pour 5 ml of *water R* and adjust the flow rate so that the water drops at a rate of about 20 drops per minute. When the level of the water comes down to near the top of the strongly acidic ion exchange resin layer, put the test stock solution into the column. After dropping 2 ml of the solution, collect 1.5 ml of the solution and use this solution as the test solution.

Reference solution. Dissolve 0.100 g of *anhydrous formic acid R* and dilute to 100.0 ml with *water R*. Dilute 1.0 ml of this solution to 100.0 ml with *water R*.

Column:
— *size*: l = 0.25-0.30 m, Ø = 4-8 mm;
— *stationary phase*: *strongly acidic ion-exchange resin R* for column chromatography (5-10 μm);
— *temperature*: 30 °C.

Mobile phase: dilute 5 ml of *perchloric acid R* to 1000 ml with *water R*.

Flow rate: adjusted so that the retention time of formic acid is about 11 min.

Detection: spectrophotometer at 210 nm.

Injection: 50 μl each of the test and reference solutions.

System suitability:
— *repeatability*: maximum relative standard deviation of 2.0 per cent after 6 injections of the reference solution.

Limits:
— *formic acid*: not more than 10 times the area of the principal peak in the chromatogram obtained with the reference solution (0.5 per cent).

Hydrazine. Thin-layer chromatography (*2.2.27*). *Use freshly prepared solutions.*

Test solution. Dissolve a quantity of the substance to be examined equivalent to 2.5 g of the anhydrous substance in 25 ml of *water R*. Add 0.5 ml of a 50 g/l solution of *salicylaldehyde R* in *methanol R*, mix and heat in a water-bath at 60 °C for 15 min. Allow to cool, add 2.0 ml of *toluene R*, shake for 2 min and centrifuge. Use the upper layer of the mixture.

Reference solution. Dissolve 90 mg of *salicylaldehyde azine R* in *toluene R* and dilute to 100 ml with the same solvent. Dilute 1 ml of this solution to 100 ml with *toluene R*.

Plate: TLC silanised silica gel plate F_{254} R.

Mobile phase: water R, methanol R (1:2 V/V).

Application: 10 μl.

Development: over 2/3 of the plate.

Drying: in air.

Detection: examine in ultraviolet light at 365 nm.

Retardation factor: salicylaldehyde azine = about 0.3.

Limit:
— *hydrazine*: any spot due to salicylaldehyde azine is not more intense than the spot in the chromatogram obtained with the reference solution (1 ppm).

Impurity A. Liquid chromatography (*2.2.29*).

Test solution. Dissolve a quantity of the substance to be examined equivalent to 0.250 g of the anhydrous substance in the mobile phase and dilute to 10.0 ml with the mobile phase.

Reference solution (a). Dissolve 50.0 mg of *1-vinylpyrrolidin-2-one R* in *methanol R* and dilute to 100.0 ml with the same solvent. Dilute 1.0 ml of the solution to 100.0 ml with *methanol R*. Dilute 5.0 ml of this solution to 100.0 ml with the mobile phase.

Reference solution (b). Dissolve 10 mg of *1-vinylpyrrolidin-2-one R* and 0.5 g of *vinyl acetate R* in *methanol R* and dilute to 100.0 ml with the same solvent. Dilute 1.0 ml of the solution to 100.0 ml with the mobile phase.

Precolumn:
— *size*: l = 0.025 m, Ø = 4 mm;
— *stationary phase*: octadecylsilyl silica gel for chromatography R (5 μm).

Column:
— *size*: l = 0.25 m, Ø = 4 mm;
— *stationary phase*: octadecylsilyl silica gel for chromatography R (5 μm);
— *temperature*: 40 °C.

Mobile phase: acetonitrile R, water R (10:90 V/V).

Flow rate: adjusted so that the retention time of the peak corresponding to impurity A is about 10 min.

Detection: spectrophotometer at 235 nm.

Injection: 50 μl. After injection of the test solution, wait for about 2 min and wash the precolumn by passing the mobile phase through the column backwards for 30 min at the same flow rate as applied in the test.

System suitability:
— *resolution*: minimum 2.0 between the peaks due to impurity A and to vinyl acetate in the chromatogram obtained with reference solution (b);

— *repeatability*: maximum relative standard deviation of 2.0 per cent after 6 injections of reference solution (a).

Limit:

— *impurity A*: not more than the area of the principal peak in the chromatogram obtained with reference solution (a) (10 ppm).

Impurity B. Liquid chromatography (*2.2.29*).

Test solution. Dissolve a quantity of the substance to be examined equivalent to 0.100 g of the anhydrous substance in *water R* and dilute to 50.0 ml with the same solvent.

Reference solution. Dissolve 0.100 g of *2-pyrrolidone R* in *water R* and dilute to 100.0 ml with the same solvent. Dilute 3.0 ml of this solution to 50.0 ml with *water R*.

Precolumn:

— *size*: l = 0.025 m, Ø = 3 mm;

— *stationary phase*: end-capped octadecylsilyl silica gel for chromatography R (5 µm).

Column:

— *size*: l = 0.25 m, Ø = 3 mm;

— *stationary phase*: end-capped octadecylsilyl silica gel for chromatography R (5 µm);

— *temperature*: 30 °C.

Mobile phase: *water R*, adjusted to pH 2.4 with *phosphoric acid R*.

Flow rate: adjusted so that the retention time of impurity B is about 11 min.

Detection: spectrophotometer at 205 nm.

Injection: 50 µl. After each injection of the test solution, wash away the polymeric material of povidone from the precolumn by passing the mobile phase through the column backwards for about 30 min at the same flow rate as applied in the test.

System suitability:

— *repeatability*: maximum relative standard deviation of 2.0 per cent after 6 injections of the reference solution.

Limit:

— *impurity B*: not more than the area of the principal peak in the chromatogram obtained with the reference solution (3.0 per cent).

Heavy metals (*2.4.8*): maximum 10 ppm.

2.0 g complies with test D. Prepare the reference solution using 2.0 ml of *lead standard solution (10 ppm Pb) R*.

Water (*2.5.12*): maximum 5.0 per cent, determined on 0.500 g.

Sulphated ash (*2.4.14*): maximum 0.1 per cent, determined on 1.0 g.

ASSAY

Place 100.0 mg of the substance to be examined (*m* mg) in a combustion flask, add 5 g of a mixture of 1 g of *copper sulphate R*, 1 g of *titanium dioxide R* and 33 g of *dipotassium sulphate R*, and 3 glass beads. Wash any adhering particles from the neck into the flask with a small quantity of *water R*. Add 7 ml of *sulphuric acid R*, allowing it to run down the insides of the flask. Heat the flask gradually until the solution has a clear, yellowish-green colour, and the inside wall of the flask is free from a carbonised material, and then heat for a further 45 min. After cooling, add cautiously 20 ml of *water R*, and connect the flask to the distillation apparatus previously washed by passing steam through it. To the absorption flask add 30 ml of a 40 g/l solution of

boric acid R, 3 drops of *bromocresol green-methyl red solution R* and sufficient water to immerse the lower end of the condenser tube. Add 30 ml of a solution of *strong sodium hydroxide solution R* through the funnel, rinse the funnel cautiously with 10 ml of *water R*, immediately close the clamp on the rubber tube, then start distillation with steam to obtain 80-100 ml of distillate. Remove the absorption flask from the lower end of the condenser tube, rinsing the end part with a small quantity of *water R*, and titrate the distillate with *0.025 M sulphuric acid* until the colour of the solution changes from green through pale greyish blue to pale greyish reddish-purple. Carry out a blank determination.

1 ml of *0.025 M sulphuric acid* is equivalent to 0.7004 mg of N.

STORAGE

In an airtight container.

LABELLING

The label indicates the nominal K-value.

IMPURITIES

A. R = CH=CH$_2$: 1-ethenylpyrrolidin-2-one (1-vinylpyrrolidin-2-one),

B. R = H: pyrrolidin-2-one (2-pyrrolidone).

07/2009:2180

PYRROLIDONE

Pyrrolidonum

C$_4$H$_7$NO
[616-45-5]

M_r 85.1

DEFINITION

Pyrrolidin-2-one.

CHARACTERS

Appearance: clear, colourless or slightly greyish liquid, or white or almost white crystals, or colourless crystal needles.

Solubility: miscible with water, with ethanol (96 per cent) and with most common organic solvents.

mp: about 25 °C; the molten substance remains liquid at temperatures below the melting point.

bp: about 245 °C.

IDENTIFICATION

First identification: A.

Second identification: B, C.

A. Infrared absorption spectrophotometry (*2.2.24*).

   Comparison: *pyrrolidone CRS*.

B. Relative density (*2.2.5*): 1.112 to 1.115.

C. Refractive index (*2.2.6*): 1.487 to 1.490.

TESTS

Use the molten substance for all tests.

Appearance. The substance to be examined is clear (*2.2.1*) and not more intensely coloured than intensity 7 of the range of reference solutions of the most appropriate colour (*2.2.2, Method II*).

Alkalinity. To 100 ml of *water R* add 1.0 ml of *bromothymol blue solution R1* and adjust to a green colour with *0.02 M potassium hydroxide* or *0.02 M hydrochloric acid*. To 50 ml of this solution add 20 ml of the substance to be examined and titrate with *0.02 M hydrochloric acid* to the initial colour. Not more than 8.0 ml of *0.02 M hydrochloric acid* is required.

Related substances. Gas chromatography (*2.2.28*): use the normalisation procedure.

Test solution. The substance to be examined.

Reference solution (a). Dissolve 1 ml of the substance to be examined and 1 ml of *N-methylpyrrolidone R* (impurity C) in *methylene chloride R* and dilute to 20 ml with the same solvent.

Reference solution (b). Dissolve 1.1 g of the substance to be examined in *methylene chloride R* and dilute to 100.0 ml with the same solvent. Dilute 1.0 ml of this solution to 20.0 ml with *methylene chloride R*.

Reference solution (c). Dissolve 1 ml of *butyrolactone R* (impurity B) and 1 ml of *butane-1,4-diol R* (impurity A) in *methylene chloride R* and dilute to 20 ml with the same solvent.

Column:
- *material*: fused silica;
- *size*: l = 30 m, Ø = 0.32 mm;
- *stationary phase*: *poly(dimethyl)siloxane R* (film thickness 5 µm).

Carrier gas: *nitrogen for chromatography R*.

Flow rate: 1.3 ml/min.

Split ratio: 1:80.

Temperature:

	Time (min)	Temperature (°C)
Column	0 - 18.75	100 → 250
	18.75 - 30	250
Injection port		250
Detector		250

Detection: flame ionisation.

Injection: 0.1 µl.

Relative retention with reference to pyrrolidone (retention time = about 13 min): impurity B = about 0.73; impurity A = about 0.76; impurity C = about 0.97.

Use the chromatogram obtained with reference solution (c) to identify the peaks due to impurities A and B; use the chromatogram obtained with reference solution (a) to identify the peak due to impurity C.

System suitability: reference solution (a):
- *resolution*: minimum 2.0 between the peaks due to impurity C and pyrrolidone.

Limits:
- *impurity B*: maximum 0.5 per cent;
- *impurities A, C*: for each impurity, maximum 0.15 per cent;
- *unspecified impurities*: for each impurity, maximum 0.10 per cent;
- *total*: maximum 0.7 per cent;
- *disregard limit*: the area of the principal peak in the chromatogram obtained with reference solution (b) (0.05 per cent).

Heavy metals (*2.4.8*): maximum 10 ppm.

Dissolve 4.0 g in *water R* and dilute to 20.0 ml with the same solvent. 12 ml of the solution complies with test A. Prepare the reference solution using *lead standard solution (2 ppm Pb) R*.

Water (*2.5.32*): maximum 0.1 per cent, determined on 1.00 g.

Sulphated ash (*2.4.14*): maximum 0.1 per cent, determined on 1.0 g.

STORAGE

Protected from light.

IMPURITIES

Specified impurities: A, B, C.

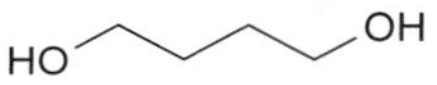

A. butane-1,4-diol,

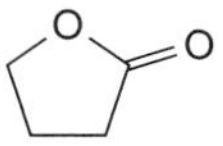

B. dihydrofuran-2(3H)-one (γ-butyrolactone),

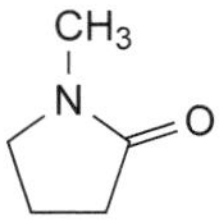

C. 1-methylpyrrolidin-2-one (*N*-methylpyrrolidone).

See the information section on general monographs (cover pages)

R

Monographs
Q-Z

07/2009:1881

RED POPPY PETALS

Papaveris rhoeados flos

DEFINITION

Dried, whole or fragmented petals of *Papaver rhoeas* L.

IDENTIFICATION

A. The petal is dark red or dark violet-brown, very thin, floppy, wrinkled, often crumpled into a ball and velvety to the touch. It is broadly ovate with an entire margin, about 6 cm long and 4-6 cm wide, narrowing at the base where there is a black spot. The vascular bundles radiate from the base and they anastomose in a continuous arc, all at the same short distance from the margin.

B. Reduce to a powder (355) (*2.9.12*). Examine under a microscope using *chloral hydrate solution R*. The powder has an intense reddish-pink colour and shows the following diagnostic characters: fragments of epidermis composed of elongated, sinuous-walled cells with small, rounded, anomocytic stomata (*2.8.3*); numerous vascular bundles with spiral vessels embedded in the parenchyma; occasional fragments of the fibrous layer of the anthers; rounded pollen grains, about 30 μm in diameter, with 3 pores and a finely verrucose exine.

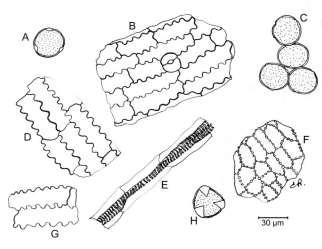

A, C and H. Pollen grains
B. Epidermis with anomocytic stoma
D and G. Epidermis of petals
E. Spiral vessels
F. Fragment of the fibrous layer of the anthers

Figure 1881.-1. — *Illustration of powdered herbal drug of red poppy petals (see Identification B)*

C. Thin-layer chromatography (*2.2.27*).

Test solution. To 1.0 g of the powdered drug (355) (*2.9.12*) add 10 ml of *ethanol (60 per cent V/V) R*. Stir for 15 min. Filter through a filter paper.

Reference solution. Dissolve 1 mg of *quinaldine red R* and 1 mg of *sulphan blue R* in 2 ml of *methanol R*.

Plate: TLC silica gel plate R.

Mobile phase: anhydrous formic acid R, water R, butanol R (10:12:40 V/V/V).

Application: 10 μl as bands.

Development: over a path of 10 cm.

Drying: in air.

Detection: examine in daylight.

Results: see below the sequence of zones present in the chromatograms obtained with the reference solution and the test solution. Furthermore, other zones may be present in the chromatogram obtained with the test solution.

Top of the plate	
	2 yellow zones
Quinaldine red: an orange-red zone	
	A violet principal zone
	A violet zone
	A yellow zone
Sulphan blue: a blue zone	
	A compact group of violet zones
Reference solution	**Test solution**

TESTS

Foreign matter (*2.8.2*): maximum 2.0 per cent of capsules and maximum 1.0 per cent of other foreign matter.

Loss on drying (*2.2.32*): maximum 12.0 per cent, determined on 1.000 g of the powdered drug (355) (*2.9.12*) by drying in an oven at 105 °C for 2 h.

Total ash (*2.4.16*): maximum 11.0 per cent.

Colouring intensity. Place 1.0 g of the powdered drug (355) (*2.9.12*) in a 250 ml flask and add 100 ml of *ethanol (30 per cent V/V) R*. Allow to macerate for 4 h with frequent stirring. Filter and discard the first 10 ml. To 10.0 ml of the filtrate add 2 ml of *hydrochloric acid R* and dilute to 100.0 ml with *ethanol (30 per cent V/V) R*. Allow to stand for 10 min. The absorbance (*2.2.25*) measured at 523 nm using *ethanol (30 per cent V/V) R* as the compensation liquid is not less than 0.6.

07/2009:2362

RIFAXIMIN

Rifaximinum

$C_{43}H_{51}N_3O_{11}$
[80621-81-4]

M_r 786

DEFINITION

(2S,16Z,18E,20S,21S,22R,23R,24R,25S,26R,27S,28E)-5,6,21,23-Tetrahydroxy-27-methoxy-2,4,11,16,20,22,24,26-octamethyl-1,15-dioxo-1,2-dihydro-2,7-(epoxypentadeca[1,11,13]trienoimino)benzofuro[4,5-*e*]pyrido[1,2-*a*]benzimidazol-25-yl acetate.

Semi-synthetic product derived from a fermentation product.

Content: 97.0 per cent to 102.0 per cent (anhydrous substance).

CHARACTERS

Appearance: red-orange, crystalline, hygroscopic powder.

Solubility: practically insoluble in water, soluble in acetone and in methanol.

It shows polymorphism (*5.9*).

IDENTIFICATION

Infrared absorption spectrophotometry (*2.2.24*).

Comparison: rifaximin CRS.

TESTS

Related substances. Liquid chromatography (*2.2.29*).

Solvent mixture: acetonitrile R, water R (40:60 V/V).

Test solution (a). Dissolve 0.100 g of the substance to be examined in 8 ml of *acetonitrile R* and dilute to 20 ml with *water R*.

Test solution (b). Dissolve 40.0 mg of the substance to be examined in the solvent mixture and dilute to 100.0 ml with the solvent mixture. Dilute 5.0 ml of this solution to 50.0 ml with the solvent mixture.

Reference solution (a). Dilute 1.0 ml of test solution (a) to 50.0 ml with the solvent mixture. Dilute 1.0 ml of this solution to 10.0 ml with the solvent mixture.

Reference solution (b). Dissolve 5 mg of *rifaximin for system suitability CRS* (containing impurity H) in 4 ml of the solvent mixture.

Reference solution (c). Dissolve 40.0 mg of *rifaximin CRS* in the solvent mixture and dilute to 100.0 ml with the solvent mixture. Dilute 5.0 ml of this solution to 50.0 ml with the solvent mixture.

Column:

— *size*: l = 0.25 m, Ø = 4.6 mm;

— *stationary phase*: end-capped octadecylsilyl silica gel for chromatography R (5 μm);

— *temperature*: 40 °C.

Mobile phase: mix 37 volumes of a 3.16 g/l solution of *ammonium formate R* adjusted to pH 7.2 with *dilute ammonia R1* and 63 volumes of a mixture of equal volumes of *acetonitrile R* and *methanol R*.

Flow rate: 1.4 ml/min.

Detection: spectrophotometer at 276 nm.

Injection: 20 μl of test solution (a) and reference solutions (a) and (b).

Run time: 3 times the retention time of rifaximin.

Relative retention with reference to rifaximin (retention time = about 12 min): impurities D and H = about 0.7.

System suitability: reference solution (b):

— *resolution*: minimum 3.0 between the peaks due to impurity H and rifaximin.

Limits:

— *sum of impurities D and H*: not more than 2.5 times the area of the principal peak in the chromatogram obtained with reference solution (a) (0.5 per cent);

— *unspecified impurities*: for each impurity, not more than 0.5 times the area of the principal peak in the chromatogram obtained with reference solution (a) (0.10 per cent);

— *total*: not more than 5 times the area of the principal peak in the chromatogram obtained with reference solution (a) (1.0 per cent);

— *disregard limit*: 0.25 times the area of the principal peak in the chromatogram obtained with reference solution (a) (0.05 per cent).

Heavy metals (*2.4.8*): maximum 20 ppm.

1.0 g complies with test C. Prepare the reference solution using 20 ml of *lead standard solution (1 ppm Pb) R*.

Water (*2.5.12*): maximum 4.5 per cent, determined on 0.50 g.

Sulphated ash (*2.4.14*): maximum 0.1 per cent, determined on 1.0 g.

ASSAY

Liquid chromatography (*2.2.29*) as described in the test for related substances with the following modification.

Injection: test solution (b) and reference solution (c).

Calculate the percentage content of $C_{43}H_{51}N_3O_{11}$ using the chromatogram obtained with reference solution (c) and the declared content of *rifaximin CRS*.

STORAGE

In an airtight container, protected from light.

IMPURITIES

Specified impurities: D, H.

Other detectable impurities (the following substances would, if present at a sufficient level, be detected by one or other of the tests in the monograph. They are limited by the general acceptance criterion for other/unspecified impurities and/or by the general monograph *Substances for pharmaceutical use (2034)*. It is therefore not necessary to identify these impurities for demonstration of compliance. See also *5.10*. *Control of impurities in substances for pharmaceutical use*): A, B, C, E, F, G.

A. 4-methylpyridin-2-amine,

B. R = CH₂-CO₂H: rifamycin B,

C. R = H: rifamycin SV,

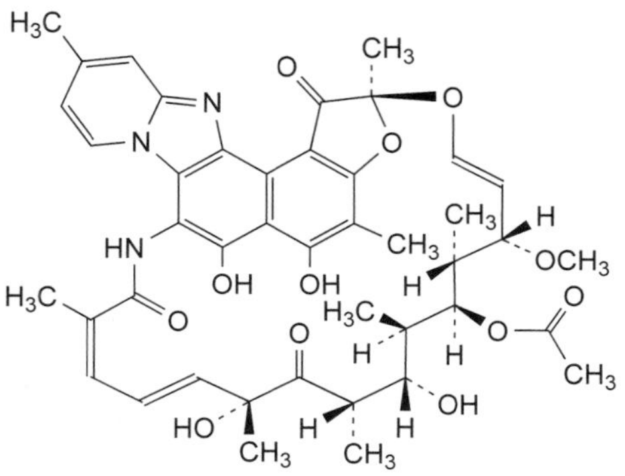

D. rifaximin Y,

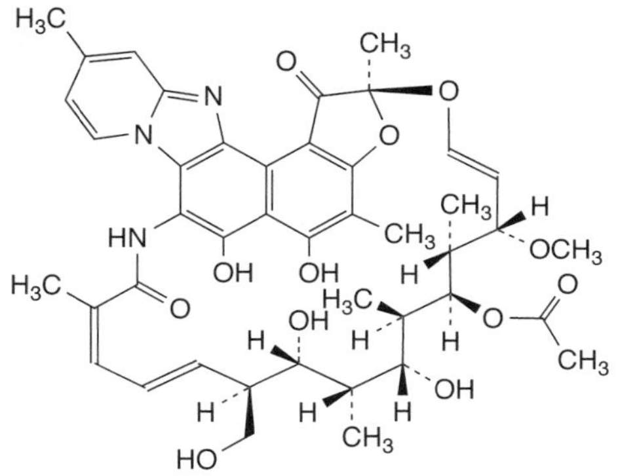

F. rifamycin O,

H. (2S,16Z,18E,20R,21S,22R,23R,24R,25S,26R,27S,28E)-
5,6,21,23-tetrahydroxy-20-(hydroxymethyl)-27-methoxy-
2,4,11,16,22,24,26-heptamethyl-1,15-dioxo-1,2-dihydro-
2,7-(epoxypentadeca[1,11,13]trienoimino)benzofuro-
[4,5-e]pyrido[1,2-a]benzimidazol-25-yl acetate
(hydroxy-rifaximin),

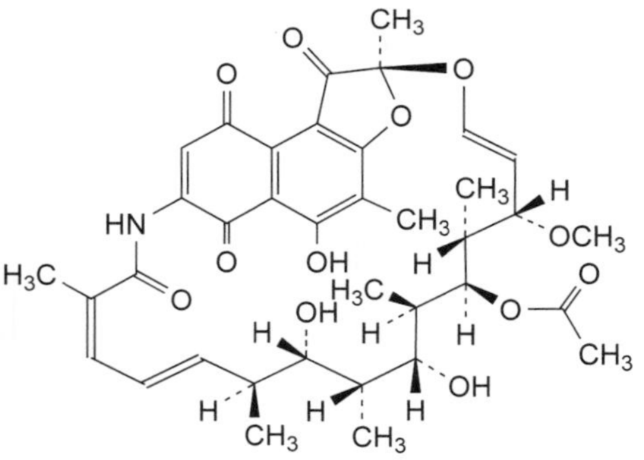

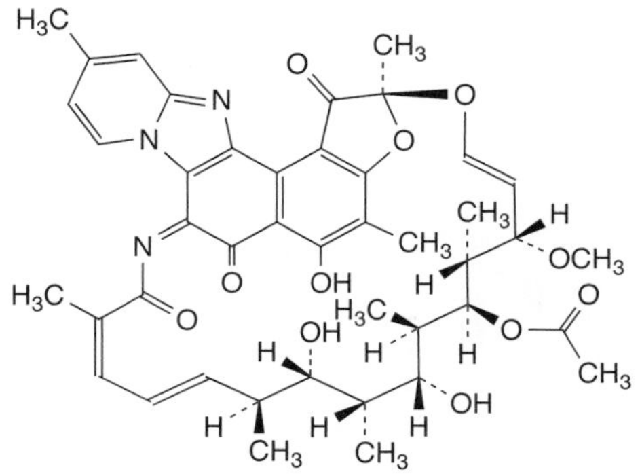

G. (2S,16Z,18E,20S,21S,22R,23R,24R,25S,26R,27S,
28E)-5,21,23-trihydroxy-27-methoxy-2,4,11,16,20,22,
24,26-octamethyl-1,6,15-trioxo-1,2,6,7-tetrahydro-2,
7-(epoxypentadeca[1,11,13]trienonitrilo)benzofuro-
[4,5-e]pyrido[1,2-a]benzimidazol-25-yl acetate (oxidised
rifaximin).

E. rifamycin S,

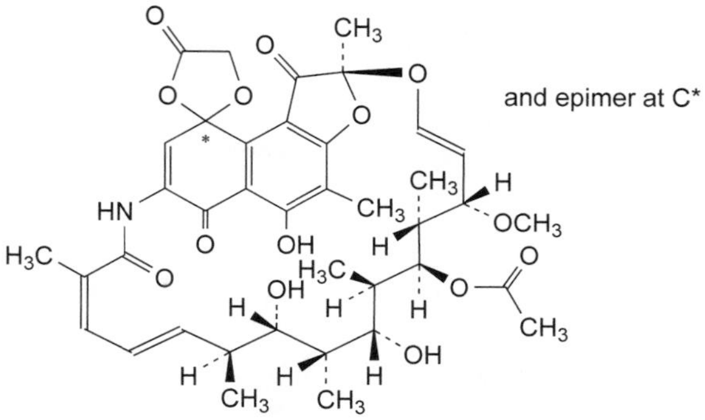

S

Monographs
Q-Z

07/2009:1031

SODIUM PICOSULFATE

Natrii picosulfas

$C_{18}H_{13}NNa_2O_8S_2,H_2O$ M_r 499.4

DEFINITION

4,4'-[(Pyridin-2-yl)methylene]diphenyl bis(sodium sulphate) monohydrate.

Content: 98.5 per cent to 100.5 per cent (anhydrous substance).

CHARACTERS

Appearance: white or almost white, crystalline powder.

Solubility: freely soluble in water, slightly soluble in ethanol 96 per cent.

IDENTIFICATION

First identification: A, E.

Second identification: B, C, D, E.

A. Infrared absorption spectrophotometry (2.2.24).

    Comparison: sodium picosulfate CRS.

B. Thin-layer chromatography (2.2.27).

    Test solution. Dissolve 20 mg of the substance to be examined in methanol R and dilute to 5 ml with the same solvent.

    Reference solution. Dissolve 20 mg of sodium picosulfate CRS in methanol R and dilute to 5 ml with the same solvent.

    Plate: TLC silica gel GF$_{254}$ plate R.

    Mobile phase: anhydrous formic acid R, water R, methanol R, ethyl acetate R (2.5:12.5:25:60 V/V/V/V).

    Application: 5 µl.

    Development: over 1/2 of the plate.

    Drying: in a current of hot air for 15 min.

    Detection: examine in ultraviolet light at 254 nm.

    Results: the principal spot in the chromatogram obtained with the test solution is similar in position and size to the principal spot in the chromatogram obtained with the reference solution.

C. To 5 ml of solution S (see Tests) add 1 ml of dilute hydrochloric acid R and heat to boiling. Add 1 ml of barium chloride solution R1. A white precipitate is formed.

D. To about 10 mg add 3 ml of sulphuric acid R and 0.1 ml of potassium dichromate solution R1. A violet colour develops.

E. Solution S gives reaction (a) of sodium (2.3.1).

TESTS

Solution S. Dissolve 2.5 g in carbon dioxide-free water R prepared from distilled water R and dilute to 50 ml with the same solvent.

Appearance of solution. Solution S is clear (2.2.1) and not more intensely coloured than reference solution GY$_7$ (2.2.2, Method II).

Acidity or alkalinity. To 10 ml of solution S add 0.05 ml of phenolphthalein solution R. The solution is colourless. Not more than 0.25 ml of 0.01 M sodium hydroxide is required to change the colour of the indicator to pink.

Related substances. Liquid chromatography (2.2.29).

Test solution. Dissolve 50 mg of the substance to be examined in the mobile phase and dilute to 100.0 ml with the mobile phase.

Reference solution (a). Dilute 1.0 ml of the test solution to 100.0 ml with the mobile phase. Dilute 10.0 ml of this solution to 100.0 ml with the mobile phase.

Reference solution (b). Dissolve the contents of a vial of picosulfate for system suitability CRS (containing impurities A and B) in 1.0 ml of the mobile phase.

Column:
- size: l = 0.25 m, Ø = 4.0 mm;
- stationary phase: spherical end-capped octadecylsilyl silica gel for chromatography R1 (5 µm);
- temperature: 40 °C.

Mobile phase: dissolve 2.3 g of disodium hydrogen phosphate dihydrate R in 800 ml of water for chromatography R, add 0.2 g of cetyltrimethylammonium bromide R, adjust to pH 7.5 with phosphoric acid R and dilute to 1000 ml with water for chromatography R; mix 550 ml of this solution and 450 ml of acetonitrile R (if necessary vary the buffer/acetonitrile proportion in 10 ml increments in order to fulfil the resolution requirement).

Flow rate: 1.0 ml/min.

Detection: spectrophotometer at 263 nm.

Injection: 40 µl.

Run time: twice the retention time of picosulfate.

Identification of impurities: use the chromatogram supplied with picosulfate for system suitability CRS and the chromatogram obtained with reference solution (b) to identify the peaks due to impurities A and B.

Relative retention with reference to picosulfate (retention time = about 7.4 min): impurity B = about 0.5; impurity A = about 0.7.

System suitability: reference solution (b):
- resolution: minimum 4.0 between the peaks due to impurities B and A.

Limits:
- correction factors: for the calculation of content, multiply the peak areas of the following impurities by the corresponding correction factor: impurity A = 0.7; impurity B = 0.5;
- impurities A, B: for each impurity, not more than twice the area of the principal peak in the chromatogram obtained with reference solution (a) (0.2 per cent);
- unspecified impurities: for each impurity, not more than the area of the principal peak in the chromatogram obtained with reference solution (a) (0.10 per cent);
- total: not more than 5 times the area of the principal peak in the chromatogram obtained with reference solution (a) (0.5 per cent);
- disregard limit: 0.5 times the area of the principal peak in the chromatogram obtained with reference solution (a) (0.05 per cent).

Chlorides (2.4.4): maximum 200 ppm.

Dilute 5 ml of solution S to 15 ml with water R.

Sulphates (*2.4.13*): maximum 400 ppm.

Dilute 7.5 ml of solution S to 15 ml with *distilled water R*.

Water (*2.5.12*): 3.0 per cent to 5.0 per cent, determined on 0.500 g.

ASSAY

Dissolve 0.400 g in 80 ml of *methanol R*. Titrate with *0.1 M perchloric acid*, determining the end-point potentiometrically (*2.2.20*).

1 ml of *0.1 M perchloric acid* is equivalent to 48.14 mg of $C_{18}H_{13}NNa_2O_8S_2$.

IMPURITIES

Specified impurities: A, B.

Other detectable impurities (the following substances would, if present at a sufficient level, be detected by one or other of the tests in the monograph. They are limited by the general acceptance criterion for other/unspecified impurities and/or by the general monograph *Substances for pharmaceutical use (2034)*. It is therefore not necessary to identify these impurities for demonstration of compliance. See also *5.10. Control of impurities in substances for pharmaceutical use): C.*

and enantiomer

A. R = SO$_3$Na: 4-[(*RS*)-(4-hydroxyphenyl)(pyridin-2-yl)methyl]phenyl sodium sulphate,

B. R = H: 4,4′-[(pyridin-2-yl)methylene]diphenol,

and enantiomer

C. 2-[(*RS*)-(pyridin-2-yl)[4-(sulphona-tooxy)phenyl]methyl]phenyl disodium sulphate.

07/2009:2419

SPIKE LAVENDER OIL

Spicae aetheroleum

DEFINITION

Essential oil obtained by steam distillation of the flowering tops of *Lavandula latifolia* Medik.

CHARACTERS

Appearance: clear, mobile, light yellow or greenish-yellow liquid.

Odour reminiscent of cineole and camphor.

IDENTIFICATION

First identification: B.

Second identification: A.

A. Thin-layer chromatography (*2.2.27*).

Test solution. Dissolve 20 µl of the substance to be examined in 1 ml of *toluene R*.

Reference solution. Dissolve 10 µl of *cineole R*, 10 µl of *linalol R* and 10 µl of *linalyl acetate R* in 1 ml of *toluene R*.

Plate: TLC silica gel plate R (5-40 µm) [or *TLC silica gel plate R* (2-10 µm)].

Mobile phase: ethyl acetate R, toluene R (5:95 *V/V*).

Application: 10 µl [or 2 µl], as bands of 10 mm [or 6 mm].

Development: over a path of 10 cm [or 8 cm].

Drying: in air.

Detection: spray with *anisaldehyde solution R* and heat at 100-105 °C for 5-10 min; examine immediately in daylight.

Results: see below the sequence of zones present in the chromatograms obtained with the reference solution and the test solution. Furthermore, other faint zones may be present in the chromatogram obtained with the test solution.

Top of the plate	
	A pink zone
Linalyl acetate: a violet or brown zone	A faint violet or brown zone may be present (linalyl acetate)
	A pink zone
Cineole: a violet-brown zone	An intense violet-brown zone (cineole)
Linalol: a violet or brown zone	An intense violet or brown zone (linalol)
	A greyish or brownish zone
	A faint violet zone
Reference solution	**Test solution**

B. Examine the chromatograms obtained in the test for chromatographic profile.

Results: the characteristic peaks in the chromatogram obtained with the test solution are similar in retention time to the peaks due to limonene, cineole, camphor, linalol, linalyl acetate, α-terpineol and *trans*-α-bisabolene in the chromatogram obtained with reference solution (a).

TESTS

Relative density (*2.2.5*): 0.894 to 0.907.

Refractive index (*2.2.6*): 1.461 to 1.468.

Optical rotation (*2.2.7*): − 7° to + 2°.

Acid value (*2.5.1*): maximum 1.5, determined on 5.00 g of the substance to be examined.

Solubility in alcohol (*2.8.10*): 1.0 ml of the substance to be examined is soluble, sometimes with opalescence, in 3.0 ml of *ethanol (70 per cent V/V) R*.

Chromatographic profile. Gas chromatography (*2.2.28*): use the normalisation procedure.

Test solution. Dissolve 200 µl of the substance to be examined in *heptane R* and dilute to 10.0 ml with the same solvent.

Reference solution (a). Dissolve 200 µl of *spike lavender oil CRS* in *heptane R* and dilute to 10.0 ml with the same solvent.

Reference solution (b). Dissolve 5 µl of *limonene R* in 50.0 ml of *heptane R*. Dilute 0.5 ml of this solution to 5.0 ml with *heptane R*.

Column:

- *material*: fused silica;
- *size*: l = 60 m, Ø = 0.25 mm;
- *stationary phase*: *macrogol 20 000 R* (film thickness 0.25 µm).

Carrier gas: *helium for chromatography R*.

Flow rate: 1.5 ml/min.

Split ratio: 1:50.

Temperature:

	Time (min)	Temperature (°C)
Column	0 - 15	70
	15 - 70	70 - 180
Injection port		220
Detector		220

Detection: flame ionisation.

Injection: 1 µl.

Identification of peaks: use the chromatogram supplied with *spike lavender oil CRS* and the chromatogram obtained with reference solution (a) to identify the peaks due to limonene, cineole, camphor, linalol, linalyl acetate, α-terpineol and *trans*-α-bisabolene.

System suitability: reference solution (a):

- the chromatogram obtained is similar to the chromatogram supplied with *spike lavender oil CRS*;
- *resolution*: minimum 1.5 between the peaks due to limonene and cineole.

Determine the percentage content of each of these components. The percentages are within the following ranges:

- *limonene*: 0.5 per cent to 3.0 per cent;
- *cineole*: 16.0 per cent to 39.0 per cent;
- *camphor*: 8.0 per cent to 16.0 per cent;
- *linalol*: 34.0 per cent to 50.0 per cent;
- *linalyl acetate*: less than 1.6 per cent;
- *α-terpineol*: 0.2 per cent to 2.0 per cent;
- *trans*-α-bisabolene: 0.4 per cent to 2.5 per cent;
- *disregard limit*: the area of the principal peak in the chromatogram obtained with reference solution (b) (0.05 per cent).

STORAGE

At a temperature not exceeding 25 °C.

07/2009:1474

STEARIC ACID

Acidum stearicum

DEFINITION

Mixture consisting mainly of stearic (octadecanoic) acid ($C_{18}H_{36}O_2$; M_r 284.5) and palmitic (hexadecanoic) acid ($C_{16}H_{32}O_2$; M_r 256.4) obtained from fats or oils of vegetable or animal origin.

Content:

Stearic acid 50	*Stearic acid*: 40.0 per cent to 60.0 per cent.
	Sum of the contents of stearic and palmitic acids: minimum 90.0 per cent.
Stearic acid 70	*Stearic acid*: 60.0 per cent to 80.0 per cent.
	Sum of the contents of stearic and palmitic acids: minimum 90.0 per cent.
Stearic acid 95	*Stearic acid*: minimum 90.0 per cent.
	Sum of the contents of stearic and palmitic acids: minimum 96.0 per cent.

CHARACTERS

Appearance: white or almost white, waxy, flaky crystals, white or almost white hard masses, or white or yellowish-white powder.

Solubility: practically insoluble in water, soluble in ethanol (96 per cent) and in light petroleum (50-70 °C).

IDENTIFICATION

A. It complies with the test for freezing point (see Tests).

B. Acid value (2.5.1): 194 to 212, determined on 0.5 g.

C. Examine the chromatograms obtained in the assay.

Results: the principal peaks in the chromatogram obtained with the test solution are similar in retention time to those in the chromatogram obtained with the reference solution.

TESTS

Appearance. Heat the substance to be examined to about 75 °C. The resulting liquid is not more intensely coloured than reference solution Y_7 or BY_7 (2.2.2, Method I).

Acidity. Melt 5.0 g, shake for 2 min with 10 ml of hot *carbon dioxide-free water R*, cool slowly and filter. To the filtrate add 0.05 ml of *methyl orange solution R*. No red colour develops.

Iodine value (2.5.4). See Table 1474.-1.

Freezing point (2.2.18). See Table 1474.-1.

Table 1474.-1.

Type	Iodine value	Freezing point (°C)
Stearic acid 50	maximum 4.0	53 - 59
Stearic acid 70	maximum 4.0	57 - 64
Stearic acid 95	maximum 1.5	64 - 69

Nickel (2.4.31): maximum 1 ppm.

ASSAY

Gas chromatography (2.2.28): use the normalisation procedure.

Test solution. In a conical flask fitted with a reflux condenser, dissolve 0.100 g of the substance to be examined in 5 ml of *boron trifluoride-methanol solution R*. Boil under reflux for 10 min. Add 4.0 ml of *heptane R* through the condenser and boil again under reflux for 10 min. Allow to cool. Add 20 ml of a saturated solution of *sodium chloride R*. Shake and allow the layers to separate. Remove about 2 ml of the organic layer and dry it over 0.2 g of *anhydrous sodium sulphate R*. Dilute 1.0 ml of this solution to 10.0 ml with *heptane R*.

Monographs Q-Z

Reference solution. Prepare the reference solution in the same manner as the test solution using 50 mg of *palmitic acid CRS* and 50 mg of *stearic acid CRS* instead of the substance to be examined.

Column:
— *material*: fused silica;
— *size*: l = 30 m, Ø = 0.32 mm;
— *stationary phase*: *macrogol 20 000 R* (film thickness 0.5 µm).

Carrier gas: *helium for chromatography R*.

Flow rate: 2.4 ml/min.

Temperature:

	Time (min)	Temperature (°C)
Column	0 - 2	70
	2 - 36	70 → 240
	36 - 41	240
Injection port		220
Detector		260

Detection: flame ionisation.

Injection: 1 µl.

Relative retention with reference to methyl stearate: methyl palmitate = about 0.9.

System suitability: reference solution:
— *resolution*: minimum 5.0 between the peaks due to methyl palmitate and methyl stearate;
— *repeatability*: maximum relative standard deviation of 3.0 per cent for the areas of the peaks due to methyl palmitate and methyl stearate, after 6 injections; maximum 1.0 per cent for the ratio of the areas of the peaks due to methyl palmitate to the areas of the peaks due to methyl stearate, after 6 injections.

LABELLING

The label states the type of stearic acid (50, 70, 95).

07/2009:2319

SUCROSE MONOPALMITATE

Sacchari monopalmitas

DEFINITION

Mixture of sucrose monoesters, mainly sucrose monopalmitate, obtained by transesterification of palmitic acid methyl esters of vegetable origin with *Sucrose (0204)*. The manufacture of the fatty acid methyl esters includes a distillation step.

It contains variable quantities of mono-, di-, tri- and polyesters.

Content:
— *monoesters*: minimum 55.0 per cent;
— *diesters*: maximum 40.0 per cent;
— *sum of triesters and polyesters*: maximum 20.0 per cent.

CHARACTERS

Appearance: white or almost white, unctuous powder.

Solubility: very slightly soluble in water, sparingly soluble in ethanol (96 per cent).

IDENTIFICATION

A. Composition of fatty acids (see Tests).

B. It complies with the limits of the assay.

TESTS

Acid value (*2.5.1*): maximum 6.0, determined on 3.00 g. Use a freshly neutralised mixture of 1 volume of *water R* and 2 volumes of *2-propanol R* as solvent and heat gently.

Composition of fatty acids (*2.4.22, Method C*). Use the mixture of calibrating substances in Table 2.4.22.-1.

Composition of the fatty-acid fraction of the substance:
— *lauric acid*: maximum 3.0 per cent;
— *myristic acid*: maximum 3.0 per cent;
— *palmitic acid*: 70.0 per cent to 85.0 per cent;
— *stearic acid*: 10.0 per cent to 25.0 per cent;
— *sum of the contents of palmitic acid and stearic acid*: minimum 90.0 per cent.

Free sucrose. Liquid chromatography (*2.2.29*).

Solvent mixture: *water for chromatography R, tetrahydrofuran for chromatography R* (12.5:87.5 *V/V*).

Test solution. Dissolve 0.200 g of the substance to be examined in the solvent mixture and dilute to 4.0 ml with the solvent mixture.

Reference solution (a). Dissolve 20.0 mg of *sucrose CRS* in the solvent mixture and dilute to 10.0 ml with the solvent mixture. Dilute 1.0 ml of this solution to 10.0 ml with the solvent mixture.

Reference solution (b). In 4 volumetric flasks, introduce respectively 5.0 mg, 10.0 mg, 20.0 mg and 25.0 mg of *sucrose CRS*, dissolve in the solvent mixture and dilute to 10.0 ml with the solvent mixture.

Column:
— *size*: l = 0.25 m, Ø = 4.6 mm;
— *stationary phase*: spherical *aminopropylsilyl silica gel for chromatography R* (4 µm).

Mobile phase:
— *mobile phase A*: 0.01 g/l solution of *ammonium acetate R* in *acetonitrile for chromatography R*;
— *mobile phase B*: 0.01 g/l solution of *ammonium acetate R* in a mixture of 10 volumes of *water for chromatography R* and 90 volumes of *tetrahydrofuran for chromatography R*;

Time (min)	Mobile phase A (per cent *V/V*)	Mobile phase B (per cent *V/V*)	Flow rate (ml/min)
0 - 1	100	0	1.0
1 - 9	100 → 0	0 → 100	1.0
9 - 16	0	100	1.0
16 - 16.01	0	100	1.0 → 2.5
16.01 - 32	0	100	2.5
32 - 33	0 → 100	100 → 0	2.5
33 - 36	100	0	2.5 → 1.0

Detection: evaporative light-scattering detector; the following settings have been found to be suitable; if the detector has different setting parameters, adjust the detector settings so as to comply with the system suitability criterion:
— *carrier gas*: *nitrogen R*;
— *flow rate*: 1.0 ml/min;
— *evaporator temperature*: 45 °C;
— *nebuliser temperature*: 40 °C.

Injection: 20 µl.

Retention time: about 26 min.

System suitability: reference solution (a):

– *signal-to-noise ratio*: minimum 10.

Limit: maximum 4.0 per cent.

Water (*2.5.12*): maximum 4.0 per cent, determined on 0.20 g.

Total ash (*2.4.16*): maximum 1.5 per cent.

ASSAY

Size-exclusion chromatography (*2.2.30*): use the normalisation procedure.

Test solution. Dissolve 60.0 mg of the substance to be examined in *tetrahydrofuran R* and dilute to 4.0 ml with the same solvent.

Column:

– *size*: l = 0.6 m, Ø = 7 mm;

– *stationary phase*: *styrene-divinylbenzene copolymer R* (5 μm) with a pore size of 10 nm.

Mobile phase: *tetrahydrofuran R*.

Flow rate: 1.2 ml/min.

Detection: differential refractometer.

Injection: 20 μl.

Relative retention with reference to monoesters (retention time = about 10 min): diesters = about 0.92; triesters and polyesters = about 0.90.

Calculations:

– *disregard limit*: disregard the peaks having a signal-to-noise ratio less than 10;

– *free fatty acids (D)*: calculate the percentage content of free fatty acids, using the following expression:

$$\frac{I_A \times 256}{561.1}$$

I_A =   acid value.

– *monoesters*: calculate the percentage content of monoesters using the following expression:

$$\frac{A \times (100 - D - S - E)}{100}$$

– *diesters*: calculate the percentage content of diesters using the following expression:

$$\frac{B \times (100 - D - S - E)}{100}$$

– *sum of triesters and polyesters*: calculate the sum of the percentage contents of triesters and polyesters using the following expression:

$$\frac{C \times (100 - D - S - E)}{100}$$

A =   percentage content of monoesters determined by the normalisation procedure;

S =   percentage content of free sucrose (see Tests);

E =   percentage content of water (see Tests);

B =   percentage content of diesters determined by the normalisation procedure;

C =   sum of the percentage contents of triesters and polyesters determined by the normalisation procedure.

STORAGE

Protected from humidity.

07/2009:2318

SUCROSE STEARATE

Sacchari stearas

DEFINITION

Mixture of sucrose esters, mainly sucrose stearate, obtained by transesterification of stearic acid methyl esters of vegetable origin with *sucrose (0204)*. The manufacture of the fatty acid methyl esters includes a distillation step.

It contains variable quantities of mono-, di-, tri- and polyesters.

Content:

Sucrose stearate type I:

– *monoesters*: minimum 50.0 per cent;

– *diesters*: maximum 40.0 per cent;

– *sum of triesters and polyesters*: maximum 25.0 per cent;

Sucrose stearate type II:

– *monoesters*: 20.0 per cent to 45.0 per cent;

– *diesters*: 30.0 per cent to 40.0 per cent;

– *sum of triesters and polyesters*: maximum 30.0 per cent;

Sucrose stearate type III:

– *monoesters*: 15.0 per cent to 25.0 per cent;

– *diesters*: 30.0 per cent to 45.0 per cent;

– *sum of triesters and polyesters*: 35.0 per cent to 50.0 per cent.

CHARACTERS

Appearance: white or almost white, unctuous powder.

Solubility: very slightly soluble in water, sparingly soluble in ethanol (96 per cent).

IDENTIFICATION

A. Composition of fatty acids (see Tests).

B. It complies with the limits of the assay.

TESTS

Acid value (*2.5.1*): maximum 6.0, determined on 3.00 g.

Use a freshly neutralised mixture of 1 volume of *water R* and 2 volumes of *2-propanol R* as solvent and heat gently.

Composition of fatty acids (*2.4.22, Method C*). Use the mixture of calibrating substances in Table 2.4.22.-1.

Composition of the fatty-acid fraction of the substance:

– *lauric acid*: maximum 3.0 per cent;

– *myristic acid*: maximum 3.0 per cent;

– *palmitic acid*: 25.0 per cent to 40.0 per cent;

– *stearic acid*: 55.0 per cent to 75.0 per cent;

– *sum of the contents of palmitic acid and stearic acid*: minimum 90.0 per cent.

Free sucrose. Liquid chromatography (*2.2.29*).

Solvent mixture: *water for chromatography R, tetrahydrofuran for chromatography R* (12.5:87.5 *V/V*).

Test solution. Dissolve 0.200 g of the substance to be examined in the solvent mixture and dilute to 4.0 ml with the solvent mixture.

Reference solution (a). Dissolve 20.0 mg of *sucrose CRS* in the solvent mixture and dilute to 10.0 ml with the solvent mixture. Dilute 1.0 ml of this solution to 10.0 ml with the solvent mixture.

General Notices (1) apply to all monographs and other texts

Reference solution (b). In 4 volumetric flasks, introduce respectively 5.0 mg, 10.0 mg, 20.0 mg and 25.0 mg of *sucrose CRS*, dissolve in the solvent mixture and dilute to 10.0 ml with the solvent mixture.

Column:
— *size*: l = 0.25 m, Ø = 4.6 mm;
— *stationary phase*: spherical *aminopropylsilyl silica gel for chromatography R* (4 μm).

Mobile phase:
— *mobile phase A*: 0.01 g/l solution of *ammonium acetate R* in *acetonitrile for chromatography R*;
— *mobile phase B*: 0.01 g/l solution of *ammonium acetate R* in a mixture of 10 volumes of *water for chromatography R* and 90 volumes of *tetrahydrofuran for chromatography R*;

Time (min)	Mobile phase A (per cent V/V)	Mobile phase B (per cent V/V)	Flow rate (ml/min)
0 - 1	100	0	1.0
1 - 9	100 → 0	0 → 100	1.0
9 - 16	0	100	1.0
16 - 16.01	0	100	1.0 → 2.5
16.01 - 32	0	100	2.5
32 - 33	0 → 100	100 → 0	2.5
33 - 36	100	0	2.5 → 1.0

Detection: evaporative light-scattering detector; the following settings have been found to be suitable; if the detector has different setting parameters, adjust the detector settings so as to comply with the system suitability criterion:
— *carrier gas*: *nitrogen R*;
— *flow rate*: 1.0 ml/min;
— *evaporator temperature*: 45 °C;
— *nebuliser temperature*: 40 °C.

Injection: 20 μl.

Retention time: about 26 min.

System suitability: reference solution (a):
— *signal-to-noise ratio*: minimum 10.

Limit:
— *sucrose*: maximum 4.0 per cent.

Water (*2.5.12*): maximum 4.0 per cent, determined on 0.20 g.

Total ash (*2.4.16*): maximum 1.5 per cent.

ASSAY

Size-exclusion chromatography (*2.2.30*): use the normalisation procedure.

Test solution. Dissolve 60.0 mg of the substance to be examined in *tetrahydrofuran R* and dilute to 4.0 ml with the same solvent.

Column:
— *size*: l = 0.6 m, Ø = 7 mm;

— *stationary phase*: *styrene-divinylbenzene copolymer R* (5 μm) with a pore size of 10 nm.

Mobile phase: *tetrahydrofuran R*.

Flow rate: 1.2 ml/min.

Detection: differential refractometer.

Injection: 20 μl.

Relative retention with reference to monoesters (retention time = about 10 min): diesters = about 0.92; triesters and polyesters = about 0.90.

Calculations:
— *disregard limit*: disregard the peaks having a signal-to-noise ratio less than 10;
— *free fatty acids (D)*: calculate the percentage content of free fatty acids, using the following expression:

$$\frac{I_A \times 284.5}{561.1}$$

I_A = acid value;

— *monoesters*: calculate the percentage content of monoesters using the following expression:

$$\frac{A \times (100 - D - S - E)}{100}$$

— *diesters*: calculate the percentage content of diesters using the following expression:

$$\frac{B \times (100 - D - S - E)}{100}$$

— *sum of triesters and polyesters*: calculate the sum of the percentage contents of triesters and polyesters using the following expression:

$$\frac{C \times (100 - D - S - E)}{100}$$

A = percentage content of monoesters determined by the normalisation procedure;

S = percentage content of free sucrose (see Tests);

E = percentage content of water (see Tests);

B = percentage content of diesters determined by the normalisation procedure;

C = sum of the percentage contents of triesters and polyesters determined by the normalisation procedure.

LABELLING

The label states the type of sucrose stearate (type I, II or III). |

STORAGE

Protected from humidity.

T

Monographs
Q-Z

01/2008:2131
corrected 6.5

TAMSULOSIN HYDROCHLORIDE

Tamsulosini hydrochloridum

$C_{20}H_{29}ClN_2O_5S$ M_r 445.0
[106463-17-6]

DEFINITION

5-[(2R)-2-[[2-(2-Ethoxyphenoxy)ethyl]amino]propyl]-2-methoxybenzenesulfonamide hydrochloride.

Content: 98.5 per cent to 101.0 per cent (dried substance).

CHARACTERS

Appearance: white or almost white powder.

Solubility: slightly soluble in water, freely soluble in formic acid, slightly soluble in anhydrous ethanol.

mp: about 230 °C.

IDENTIFICATION

Carry out either tests A, C, D or tests A, B, D.

A. Infrared absorption spectrophotometry (*2.2.24*).
   Comparison: tamsulosin hydrochloride CRS.

B. Specific optical rotation (*2.2.7*): – 17.5 to – 20.5 (dried substance).
   Dissolve with heating 0.15 g in *water R* and dilute to 20.0 ml with the same solvent.

C. Enantiomeric purity (see Tests).

D. Dissolve with heating 0.75 g in *water R* and dilute to 100.0 ml with the same solvent. Take 5 ml of the solution and cool in an ice-bath. Add 3 ml of *dilute nitric acid R* and shake. Allow to stand at room temperature for 30 min and filter. The filtrate gives reaction (a) of chlorides (*2.3.1*).

TESTS

Related substances.

A. Impurities eluting before tamsulosin. Liquid chromatography (*2.2.29*).

Test solution. Dissolve 50.0 mg of the substance to be examined in the mobile phase and dilute to 10.0 ml with the mobile phase.

Reference solution (a). Dilute 1.0 ml of the test solution to 100.0 ml with the mobile phase. Dilute 1.0 ml of this solution to 10.0 ml with the mobile phase.

Reference solution (b). Dissolve 4 mg of *tamsulosin impurity D CRS* and 4 mg of the substance to be examined in the mobile phase and dilute to 20.0 ml with the mobile phase. Dilute 2.0 ml of this solution to 20.0 ml with the mobile phase.

Reference solution (c). Dissolve 4 mg of *tamsulosin impurity H CRS* and 4 mg of the substance to be examined in the mobile phase and dilute to 20.0 ml with the mobile phase. Dilute 2.0 ml of this solution to 20.0 ml with the mobile phase.

Column:
— *size*: l = 0.15 m, Ø = 4.6 mm;

— *stationary phase*: octadecylsilyl silica gel for chromatography R (5 µm);
— *temperature*: 40 °C.

Mobile phase: dissolve 3.0 g of *sodium hydroxide R* in a mixture of 8.7 ml of *perchloric acid R* and 1.9 litres of *water R*; adjust to pH 2.0 with *0.5 M sodium hydroxide* and dilute to 2 litres with *water R*; to 1.4 litres of this solution, add 600 ml of *acetonitrile R*.

Flow rate: 1.3 ml/min.

Detection: spectrophotometer at 225 nm.

Injection: 10 µl of the test solution and reference solutions (a) and (b).

Run time: 1.5 times the retention time of tamsulosin (retention time = about 6 min).

System suitability: reference solution (b):
— *resolution*: minimum 6 between the peaks due to impurity D and tamsulosin.

Limits:
— *unspecified impurities*: for each impurity, not more than the area of the principal peak in the chromatogram obtained with reference solution (a) (0.10 per cent);
— *disregard limit*: 0.5 times the area of the principal peak in the chromatogram obtained with reference solution (a) (0.05 per cent).

B. Impurities eluting after tamsulosin. Liquid chromatography (*2.2.29*) as described in test A with the following modifications.

Mobile phase: dissolve 3.0 g of *sodium hydroxide R* in a mixture of 8.7 ml of *perchloric acid R* and 1.9 litres of *water R*; adjust to pH 2.0 with *0.5 M sodium hydroxide* and dilute to 2 litres with *water R*; add 2 litres of *acetonitrile R*.

Flow rate: 1.0 ml/min.

Injection: 10 µl of the test solution and reference solutions (a) and (c).

Run time: 5 times the retention time of tamsulosin (retention time = about 2.5 min).

System suitability: reference solution (c):
— *resolution*: minimum 2 between the peaks due to tamsulosin and impurity H.

Limits:
— *unspecified impurities*: for each impurity, not more than the area of the principal peak in the chromatogram obtained with reference solution (a) (0.10 per cent);
— *sum of impurities eluting before tamsulosin in test A and after tamsulosin in test B*: not more than twice the area of the principal peak in the chromatogram obtained with reference solution (a) (0.2 per cent);
— *disregard limit*: 0.5 times the area of the principal peak in the chromatogram obtained with reference solution (a) (0.05 per cent).

Enantiomeric purity. Liquid chromatography (*2.2.29*).

Test solution. Dissolve 50.0 mg of the substance to be examined in *methanol R* and dilute to 25.0 ml with the same solvent.

Reference solution (a). Dilute 1.0 ml of the test solution to 100.0 ml with *methanol R*. Dilute 1.0 ml of this solution to 10.0 ml with *methanol R*.

Reference solution (b). Dissolve 5.0 mg of *tamsulosin racemate CRS* in *methanol R* and dilute to 25.0 ml with the same solvent. Dilute 2.0 ml of this solution to 10.0 ml with *methanol R*.

Column:

— *size*: l = 0.25 m, Ø = 4.6 mm;

— *stationary phase*: *silica gel AD for chiral separation R*;

— *temperature*: 40 °C.

Mobile phase: *diethylamine R, methanol R, anhydrous ethanol R, hexane R* (1:150:200:650 *V/V/V/V*).

Flow rate: 0.5 ml/min.

Detection: spectrophotometer at 225 nm.

Injection: 10 µl.

Relative retention with reference to tamsulosin (retention time = about 14 min): impurity G = about 0.8.

System suitability: reference solution (b):

— *resolution*: minimum 2 between the peaks due to impurity G and tamsulosin.

Limit:

— *impurity G*: not more than the area of the principal peak in the chromatogram obtained with reference solution (a) (0.1 per cent).

Heavy metals (*2.4.8*): maximum 20 ppm.

1.0 g complies with test C. Prepare the reference solution using 2 ml of *lead standard solution (10 ppm Pb) R*.

Loss on drying (*2.2.32*): maximum 0.5 per cent, determined on 1.000 g by drying in an oven at 105 °C for 2 h.

Sulphated ash (*2.4.14*): maximum 0.1 per cent, determined on 1.0 g.

ASSAY

Dissolve 0.350 g in 5.0 ml of *anhydrous formic acid R*, add 75 ml of a mixture of 2 volumes of *acetic anhydride R* and 3 volumes of *glacial acetic acid R*. Titrate immediately with *0.1 M perchloric acid*, determining the end-point potentiometrically (*2.2.20*). Carry out a blank titration.

1 ml of *0.1 M perchloric acid* is equivalent to 44.50 mg of $C_{20}H_{29}ClN_2O_5S$.

IMPURITIES

Specified impurities: G.

Other detectable impurities (the following substances would, if present at a sufficient level, be detected by one or other of the tests in the monograph. They are limited by the general acceptance criterion for other/unspecified impurities and/or by the general monograph *Substances for pharmaceutical use (2034)*. It is therefore not necessary to identify these impurities for demonstration of compliance. See also *5.10*. *Control of impurities in substances for pharmaceutical use*): A, B, C, D, E, F, H, I.

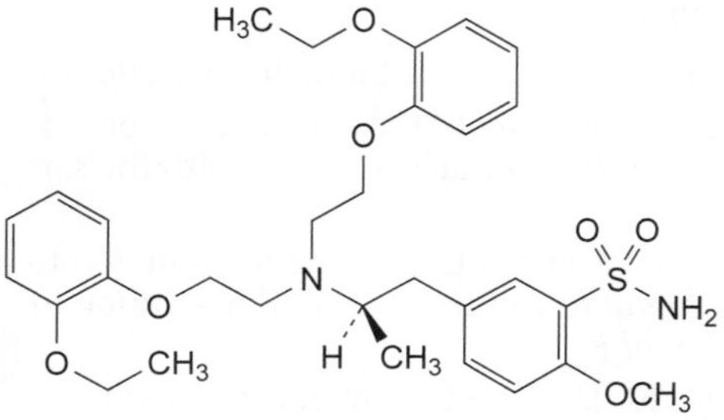

A. 5-[(2R)-2-[bis[2-(2-ethoxyphenoxy)ethyl]amino]propyl]-2-methoxybenzenesulfonamide,

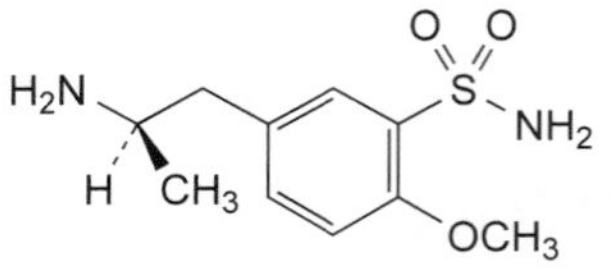

B. 5-[(2R)-2-aminopropyl]-2-methoxybenzenesulfonamide,

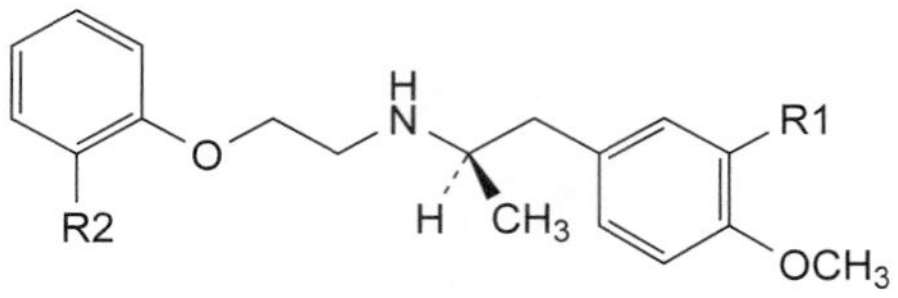

C. R1 = SO₂-NH₂, R2 = H: 2-methoxy-5-[(2R)-2-[(2-phenoxyethyl)amino]propyl]benzenesulfonamide,

D. R1 = SO₂-NH₂, R2 = OCH₃: 2-methoxy-5-[(2R)-2-[[2-(2-methoxyphenoxy)ethyl]amino]propyl]benzenesulfon-amide,

H. R1 = H, R2 = OC₂H₅: (2R)-N-[2-(2-ethoxyphenoxy)ethyl]-1-(4-methoxyphenyl)propan-2-amine,

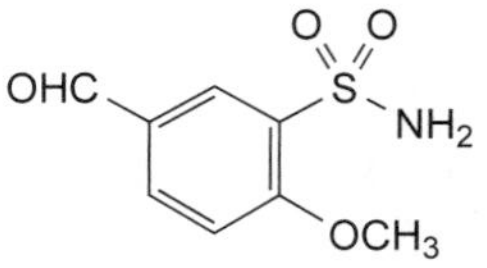

E. 5-formyl-2-methoxybenzenesulfonamide,

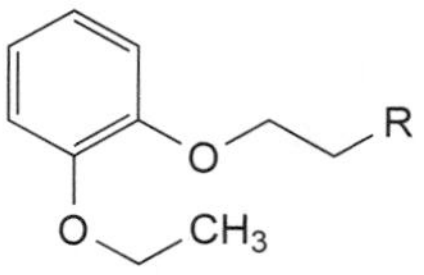

F. R = NH₂: 2-(2-ethoxyphenoxy)ethanamine,

I. R = Br: 1-(2-bromoethoxy)-2-ethoxybenzene,

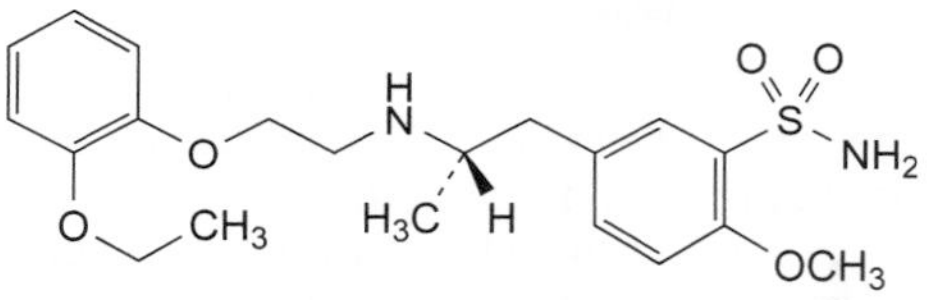

G. 5-[(2S)-2-[[2-(2-ethoxyphenoxy)ethyl]amino]propyl]-2-methoxybenzenesulfonamide.

07/2009:1156

TENOXICAM

Tenoxicamum

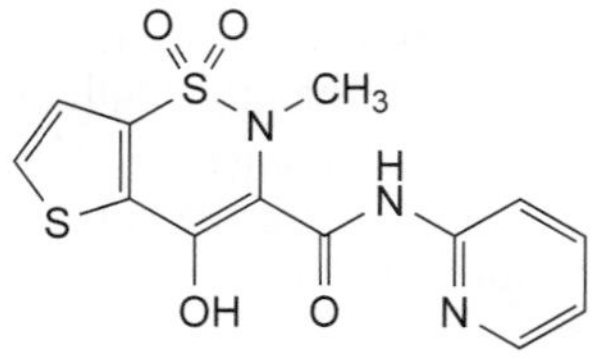

$C_{13}H_{11}N_3O_4S_2$ M_r 337.4
[59804-37-4]

DEFINITION

4-Hydroxy-2-methyl-*N*-(pyridin-2-yl)-2*H*-thieno[2,3-*e*]1,2-thiazine-3-carboxamide 1,1-dioxide.

Content: 99.0 per cent to 101.0 per cent (anhydrous substance).

CHARACTERS

Appearance: yellow, crystalline powder.

Solubility: practically insoluble in water, sparingly soluble in methylene chloride, very slightly soluble in anhydrous ethanol. It dissolves in solutions of acids and alkalis.

It shows polymorphism (*5.9*).

IDENTIFICATION

Infrared absorption spectrophotometry (*2.2.24*).

Comparison: tenoxicam CRS.

If the spectra obtained in the solid state show differences, dissolve the substance to be examined and the reference substance separately in the minimum volume of *methylene chloride R*, evaporate to dryness and record new spectra using the residues.

TESTS

Appearance of solution. The solution is clear (*2.2.1*).

Dissolve 0.10 g in *methylene chloride R* and dilute to 20 ml with the same solvent.

Related substances. Liquid chromatography (*2.2.29*). *Carry out the test protected from light.*

Solvent mixture. Mix equal volumes of *acetonitrile R* and *water R*. Adjust to apparent pH 3.2 with *dilute phosphoric acid R1*.

Test solution. Dissolve 35 mg of the substance to be examined in the solvent mixture, sonicate and dilute to 50.0 ml with the solvent mixture.

Reference solution (a). Dilute 1.0 ml of the test solution to 100.0 ml with the solvent mixture. Dilute 1.0 ml of this solution to 10.0 ml with the solvent mixture.

Reference solution (b). Dissolve 7 mg of *pyridin-2-amine R* (impurity A) in the solvent mixture and dilute to 100.0 ml with the solvent mixture. Dilute 1.0 ml of this solution to 100.0 ml with the solvent mixture.

Reference solution (c). Dissolve the contents of a vial of *tenoxicam impurity mixture CRS* (impurities B, G and H) in 1.0 ml of the test solution.

Column:
– *size*: l = 0.15 m, Ø = 4.6 mm;
– *stationary phase*: *cyanosilyl silica gel for chromatography R* (3.5 µm);
– *temperature*: 35 °C.

Mobile phase:
– *mobile phase A*: mix 25 volumes of *methanol R2* and 75 volumes of *water R* and adjust to apparent pH 3.2 with *dilute phosphoric acid R1*;
– *mobile phase B*: mix 25 volumes of *water R* and 75 volumes of *methanol R2* and adjust to apparent pH 3.2 with *dilute phosphoric acid R1*;

Time (min)	Mobile phase A (per cent *V/V*)	Mobile phase B (per cent *V/V*)
0 - 5	96	4
5 - 16	96 → 76	4 → 24
16 - 25	76	24

Flow rate: 1.0 ml/min.

Detection: spectrophotometer at 230 nm.

Injection: 20 µl.

Identification of impurities:
– use the chromatogram obtained with reference solution (b) to identify the peak due to impurity A;

– use the chromatogram supplied with *tenoxicam impurity mixture CRS* and the chromatogram obtained with reference solution (c) to identify the peaks due to impurities B, G and H; for identification of impurities G and H, which may be inverted in the elution order, take into account the heights of the corresponding peaks in the chromatogram supplied with *tenoxicam impurity mixture CRS*.

Relative retention with reference to tenoxicam (retention time = about 12 min): impurity A = about 0.1; impurity G = about 0.85; impurity H = about 0.9; impurity B = about 1.3.

System suitability: reference solution (c):
– *resolution*: minimum 1.3 between the peaks due to impurity H (or G if peaks are inverted) and tenoxicam, and between the peaks due to impurities G and H; if necessary, optimise the apparent pH of the mobile phases within the range 3.0-3.4.

Limits:
– *correction factors*: for the calculation of content, multiply the peak areas of the following impurities by the corresponding correction factor: impurity A = 0.2; impurity B = 2.0;
– *impurities A, B*: for each impurity, not more than 1.5 times the area of the principal peak in the chromatogram obtained with reference solution (a) (0.15 per cent);
– *unspecified impurities*: for each impurity, not more than the area of the principal peak in the chromatogram obtained with reference solution (a) (0.10 per cent);
– *total*: not more than 3 times the area of the principal peak in the chromatogram obtained with reference solution (a) (0.3 per cent);
– *disregard limit*: 0.5 times the area of the principal peak in the chromatogram obtained with reference solution (a) (0.05 per cent).

Heavy metals (*2.4.8*): maximum 20 ppm.

0.5 g complies with test C. Prepare the reference solution using 5 ml of *lead standard solution (2 ppm Pb) R*.

Water (*2.5.12*): maximum 0.5 per cent, determined on 1.000 g.

Sulphated ash (*2.4.14*): maximum 0.1 per cent, determined on 1.0 g.

ASSAY

Dissolve 0.250 g in 5 ml of *anhydrous formic acid R*. Add 70 ml of *anhydrous acetic acid R*. Titrate with *0.1 M perchloric acid*, determining the end-point potentiometrically (*2.2.20*).

1 ml of *0.1 M perchloric acid* is equivalent to 33.74 mg of $C_{13}H_{11}N_3O_4S_2$.

STORAGE

Protected from light.

IMPURITIES

Specified impurities: A, B.

Other detectable impurities (the following substances would, if present at a sufficient level, be detected by one or other of the tests in the monograph. They are limited by the general acceptance criterion for other/unspecified impurities and/or by the general monograph *Substances for pharmaceutical use (2034)*. It is therefore not necessary to identify these impurities for demonstration of compliance. See also *5.10*. *Control of impurities in substances for pharmaceutical use*): *C, D, E, F, G, H.*

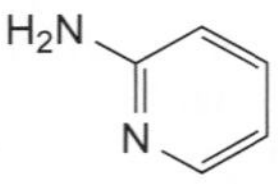

A. pyridin-2-amine,

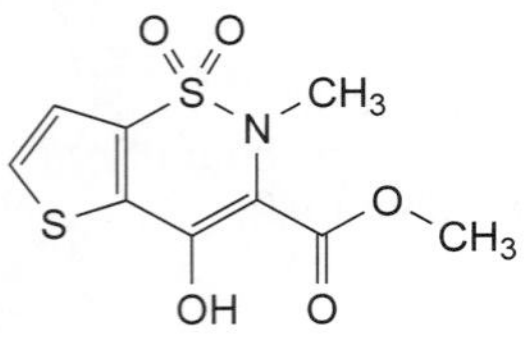

B. methyl 4-hydroxy-2-methyl-2H-thieno[2,3-e]1,2-thiazine-3-carboxylate 1,1-dioxide,

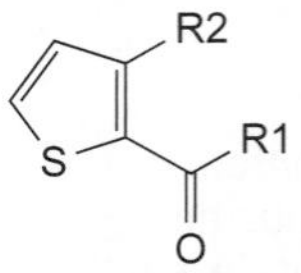

C. R1 = NH-CH₃, R2 = H: N-methylthiophene-2-carboxamide,

H. R1 = OH, R2 = SO₂-NH-CH₃: 3-[(methylamino)sulphonyl]-thiophene-2-carboxylic acid,

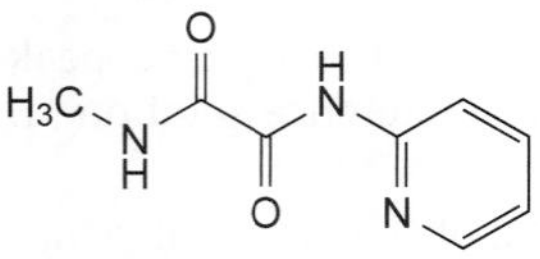

D. N-methyl-N'-(pyridin-2-yl)-ethanediamide,

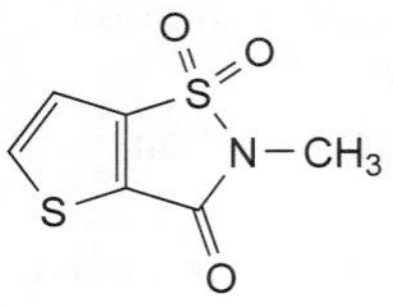

E. 2-methylthieno[2,3-d]isothiazol-3(2H)-one 1,1-dioxide,

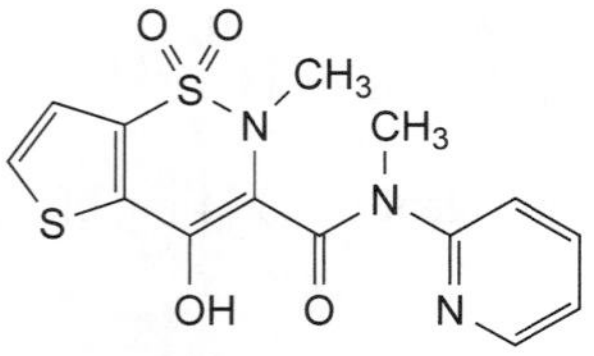

F. 4-hydroxy-N,2-dimethyl-N-(pyridin-2-yl)-2H-thieno[2,3-e]1,2-thiazine-3-carboxamide 1,1-dioxide,

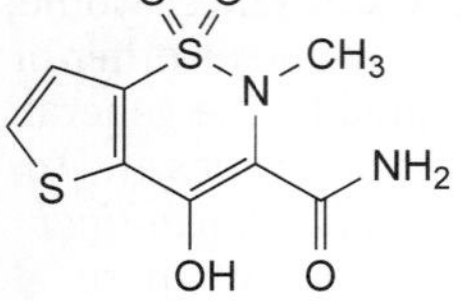

G. 4-hydroxy-2-methyl-2H-thieno[2,3-e]1,2-thiazine-3-carboxamide 1,1-dioxide.

01/2008:1738
corrected 6.5

TETRAZEPAM

Tetrazepamum

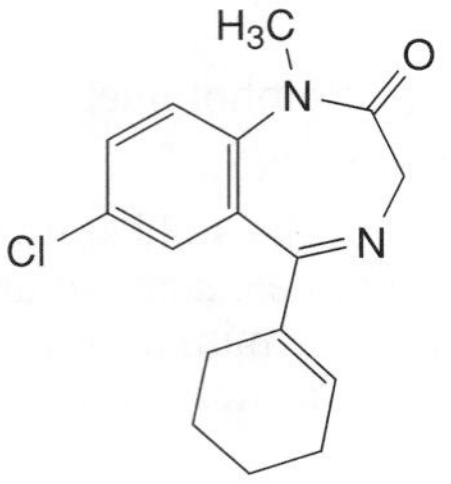

$C_{16}H_{17}ClN_2O$ $\qquad$ M_r 288.8
[10379-14-3]

DEFINITION

7-Chloro-5-(cyclohex-1-enyl)-1-methyl-1,3-dihydro-2H-1,4-benzodiazepin-2-one.

Content: 99.0 per cent to 101.0 per cent (dried substance).

CHARACTERS

Appearance: light yellow or yellow crystalline powder.

Solubility: practically insoluble in water, freely soluble in methylene chloride, soluble in acetonitrile.

IDENTIFICATION

Infrared absorption spectrophotometry (*2.2.24*).

Comparison: Ph. Eur. reference spectrum of tetrazepam.

TESTS

Related substances. Liquid chromatography (*2.2.29*).

Test solution. Dissolve 25.0 mg of the substance to be examined in *acetonitrile R* and dilute to 25.0 ml with the same solvent.

Reference solution (a). Dissolve 5.0 mg of the substance to be examined and 5.0 mg of *tetrazepam impurity C CRS* in *acetonitrile R* and dilute to 10.0 ml with the same solvent. Dilute 1.0 ml of the solution to 10.0 ml with *acetonitrile R*.

Reference solution (b). Dilute 1.0 ml of the test solution to 50.0 ml with *acetonitrile R*. Dilute 1.0 ml of this solution to 10.0 ml with *acetonitrile R*.

Column:
— *size*: l = 0.25 m, Ø = 4.6 mm;
— *stationary phase*: octadecylsilyl silica gel for chromatography R (5 µm).

Mobile phase:
— *mobile phase A*: mix 40 volumes of *acetonitrile R* and 60 volumes of a 3.4 g/l solution of *potassium dihydrogen phosphate R*;
— *mobile phase B*: *acetonitrile R*;

Time (min)	Mobile phase A (per cent V/V)	Mobile phase B (per cent V/V)
0 - 35	100	0
35 - 40	100 → 55	0 → 45
40 - 50	55	45
50 - 60	55 → 100	45 → 0

Flow rate: 1.5 ml/min.

Detection: a spectrophotometer at 229 nm.

Injection: 20 µl.

System suitability: reference solution (a):

- *resolution*: minimum 2.0 between the peaks due to tetrazepam and to impurity C.

Limits:

- *any impurity*: not more than the area of the principal peak in the chromatogram obtained with reference solution (b) (0.2 per cent);
- *total*: not more than 5 times the area of the principal peak in the chromatogram obtained with reference solution (b) (1.0 per cent);
- *disregard limit*: 0.25 times the area of the principal peak in the chromatogram obtained with reference solution (b) (0.05 per cent).

Chlorides (*2.4.4*): maximum 100 ppm.

Dissolve 0.750 g in 10 ml of *methylene chloride R* and add 15 ml of *water R*. Shake and separate the 2 layers. Dilute 10 ml of the aqueous layer to 15 ml with *water R*. The solution obtained complies with the limit test for chlorides.

Loss on drying (*2.2.32*): maximum 0.5 per cent, determined on 1.000 g by drying in an oven at 105 °C.

Sulphated ash (*2.4.14*): maximum 0.1 per cent, determined on 1.0 g.

ASSAY

Dissolve 0.230 g in 50.0 ml of *anhydrous acetic acid R*. Titrate with *0.1 M perchloric acid*, determining the end-point potentiometrically (*2.2.20*).

1 ml of *0.1 M perchloric acid* is equivalent to 28.88 mg of $C_{16}H_{17}ClN_2O$.

STORAGE

Protected from light.

IMPURITIES

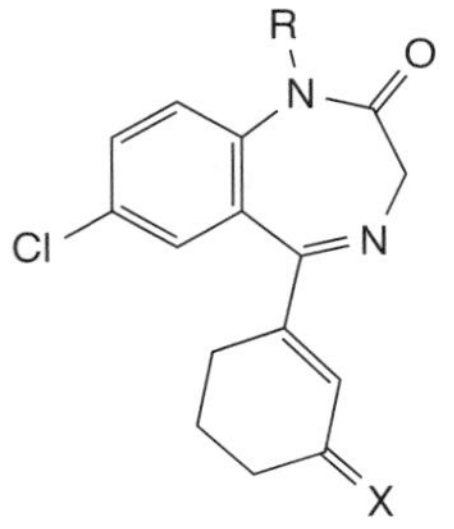

A. R = CH_3, X = O: 7-chloro-1-methyl-5-(3-oxocyclohex-1-enyl)-1,3-dihydro-2*H*-1,4-benzodiazepin-2-one,

E. R = H, X = H_2: 7-chloro-5-(cyclohex-1-enyl)-1,3-dihydro-2*H*-1,4-benzodiazepin-2-one,

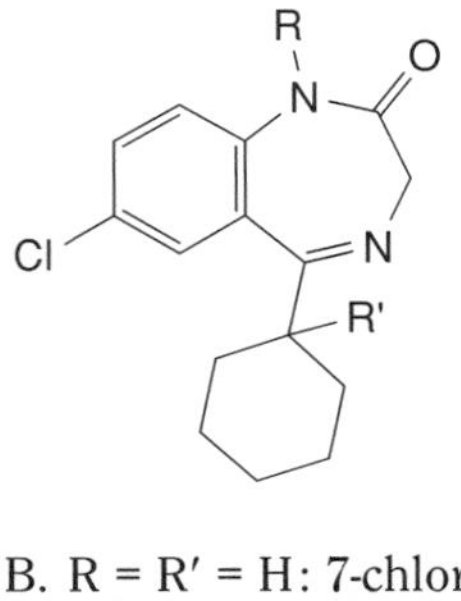

B. R = R′ = H: 7-chloro-5-cyclohexyl-1,3-dihydro-2*H*-1,4-benzodiazepin-2-one,

C. R = CH_3, R′ = H: 7-chloro-5-cyclohexyl-1-methyl-1,3-dihydro-2*H*-1,4-benzodiazepin-2-one,

D. R = CH_3, R′ = Cl: 7-chloro-5-(1-chlorocyclohexyl)-1-methyl-1,3-dihydro-2*H*-1,4-benzodiazepin-2-one.

01/2008:1660
corrected 6.5

TIAMULIN FOR VETERINARY USE

Tiamulinum ad usum veterinarium

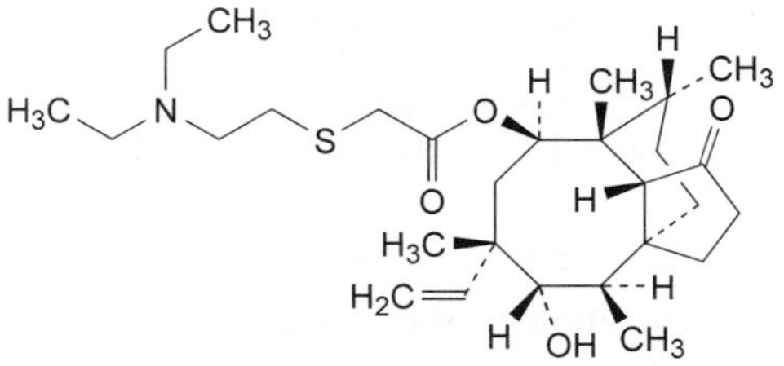

$C_{28}H_{47}NO_4S$
[55297-95-5]

M_r 493.8

DEFINITION

(3a*S*,4*R*,5*S*,6*S*,8*R*,9*R*,9a*R*,10*R*)-6-Ethenyl-5-hydroxy-4,6,9,10-tetramethyl-1-oxodecahydro-3a,9-propano-3a*H*-cyclopentacycloocten-8-yl [[2-(diethylamino)ethyl]sulphanyl]acetate.

Semi-synthetic product derived from a fermentation product.

Content: 96.5 per cent to 102.0 per cent (dried substance).

CHARACTERS

Appearance: sticky, translucent yellowish mass, slightly hygroscopic.

Solubility: practically insoluble in water, very soluble in methylene chloride, freely soluble in anhydrous ethanol.

IDENTIFICATION

Infrared absorption spectrophotometry (*2.2.24*).

Comparison: *Ph. Eur. reference spectrum of tiamulin*.

TESTS

Appearance of solution. The solution is clear (*2.2.1*) and its absorbance (*2.2.25*) at 420 nm is not greater than 0.050.

Dissolve 2.5 g in 50 ml of *methanol R*.

Related substances. Liquid chromatography (*2.2.29*).

Ammonium carbonate buffer solution pH 10.0. Dissolve 10.0 g of *ammonium carbonate R* in *water R*, add 22 ml of *perchloric acid solution R* and dilute to 1000.0 ml with *water R*. Adjust to pH 10.0 with *concentrated ammonia R1*.

Solvent mixture: acetonitrile R1, ammonium carbonate buffer solution pH 10.0 (50:50 *V/V*).

Test solution. Dissolve 0.200 g of the substance to be examined in the solvent mixture and dilute to 50.0 ml with the solvent mixture.

Reference solution (a). Dissolve 0.250 g of *tiamulin hydrogen fumarate CRS* in the solvent mixture and dilute to 50.0 ml with the solvent mixture.

Reference solution (b). Dilute 1.0 ml of the test solution to 100.0 ml with the solvent mixture.

Reference solution (c). Dilute 0.1 ml of *toluene R* to 100 ml with *acetonitrile R*. Dilute 0.1 ml of this solution to 100.0 ml with the solvent mixture.

Column:

- *size*: *l* = 0.15 m, Ø = 4.6 mm;

— *stationary phase*: end-capped octadecylsilyl silica gel for chromatography R (5 µm);

— *temperature*: 30 °C.

Mobile phase: acetonitrile R1, ammonium carbonate buffer solution pH 10.0, *methanol R1* (21:30:49 V/V/V).

Flow rate: 1.0 ml/min.

Detection: spectrophotometer at 212 nm.

Injection: 20 µl.

Run time: 3 times the retention time of tiamulin.

Relative retention with reference to tiamulin (retention time = about 18 min): impurity A = about 0.22; impurity B = about 0.5; impurity C = about 0.66; impurity D = about 1.1; impurity F = about 1.6; impurity E = about 2.4.

System suitability: reference solution (a):

— baseline separation between the peaks due to tiamulin and impurity D.

Limits:

— *impurities A, B, C, D, E, F*: for each impurity, not more than the area of the principal peak in the chromatogram obtained with reference solution (b) (1.0 per cent);

— *any other impurity*: for each impurity, not more than 0.2 times the area of the principal peak in the chromatogram obtained with reference solution (b) (0.2 per cent);

— *total*: not more than 3 times the area of the principal peak in the chromatogram obtained with reference solution (b) (3.0 per cent);

— *disregard limit*: 0.1 times the area of the principal peak in the chromatogram obtained with reference solution (b) (0.1 per cent); disregard any peak present in the chromatogram obtained with reference solution (c).

Loss on drying (*2.2.32*): maximum 1.0 per cent, determined on 1.000 g by drying in an oven at 80 °C.

Bacterial endotoxins (*2.6.14, Method D*): less than 0.4 IU/mg, determined in a 1 mg/ml solution in *anhydrous ethanol R* (endotoxin free) diluted 1:40 with water for bacterial endotoxins test.

ASSAY

Liquid chromatography (*2.2.29*) as described in the test for related substances with the following modification.

Injection: test solution and reference solution (a).

Calculate the percentage content of $C_{28}H_{47}NO_4S$, from the declared content of *tiamulin hydrogen fumarate CRS*.

STORAGE

Protected from light.

IMPURITIES

Specified impurities: A, B, C, D, E, F.

Other detectable impurities (the following substances would, if present at a sufficient level, be detected by one or other of the tests in the monograph. They are limited by the general acceptance criterion for other/unspecified impurities and/or by the general monograph *Substances for pharmaceutical use (2034)*. It is therefore not necessary to identify these impurities for demonstration of compliance. See also *5.10. Control of impurities in substances for pharmaceutical use*): G, H, I, J, K, L, M, N, O, P, Q, R.

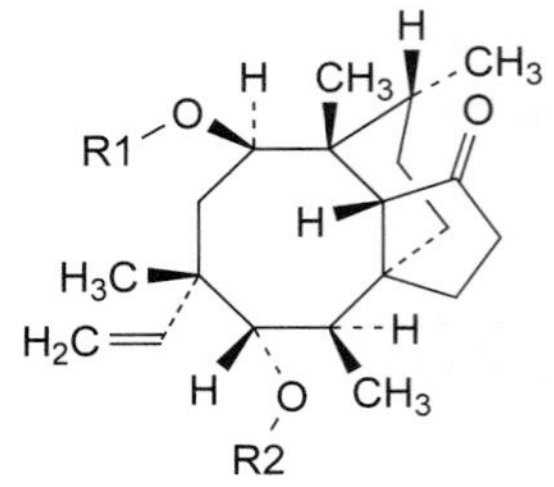

A. R1 = R2 = H: (3a*S*,4*R*,5*S*,6*S*,8*R*,9*R*,9a*R*,10*R*)-6-ethenyl-5, 8-dihydroxy-4,6,9,10-tetramethyloctahydro-3a,9-propano-3a*H*-cyclopentacycloocten-1(4*H*)-one (mutilin),

G. R1 = CO-CH₂OH, R2 = H: (3a*S*,4*R*,5*S*,6*S*,8*R*,9*R*,9a*R*,10*R*)-6-ethenyl-5-hydroxy-4,6,9,10-tetramethyl-1-oxodecahydro-3a,9-propano-3a*H*-cyclopentacycloocten-8-yl hydroxyacetate (pleuromutilin),

J. R1 = CO-CH₃, R2 = H: (3a*S*,4*R*,5*S*,6*S*,8*R*,9*R*,9a*R*,10*R*)-6-ethenyl-5-hydroxy-4,6,9,10-tetramethyl-1-oxodecahydro-3a, 9-propano-3a*H*-cyclopentacycloocten-8-yl acetate (mutilin 14-acetate),

K. R1 = H, R2 = CO-CH₃: (3a*S*,4*R*,5*S*,6*S*,8*R*,9*R*,9a*R*,10*R*)-6-ethenyl-8-hydroxy-4,6,9,10-tetramethyl-1-oxodecahydro-3a, 9-propano-3a*H*-cyclopentacycloocten-5-yl acetate (mutilin 11-acetate),

L. R1 = CO-CH₂-O-SO₂-C₆H₄-*p*CH₃, R2 = H: (3a*S*,4*R*,5*S*,6*S*,8*R*,9*R*,9a*R*,10*R*)-6-ethenyl-5-hydroxy-4,6,9,10-tetramethyl-1-oxodecahydro-3a,9-propano-3a*H*-cyclopentacycloocten-8-yl [[(4-methylphenyl)sulphonyl]oxy]acetate (pleuromutilin 22-tosylate),

M. R1 = R2 = CO-CH₃: (3a*S*,4*R*,5*S*,6*S*,8*R*,9*R*,9a*R*,10*R*)-6-ethenyl-4,6,9,10-tetramethyl-1-oxodecahydro-3a,9-propano-3a*H*-cyclopentacycloocten-5,8-diyl diacetate (mutilin 11,14-diacetate),

P. R1 = CO-CH₂-O-SO₂-C₆H₅, R2 = H: (3a*S*,4*R*,5*S*,6*S*,8*R*, 9*R*,9a*R*,10*R*)-6-ethenyl-5-hydroxy-4,6,9,10-tetramethyl-1-oxodecahydro-3a,9-propano-3a*H*-cyclopentacycloocten-8-yl [(phenylsulphonyl)oxy]acetate,

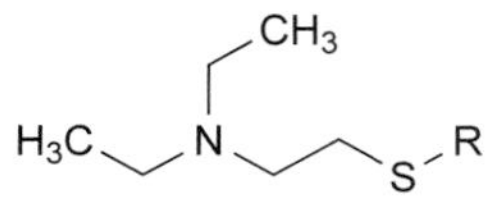

B. R = CH₂-C₆H₅: 2-(benzylsulphanyl)-*N,N*-diethylethanamine,

C. R = S-CH₂-CH₂-N(C₂H₅)₂: 2,2'-(disulphane-1,2-diyl)bis(*N,N*-diethylethanamine),

O. R = H: 2-(diethylamino)ethanethiol,

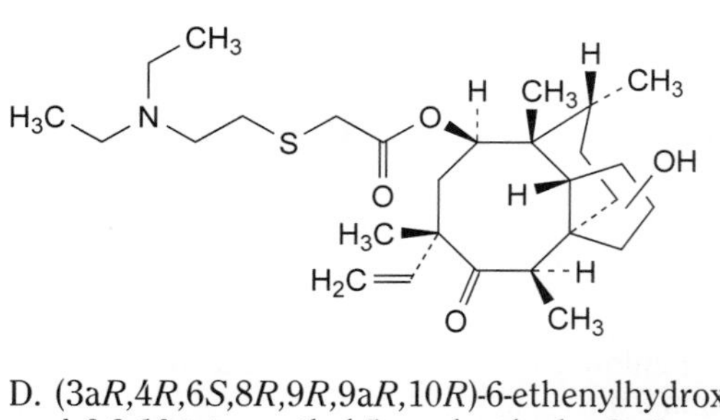

D. (3a*R*,4*R*,6*S*,8*R*,9*R*,9a*R*,10*R*)-6-ethenylhydroxy-4,6,9,10-tetramethyl-5-oxodecahydro-3a,9-propano-3a*H*-cyclopentacycloocten-8-yl [[2-(diethylamino)ethyl]sulphanyl]acetate,

E. (3aS,4R,6S,8R,9R,9aR,10R)-6-ethenyl-4,6,9,10-tetramethyl-1,5-dioxodecahydro-3a,9-propano-3aH-cyclopentacycloocten-8-yl [[2-(diethylamino)ethyl]sulphanyl]acetate (11-oxotiamulin),

F. (1RS,3aR,4R,6S,8R,9R,9aR,10R)-6-ethenyl-1-hydroxy-4,6,9,10-tetramethyl-5-oxodecahydro-3a,9-propano-3aH-cyclopentacycloocten-8-yl [[2-(diethylamino)ethyl]sulphanyl]acetate (1-hydroxy-11-oxotiamulin),

H. (2E)-4-[(2RS)-2-[(3aS,4R,5S,6R,8R,9R,9aR,10R)-8-[[[[2-(diethylamino)ethyl]sulphanyl]acetyl]oxy]-5-hydroxy-4,6,9,10-tetramethyl-1-oxodecahydro-3a,9-propano-3aH-cyclopentacycloocten-6-yl]-2-hydroxyethoxy]-4-oxobut-2-enoic acid (19,20-dihydroxytiamulin 20-fumarate),

I. (2E)-4-[[(3aS,4R,5S,6S,8R,9R,9aR,10R)-8-[[[[2-(diethylamino)ethyl]sulphanyl]acetyl]oxy]-6-ethenyl-1,5-dihydroxy-4,6,9,10-tetramethyldecahydro-3a,9-propano-3aH-cyclopentacycloocten-2-yl]oxy]-4-oxobut-2-enoic acid (2,3-dihydroxytiamulin 2-fumarate),

N. (2E)-4-[2-[[(3aS,4R,5S,6S,8R,9R,9aR,10R)-6-ethenyl-5-hydroxy-4,6,9,10-tetramethyl-1-oxodecahydro-3a,9-propano-3aH-cyclopentacycloocten-8-yl]oxy]-2-oxoethoxy]-4-oxobut-2-enoic acid (pleuromutilin 22-fumarate),

Q. (3aS,4R,5S,6S,8R,9R,10R)-6-ethenyl-2,5-dihydroxy-4,6,9,10-tetramethyl-2,3,4,5,6,7,8,9-octahydro-3a,9-propano-3aH-cyclopentacycloocten-8-yl [[2-(diethylamino)ethyl]sulphanyl]acetate (3,4-didehydro-2-hydroxytiamulin),

R. N-benzyl-N,N-dibutylbutan-1-aminium.

07/2009:1158

TOLNAFTATE

Tolnaftatum

$C_{19}H_{17}NOS$ M_r 307.4
[2398-96-1]

DEFINITION

O-Naphthalen-2-yl methyl(3-methylphenyl)carbamothioate.

Content: 97.0 per cent to 103.0 per cent (dried substance).

CHARACTERS

Appearance: white or yellowish-white powder.

Solubility: practically insoluble in water, freely soluble in acetone and in methylene chloride, very slightly soluble in ethanol (96 per cent).

IDENTIFICATION

Infrared absorption spectrophotometry (*2.2.24*).

Comparison: tolnaftate CRS.

TESTS

Impurity D. Liquid chromatography (*2.2.29*).

Test solution. Dissolve 0.400 g of the substance to be examined in 2 ml of *methylene chloride R*. Extract with 3 quantities, each of 3 ml, of *0.01 M hydrochloric acid*. Combine the aqueous phases and dilute to 10.0 ml with *0.01 M hydrochloric acid*.

Reference solution (a). Dissolve 20.0 mg of *N-methyl-m-toluidine R* (impurity D) in 50.0 ml of *methylene chloride R*.

Reference solution (b). Dilute 1.0 ml of reference solution (a) to 100.0 ml with *methylene chloride R*. Take 2.0 ml of this solution and extract with 3 quantities, each of 3 ml, of *0.01 M hydrochloric acid*. Combine the aqueous phases and dilute to 10.0 ml with *0.01 M hydrochloric acid*.

Reference solution (c). Dissolve 10 mg of the substance to be examined in 25 ml of *methanol R*. Add 2 ml of this solution to 2 ml of reference solution (a) and dilute to 25 ml with *methanol R*.

Column:
— *size*: l = 0.15 m, Ø = 4.6 mm;
— *stationary phase*: octadecylsilyl silica gel for chromatography R (5 µm).

Mobile phase:
— *mobile phase A*: *trifluoroacetic acid R, methanol R, water R* (0.1:10:90 *V/V/V*);
— *mobile phase B*: *trifluoroacetic acid R, water R, methanol R* (0.1:10:90 *V/V/V*);

Time (min)	Mobile phase A (per cent *V/V*)	Mobile phase B (per cent *V/V*)
0 - 3	70	30
3 - 8	70 → 0	30 → 100
8 - 20	0	100

Flow rate: 1.0 ml/min.

Detection: spectrophotometer at 254 nm.

Injection: 100 µl of the test solution and reference solution (b); 10 µl of reference solution (c).

Relative retention with reference to tolnaftate (retention time = about 15 min): impurity D = about 0.25.

System suitability: reference solution (c):
— *resolution*: minimum 5.0 between the peaks due to impurity D and tolnaftate.

Limit:
— *impurity D*: not more than the area of the principal peak in the chromatogram obtained with reference solution (b) (20 ppm).

Related substances. Liquid chromatography (*2.2.29*).

Test solution. Dissolve 25 mg of the substance to be examined in 5 ml of *methanol R* and dilute to 25.0 ml with the same solvent.

Reference solution (a). Dilute 1.0 ml of the test solution to 100.0 ml with *methanol R*. Dilute 1.0 ml of this solution to 10.0 ml with *methanol R*.

Reference solution (b). Dissolve 5 mg of *tolnaftate for system suitability CRS* (containing resolution component A) in 5.0 ml of *methanol R*.

Column:
— *size*: l = 0.15 m, Ø = 4.6 mm;
— *stationary phase*: octadecylsilyl silica gel for chromatography R (5 µm).

Mobile phase:
— *mobile phase A*: *trifluoroacetic acid R, water R, methanol R* (0.1:30:70 *V/V/V*);
— *mobile phase B*: *trifluoroacetic acid R, water R, methanol R* (0.1:10:90 *V/V/V*);

Time (min)	Mobile phase A (per cent *V/V*)	Mobile phase B (per cent *V/V*)
0 - 12	100	0
12 - 30	100 → 0	0 → 100
30 - 33	0	100

Flow rate: 1.0 ml/ min.

Detection: spectrophotometer at 254 nm.

Injection: 10 µl.

Relative retention with reference to tolnaftate (retention time = about 18 min): resolution component A = about 0.7.

System suitability: reference solution (b):
— *resolution*: minimum 5.0 between the peaks due to resolution component A and tolnaftate.

Limits:
— *unspecified impurities*: for each impurity, not more than the area of the principal peak in the chromatogram obtained with reference solution (a) (0.10 per cent);
— *total*: not more than twice the area of the principal peak in the chromatogram obtained with reference solution (a) (0.2 per cent);
— *disregard limit*: 0.5 times the area of the principal peak in the chromatogram obtained with reference solution (a) (0.05 per cent).

Loss on drying (*2.2.32*): maximum 0.5 per cent, determined on 1.000 g by drying at 60 °C at a pressure not exceeding 0.7 kPa for 3 h.

Sulphated ash (*2.4.14*): maximum 0.1 per cent, determined on 1.0 g.

ASSAY

Dissolve 50.0 mg in *methanol R* and dilute to 250.0 ml with the same solvent. Dilute 2.0 ml of this solution to 50.0 ml with *methanol R*. Measure the absorbance (*2.2.25*) at the absorption maximum at 257 nm.

Calculate the content of $C_{19}H_{17}NOS$ taking the specific absorbance to be 720.

STORAGE

Protected from light.

IMPURITIES

Specified impurities: D.

Other detectable impurities (the following substances would, if present at a sufficient level, be detected by one or other of the tests in the monograph. They are limited by the general acceptance criterion for other/unspecified impurities and/or by the general monograph *Substances for pharmaceutical use (2034)*. It is therefore not necessary to identify these impurities for demonstration of compliance. See also *5.10. Control of impurities in substances for pharmaceutical use*): A, B.

A. naphthalen-2-ol (β-naphthol),

B. *O,O*-dinaphthalen-2-yl carbonothioate,

D. *N*,3-dimethylaniline (*N*-methyl-*m*-toluidine).

V

Monographs
Q-Z

See the information section on general monographs (cover pages)

07/2009:2248

VEDAPROFEN FOR VETERINARY USE

Vedaprofenum ad usum veterinarium

and enantiomer

$C_{19}H_{22}O_2$ M_r 282.4
[71109-09-6]

DEFINITION

(2RS)-2-(4-Cyclohexyl-1-naphthyl)propanoic acid.

Content: 98.5 per cent to 101.0 per cent (dried substance).

CHARACTERS

Appearance: white or almost white powder.

Solubility: practically insoluble in water, freely soluble in acetone, soluble in methanol. It dissolves in dilute solutions of alkali hydroxides.

IDENTIFICATION

Infrared absorption spectrophotometry (2.2.24).

Comparison: vedaprofen CRS.

TESTS

Appearance of solution. The solution is clear (2.2.1) and not more intensely coloured than reference solution Y_5 (2.2.2, Method II).

Dissolve 2.0 g in acetone R and dilute to 20.0 ml with the same solvent.

Related substances. Liquid chromatography (2.2.29).

Test solution. Dissolve 25 mg of the substance to be examined in methanol R and dilute to 50.0 ml with the same solvent.

Reference solution (a). Dilute 1.0 ml of the test solution to 50.0 ml with methanol R. Dilute 1.0 ml of this solution to 10.0 ml with methanol R.

Reference solution (b). Dissolve the contents of a vial of vedaprofen impurity mixture CRS (impurities A, B and C) in 1.0 ml of reference solution (a).

Column:

— size: l = 0.10 m, Ø = 3.0 mm;

— stationary phase: octadecylsilyl silica gel for chromatography R (5 µm);

— temperature: 35 °C.

Mobile phase: dissolve 1.70 g of tetrabutylammonium hydrogen sulphate R in 1000 ml of a mixture of 20 volumes of water R and 80 volumes of methanol R.

Flow rate: 0.4 ml/min.

Detection: spectrophotometer at 288 nm.

Injection: 10 µl.

Run time: 5 times the retention time of vedaprofen.

Identification of impurities: use the chromatogram supplied with vedaprofen impurity mixture CRS and the chromatogram obtained with reference solution (b) to identify the peaks due to impurities A, B and C.

Relative retention with reference to vedaprofen (retention time = about 6 min): impurity C = about 0.8; impurity A = about 1.8; impurity B = about 3.7.

System suitability: reference solution (b):

— resolution: minimum 2.0 between the peaks due to impurity C and vedaprofen.

Limits:

— correction factor: for the calculation of content, multiply the peak area of impurity B by 0.7;

— impurities A, B: for each impurity, not more than twice the area of the principal peak in the chromatogram obtained with reference solution (a) (0.4 per cent);

— unspecified impurities: for each impurity, not more than the area of the principal peak in the chromatogram obtained with reference solution (a) (0.20 per cent);

— total: not more than 2.5 times the area of the principal peak in the chromatogram obtained with reference solution (a) (0.5 per cent);

— disregard limit: 0.5 times the area of the principal peak in the chromatogram obtained with reference solution (a) (0.1 per cent).

Heavy metals (2.4.8): maximum 10 ppm.

Dissolve 1.0 g in a mixture of 15 volumes of water R and 85 volumes of acetone R and dilute to 20 ml with the same mixture of solvents. 12 ml of the solution complies with test B. Prepare the reference solution using lead standard solution (0.5 ppm Pb) obtained by diluting lead standard solution (100 ppm Pb) R with a mixture of 15 volumes of water R and 85 volumes of acetone R.

Loss on drying (2.2.32): maximum 0.5 per cent, determined on 1.000 g by drying in an oven at 105 °C.

Sulphated ash (2.4.14): maximum 0.3 per cent, determined on 0.500 g.

ASSAY

Dissolve 0.200 g in 50 ml of ethanol (96 per cent) R and add 1.0 ml of 0.1 M hydrochloric acid. Carry out a potentiometric titration (2.2.20), using 0.1 M sodium hydroxide. Read the volume added between the 2 points of inflexion.

1 ml of 0.1 M sodium hydroxide is equivalent to 28.24 mg of $C_{19}H_{22}O_2$.

IMPURITIES

Specified impurities: A, B.

Other detectable impurities (the following substances would, if present at a sufficient level, be detected by one or other of the tests in the monograph. They are limited by the general acceptance criterion for other/unspecified impurities and/or by the general monograph Substances for pharmaceutical use (2034). It is therefore not necessary to identify these impurities for demonstration of compliance. See also 5.10. Control of impurities in substances for pharmaceutical use): C, D.

and enantiomer

A. R = CH$_3$: methyl (2RS)-2-(4-cyclohexyl-1-naphthyl)propanoate,

B. R = C(CH$_3$)$_3$: 1,1-dimethylethyl (2RS)-2-(4-cyclohexyl-1-naphthyl)propanoate,

C. R = H: (4-cyclohexyl-1-naphthyl)acetic acid,

D. R = CH$_3$: methyl (2RS)-2-(4-cyclohexyl-1-naphthyl)acetate.

Z

See the information section on general monographs (cover pages)

07/2009:1059

ZIDOVUDINE

Zidovudinum

C$_{10}$H$_{13}$N$_5$O$_4$
[30516-87-1]

M_r 267.2

DEFINITION

1-(3-Azido-2,3-dideoxy-β-D-*erythro*-pentofuranosyl)-5-methylpyrimidine-2,4(1*H*,3*H*)-dione.

Content: 97.0 per cent to 102.0 per cent (dried substance).

CHARACTERS

Appearance: white or brownish powder.

Solubility: sparingly soluble in water, soluble in anhydrous ethanol.

mp: about 124 °C.

It shows polymorphism (*5.9*).

IDENTIFICATION

Infrared absorption spectrophotometry (*2.2.24*).

Comparison: zidovudine CRS.

If the spectra obtained in the solid state show differences, dissolve the substance to be examined and the reference substance separately in the minimum volume of *water R*, evaporate to dryness in a desiccator, under high vacuum over *diphosphorus pentoxide R* and record new spectra using the residues.

TESTS

Appearance of solution. The solution is not more intensely coloured than reference solution BY$_5$ (*2.2.2, Method II*).

Dissolve 0.5 g in 50 ml of *water R*, heating if necessary.

Specific optical rotation (*2.2.7*): + 60.5 to + 63.0 (dried substance).

Dissolve 0.50 g in *anhydrous ethanol R* and dilute to 50.0 ml with the same solvent. Carry out the determination at 25 °C.

Related substances

A. Thin-layer chromatography (*2.2.27*).

Test solution. Dissolve 0.20 g of the substance to be examined in *methanol R* and dilute to 10 ml with the same solvent.

Reference solution (a). Dissolve 5 mg of *thymine R* (impurity C), 5 mg of *zidovudine impurity A CRS* and 5 mg of *triphenylmethanol R* (impurity D) in *methanol R*, add 0.25 ml of the test solution and dilute to 25 ml with *methanol R*.

Reference solution (b). Dilute 5.0 ml of reference solution (a) to 10 ml with *methanol R*.

Plate: TLC silica gel F$_{254}$ plate R.

Mobile phase: methanol R, methylene chloride R (10:90 *V/V*).

Application: 10 µl.

Development: over a path of 12 cm.

Drying: in air.

Detection A: examine in ultraviolet light at 254 nm.

Limits:

— *impurity A*: any spot due to impurity A is not more intense than the corresponding spot in the chromatogram obtained with reference solution (b) (0.5 per cent);

— *any other impurity*: any other spot apart from the principal spot and any spot due to impurity C (which is limited by liquid chromatography) is not more intense than the spot due to zidovudine in the chromatogram obtained with reference solution (b) (0.5 per cent).

Detection B: spray with a 10 g/l solution of *vanillin R* in *sulphuric acid R*.

Limit:

— *impurity D*: any spot due to impurity D is not more intense than the corresponding spot in the chromatogram obtained with reference solution (b) (0.5 per cent).

System suitability: reference solution (a):

— the chromatogram shows 4 clearly separated spots, due to impurity C, impurity A, zidovudine and impurity D, in order of increasing R_F value.

B. Liquid chromatography (*2.2.29*).

Test solution (a). Dissolve 50.0 mg of the substance to be examined in the mobile phase and dilute to 50.0 ml with the mobile phase.

Test solution (b). Dilute 10.0 ml of test solution (a) to 50.0 ml with the mobile phase.

Reference solution (a). Dissolve 10.0 mg of *zidovudine CRS* in the mobile phase and dilute to 50.0 ml with the mobile phase.

Reference solution (b). Dissolve 10.0 mg of *thymine R* (impurity C) in *methanol R* and dilute to 50.0 ml with the same solvent. Dilute 5.0 ml of this solution to 50.0 ml with the mobile phase.

Reference solution (c). Dissolve 5 mg of *zidovudine impurity B CRS* in 25.0 ml of reference solution (a) and dilute to 50.0 ml with the mobile phase.

Reference solution (d). Dilute 5.0 ml of reference solution (c) to 50.0 ml with the mobile phase.

Reference solution (e). Dilute 0.25 ml of test solution (a) to 50.0 ml with the mobile phase.

Column:

— *size*: l = 0.25 m, Ø = 4.6 mm;

— *stationary phase*: octadecylsilyl silica gel for chromatography R (5 µm).

Mobile phase: methanol R, water R (20:80 *V/V*).

Flow rate: 1.2 ml/min.

Detection: spectrophotometer at 265 nm.

Equilibration: with the mobile phase for about 45 min.

Injection: 10 µl of test solution (a) and reference solutions (b), (c), (d) and (e).

Run time: 1.5 times the retention time of zidovudine.

Elution order: impurity C, zidovudine, impurity B.

System suitability: reference solution (c):

— *resolution*: minimum 1.5 between the peaks due to zidovudine and impurity B.

Limits:

— *impurity C*: not more than the area of the corresponding peak in the chromatogram obtained with reference solution (b) (2 per cent);

— *impurity B*: not more than the area of the corresponding peak in the chromatogram obtained with reference solution (d) (1 per cent);

— *any other impurity*: for each impurity, not more than the area of the principal peak in the chromatogram obtained with reference solution (e) (0.5 per cent);

— *total*: not more than 6 times the area of the principal peak in the chromatogram obtained with reference solution (e) (3.0 per cent);

— *disregard limit*: 0.1 times the area of the principal peak in the chromatogram obtained with reference solution (e) (0.05 per cent).

Heavy metals (*2.4.8*): maximum 20 ppm.

1.00 g complies with test D. Prepare the reference solution using 2 ml of *lead standard solution (10 ppm Pb) R*.

Loss on drying (*2.2.32*): maximum 1.0 per cent, determined on 1.000 g by drying in an oven at 105 °C.

Sulphated ash (*2.4.14*): maximum 0.25 per cent, determined on 1.00 g.

ASSAY

Liquid chromatography (*2.2.29*) as described in the test for related substances with the following modification.

Injection: test solution (b) and reference solution (a).

Calculate the content of $C_{10}H_{13}N_5O_4$ from the declared content of *zidovudine CRS*.

STORAGE

Protected from light.

IMPURITIES

Specified impurities: A, B, C, D.

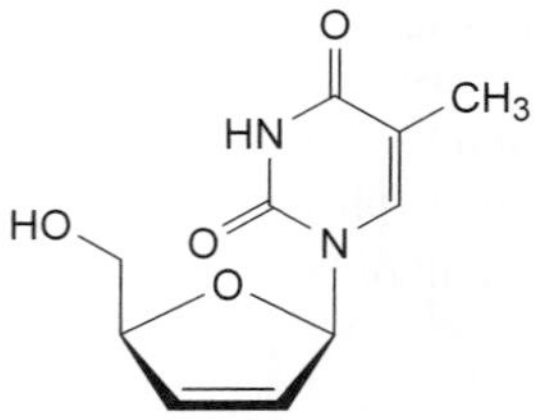

A. 1-[(2R,5S)-5-(hydroxymethyl)-2,5-dihydrofuran-2-yl)-5-methylpyrimidine-2,4(1H,3H)-dione,

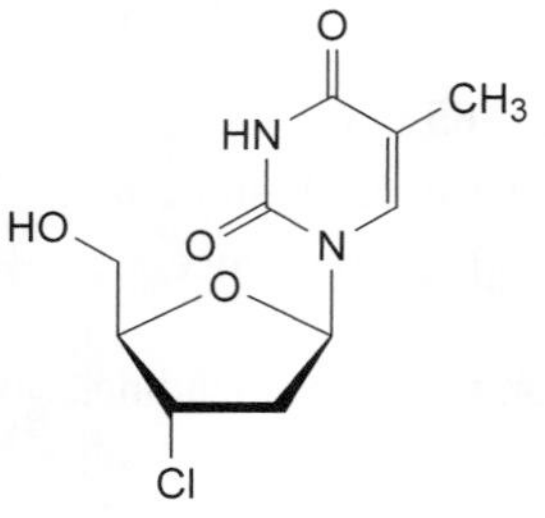

B. 1-(3-chloro-2,3-dideoxy-β-D-*erythro*-pentofuranosyl)-5-methylpyrimidine-2,4(1H,3H)-dione,

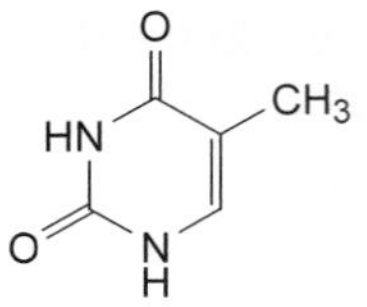

C. 5-methylpyrimidine-2,4(1H,3H)-dione (thymine),

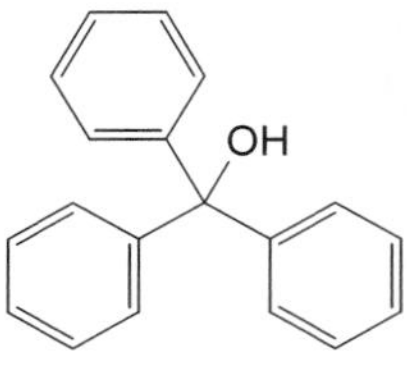

D. triphenylmethanol.

07/2009:2164

ZINC GLUCONATE

Zinci gluconas

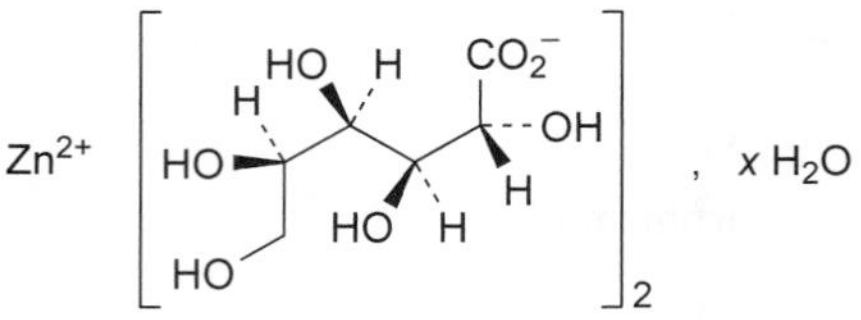

$$Zn^{2+} \left[\begin{array}{c} \end{array} \right]_2 , \ x H_2O$$

$C_{12}H_{22}ZnO_{14}$,xH_2O M_r 455.7 (anhydrous substance)

DEFINITION

Anhydrous or hydrated zinc D-gluconate.

Content: 98.0 per cent to 102.0 per cent (anhydrous substance).

CHARACTERS

Appearance: white or almost white, hygroscopic, crystalline powder.

Solubility: soluble in water, practically insoluble in anhydrous ethanol and in methylene chloride.

IDENTIFICATION

A. Thin-layer chromatography (*2.2.27*).

Test solution. Dissolve 20 mg of the substance to be examined in 1 ml of *water R*.

Reference solution. Dissolve 20 mg of *calcium gluconate CRS* in 1 ml of *water R*, heating if necessary in a water-bath at 60 °C.

Plate: *TLC silica gel plate R* (5-40 μm) [or *TLC silica gel plate R* (2-10 μm)].

Mobile phase: *concentrated ammonia R, ethyl acetate R, water R, ethanol (96 per cent) R* (10:10:30:50 *V/V/V/V*).

Application: 1 μl.

Development: over 3/4 of the plate.

Drying: at 100-105 °C for 20 min, then allow to cool to room temperature.

Detection: spray with a solution containing 25 g/l of *ammonium molybdate R* and 10 g/l of *cerium sulphate R* in *dilute sulphuric acid R*, and heat at 100-105 °C for about 10 min.

Results: the principal spot in the chromatogram obtained with the test solution is similar in position, colour and size to the principal spot in the chromatogram obtained with the reference solution.

B. Dissolve 0.1 g in 5 ml of *water R*. Add 0.5 ml of *potassium ferrocyanide solution R*. A white precipitate is formed that does not dissolve upon the addition of 5 ml of *hydrochloric acid R*.

TESTS

Solution S. Dissolve 1.0 g in *water R* and dilute to 50 ml with the same solvent.

Appearance of solution. Solution S is not more opalescent than reference suspension II (*2.2.1*) and not more intensely coloured than reference solution Y_6 (*2.2.2, Method II*).

Sucrose and reducing sugars. Dissolve 0.5 g in a mixture of 2 ml of *hydrochloric acid R1* and 10 ml of *water R*. Boil for 5 min, allow to cool, add 10 ml of *sodium carbonate solution R* and allow to stand for 10 min. Dilute to 25 ml with *water R* and filter. To 5 ml of the filtrate add 2 ml of *cupri-tartaric solution R* and boil for 1 min. Allow to stand for 2 min. No red precipitate is formed.

Chlorides (*2.4.4*): maximum 500 ppm.

Dilute 5 ml of solution S to 15 ml with *water R*.

Sulphates (*2.4.13*): maximum 500 ppm.

Dissolve 2.0 g in a mixture of 10 ml of *acetic acid R* and 90 ml of *distilled water R*.

Cadmium: maximum 2.0 ppm.

Atomic absorption spectrometry (*2.2.23, Method II*).

Test solution. Dissolve 5.00 g in 20 ml of *deionised distilled water R* with the aid of ultrasound and dilute to 25.0 ml with the same solvent.

Reference solutions. Prepare the reference solutions using *cadmium standard solution (0.1 per cent Cd) R*, diluting with *deionised distilled water R*.

Source: cadmium hollow-cathode lamp.

Wavelength: 228.8 nm.

Atomisation device: air-acetylene flame.

Heavy metals (*2.4.8*): maximum 10 ppm.

Dissolve 2.0 g in 20 ml of *water R*, heating in a water-bath at 60 °C. 12 ml of the solution complies with test A. Prepare the reference solution using *lead standard solution (1 ppm Pb) R*.

Water (*2.5.32*): maximum 12.0 per cent, determined on 80.0 mg.

Microbial contamination

TAMC: acceptance criterion 10^3 CFU/g (*2.6.12*).

TYMC: acceptance criterion 10^2 CFU/g (*2.6.12*).

ASSAY

Dissolve 0.400 g in 5 ml of *dilute acetic acid R*. Carry out the complexometric titration of zinc (*2.5.11*).

1 ml of *0.1 M sodium edetate* is equivalent to 45.57 mg of $C_{12}H_{22}ZnO_{14}$.

STORAGE

In a non-metallic, airtight container.

See the information section on general monographs (cover pages)

INDEX

To aid users the index includes a reference to the supplement where the latest version of a text can be found.

For example: Amikacin...**6.1**-3396

means the monograph Amikacin can be found on page 3396 of Supplement 6.1.

Note that where no reference to a supplement is made, the text can be found in the principal volume.

Monographs deleted from the 6th Edition are not included in the index; a list of deleted texts is found in the Contents of this supplement, page xliv.

Index

See the information section on general monographs (cover pages)

Index

Index

Index

Index

Index

See the information section on general monographs (cover pages)

General Notices (1) apply to all monographs and other texts

Index

Index

Index

Index

Index

Index

Index

Index

See the information section on general monographs (cover pages)

Index

Index

See the information section on general monographs (cover pages)

Index

Index

Index

Index

Index

Index

See the information section on general monographs (cover pages)

Version date of the text ——————— **01/2008:0884**

corrected 6.5

Text reference number

CARBIMAZOLE

Carbimazolum

Modification to be taken into account from the publication date of Supplement 6.5

$C_7H_{10}N_2O_2S$

CAS number — [22232-54-8]

M_r 186.2

DEFINITION

Chemical name in accordance with IUPAC nomenclature rules

Ethyl 3-methyl-2-thioxo-2,3-dihydro-1*H*-imidazole-1-carboxylate.

Content: 98.0 per cent to 102.0 per cent (dried substance).

CHARACTERS

Appearance: white or yellowish-white, crystalline powder.

Solubility: slightly soluble in water, soluble in acetone and in ethanol (96 per cent).

IDENTIFICATION

Application of the first and second identification is defined in the General Notices (chapter 1)

First identification: B.

Second identification: A, C.

A. Melting point (*2.2.14*): 122 °C to 125 °C.

B. Infrared absorption spectrophotometry (*2.2.24*).

Preparation: discs.

Reference standard available from the Secretariat (see www.edqm.eu)

Comparison: carbimazole CRS.

C. Thin-layer chromatography (*2.2.27*).

Test solution. Dissolve 10 mg of the substance to be examined in *methylene chloride R* and dilute to 10 ml with the same solvent.

Reference solution. Dissolve 10 mg of *carbimazole CRS* in *methylene chloride R* and dilute to 10 ml with the same solvent.

Plate: TLC silica gel GF$_{254}$ plate R.

Reagents described in chapter 4

Mobile phase: acetone R, methylene chloride R (20:80 *V/V*).

Application: 10 μl.

Development: over a path of 15 cm.

Drying: in air for 30 min.

Detection: examine in ultraviolet light at 254 nm.

Further information available on www.edqm.eu (KNOWLEDGE)

Results: the principal spot in the chromatogram obtained with the test solution is similar in position and size to the principal spot in the chromatogram obtained with the reference solution.

TESTS

Reference to a general chapter

Related substances. Liquid chromatography (*2.2.29*).

Line in the margin indicating where part of the text has been modified (technical modification)

Test solution. Dissolve 5.0 mg of the substance to be examined in 10.0 ml of a mixture of 20 volumes of *acetonitrile R* and 80 volumes of *water R*. Use this solution within 5 min of preparation.

Reference solution (a). Dissolve 5 mg of *thiamazole R* and 0.10 g of *carbimazole CRS* in a mixture of 20 volumes of *acetonitrile R* and 80 volumes of *water R* and dilute to 100.0 ml with the same mixture of solvents. Dilute 1.0 ml

of this solution to 10.0 ml with a mixture of 20 volumes of *acetonitrile R* and 80 volumes of *water R*.

Reference solution (b). Dissolve 5.0 mg of *thiamazole R* in a mixture of 20 volumes of *acetonitrile R* and 80 volumes of *water R* and dilute to 10.0 ml with the same mixture of solvents. Dilute 1.0 ml of this solution to 100.0 ml with a mixture of 20 volumes of *acetonitrile R* and 80 volumes of *water R*.

Column:

– *size*: *l* = 0.15 m, Ø = 3.9 mm,

– *stationary phase*: octadecylsilyl silica gel for chromatography R (5 μm).

Mobile phase: acetonitrile R, water R (10:90 *V/V*).

Flow rate: 1 ml/min.

Detection: spectrophotometer at 254 nm.

Injection: 10 μl.

Run time: 1.5 times the retention time of carbimazole.

Retention time: carbimazole = about 6 min.

System suitability: reference solution (a):

– *resolution*: minimum 5.0 between the peaks due to impurity A and carbimazole.

Limits:

– *impurity A*: not more than 0.5 times the area of the principal peak in the chromatogram obtained with reference solution (b) (0.5 per cent),

– *unspecified impurities*: for each impurity, not more than 0.1 times the area of the principal peak in the chromatogram obtained with reference solution (b) (0.10 per cent).

Loss on drying (*2.2.32*): maximum 0.5 per cent, determined on 1.000 g by drying in a desiccator over *diphosphorus pentoxide R* at a pressure not exceeding 0.7 kPa for 24 h.

Sulphated ash (*2.4.14*): maximum 0.1 per cent, determined on 1.0 g.

ASSAY

Dissolve 50.0 mg in *water R* and dilute to 500.0 ml with the same solvent. To 10.0 ml add 10 ml of *dilute hydrochloric acid R* and dilute to 100.0 ml with *water R*. Measure the absorbance (*2.2.25*) at the absorption maximum at 291 nm.

Calculate the content of $C_7H_{10}N_2O_2S$ taking the specific absorbance to be 557.

IMPURITIES

Specified impurities: A.

Other detectable impurities (the following substances would, if present at a sufficient level, be detected by one or other of the tests in the monograph. They are limited by the general acceptance criterion for other/unspecified impurities and/or by the general monograph *Substances for pharmaceutical use* (2034). It is therefore not necessary to identify these impurities for demonstration of compliance. See also *5.10. Control of impurities in substances for pharmaceutical use*): B.

A. 1-methyl-1*H*-imidazole-2-thiol (thiamazole),